Fundamentals of Diabetes

Fundamentals of Diabetes

Editor-in-Chief
Kamlakar Tripathi
Professor
Department of Medicine
Institute of Medical Sciences, Banaras Hindu University
Varanasi (UP), India

Editors

Anuj Maheshwari
Professor and Head
Department of General Medicine
BBDCODS, BBD University
Faizabad Road, Lucknow (UP), India

Brij Mohan
Physician Diabetologist
Director
BMC Hospital, Kanpur (UP)
Brij Medical Centre Pvt Ltd, Kanpur (UP), India

Narsingh Verma
Professor, Department of Physiology
King George's Medical University
Lucknow (UP), India

Sarita Bajaj
Director-Professor and Head
Department of Medicine
MLN Medical College
Allahabad (UP), India

Associate Editors

Amit N Dwivedi
Associate Professor
Department of Radiodiagnosis
and Imaging
Institute of Medical Sciences
Banaras Hindu University
Varanasi (UP), India

Richik Tripathi
Service Senior Resident
Department of Oral and
Maxillofacial Surgery
Faculty of Dental Sciences
Institute of Medical Sciences
Banaras Hindu University
Varanasi (UP), India

Forewords
HS Bajpai
Amulya Ranjan Sircar

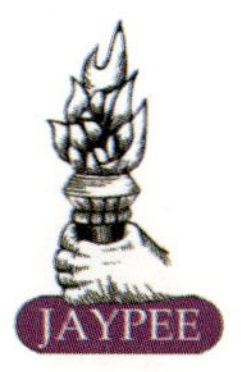

The Health Sciences Publisher

New Delhi | London | Philadelphia | Panama

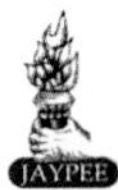

Jaypee Brothers Medical Publishers (P) Ltd

Headquarters

Jaypee Brothers Medical Publishers (P) Ltd
4838/24, Ansari Road, Daryaganj
New Delhi 110 002, India
Phone: +91-11-43574357
Fax: +91-11-43574314
Email: jaypee@jaypeebrothers.com

Overseas Offices

J.P. Medical Ltd
83 Victoria Street, London
SW1H 0HW (UK)
Phone: +44 20 3170 8910
Fax: +44 (0)20 3008 6180
Email: info@jpmedpub.com

Jaypee-Highlights Medical Publishers Inc
City of Knowledge, Bld. 237, Clayton
Panama City, Panama
Phone: +1 507-301-0496
Fax: +1 507-301-0499
Email: cservice@jphmedical.com

Jaypee Medical Inc
325 Chestnut Street
Suite 412, Philadelphia,
PA 19106, USA
Phone: +1 267-519-9789
Email: jpmed.us@gmail.com

Jaypee Brothers Medical Publishers (P) Ltd
17/1-B Babar Road, Block-B, Shaymali
Mohammadpur, Dhaka-1207
Bangladesh
Mobile: +08801912003485
Email: jaypeedhaka@gmail.com

Jaypee Brothers Medical Publishers (P) Ltd
Bhotahity, Kathmandu, Nepal
Phone: +977-9741283608
Email: kathmandu@jaypeebrothers.com

Website: www.jaypeebrothers.com
Website: www.jaypeedigital.com

Inquiries for bulk sales may be solicited at: jaypee@jaypeebrothers.com

Fundamentals of Diabetes

First Edition: **2016**

ISBN: 978-93-5250-151-9

Printed at Sanat Printers

Dedicated to

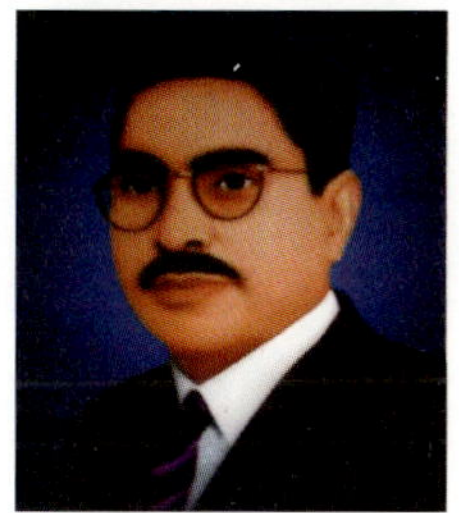

Prof KN Gaur

MD FRCP (Ed)

Former Professor and Head

Department of Medicine, Sarojini Naidu Medical College, Agra, 1950–1957

Department of Medicine, GSVM Medical College, Kanpur, 1957–1962

Department of Medicine, College of Medical Sciences

(now Institute of Medical Sciences),

Banaras Hindu University, Varanasi, 1962–1965

Department of Medicine, Aligarh Muslim University, 1965–1968

The Founder President of Endocrine Society of India

and

Father of Clinical Endocrinology and Diabetes in India

CONTRIBUTORS

Amit Kumar Singh
Resident
Department of Medicine
Institute of Medical Sciences
Banaras Hindu University
Varanasi (UP), India

Amit Nandan Dwivedi
Associate Professor
Department of Radiodiagnosis and Imaging
Institute of Medical Sciences
Banaras Hindu University
Varanasi (UP), India

Amita Diwaker
Department of Medicine
Institute of Medical Sciences
Banaras Hindu University
Varanasi (UP), India

Anuj Maheshwari
Professor and Head
Department of General Medicine
BBDCODS, BBD University
Faizabad Road, Lucknow (UP), India

Arpit Agrawal
Resident
Department of Endocrinology
Institute of Medical Sciences
Banaras Hindu University
Varanasi (UP), India

Ashutosh Jain
Resident
Department of Medicine
Institute of Medical Sciences
Banaras Hindu University
Varanasi (UP), India

Asim Siddiqui
Apollo Centre for Obesity,
Diabetes and Endocrinology
Indraprastha Apollo Hospital
Sarita Vihar, New Delhi, India

Banshi Saboo
Dia Care - A Complete Diabetes Care Centre
Gandhi Park Nehru Nagar Road, Ambavadi
Ahmedabad (Gujarat), India

Bhavana Sole
Consultant Diabetologist- Division Hospital
Bengaluru, Karnataka, India

DK Hazra
Boston Medical Centre, Soami Bagh
Agra (UP), India

Dheeraj Kapoor
Senior Consultant Endocrinology
Artemis Health Institute
Gurgaon, Haryana, India

Dheeraj Kishore
Associate Professor
Department of Medicine
Institute of Medical Sciences
Banaras Hindu University
Varanasi (UP), India

Jamal Ahmad
Director and Professor
Rajiv Gandhi Centre for Diabetes and Endocrinology
Faculty of Medicine
Aligarh Muslim University
Aligarh (UP), India

Kamlakar Tripathi
Professor
Department of Medicine
Institute of Medical Sciences
Banaras Hindu University
Varanasi (UP), India

Madhukar Rai
Professor, Department of Medicine
Institute of Medical Sciences
Banaras Hindu University
Varanasi (UP), India

MK Singh
Professor, Department of Ophthalmology
Institute of Medical Sciences
Banaras Hindu University
Varanasi (UP), India

Mumtaz Ahmad Ansari
Professor, Department of General Surgery
Institute of Medical Sciences
Banaras Hindu University
Varanasi (UP), India

Murlidhar S Rao
Former President
Association of Physicians of India, RSSDI and HIS
Former Professor and HOD of Medicine
M R Medical College
Gulbarga, Karnataka, India

Nandita Hazra
Boston Medical Centre
Soami Bagh
Agra (UP), India

Narsingh Verma
Professor
Department of Physiology
King George's Medical University
Lucknow (UP), India

Neeraj Agrawal
Professor and Head
Department of Endocrinology
Institute of Medical Sciences
Banaras Hindu University
Varanasi (UP), India

Niti Singh
Assistant Professor
Department of Medicine
Institute of Medical Sciences
Banaras Hindu University
Varanasi (UP), India

Padmamalika Khanna-Hazra
Boston Medical Centre
Soami Bagh
Agra (UP), India

Pankaj Kanaujia
Resident, Department of Medicine
Institute of Medical Sciences
Banaras Hindu University
Varanasi (UP), India

Prasanna Kumar KM
Consultant Endocrinologist
Bangalore Diabetes Hospital and CDEC
Bengaluru, Karnataka, India

Prashant Bhushan
Associate Professor
Department of Ophthalmology
Institute of Medical Sciences
Banaras Hindu University
Varanasi (UP), India

Radhika Jindal
Apollo Centre for Obesity,
Diabetes and Endocrinology
Indraprastha Apollo Hospital
Sarita Vihar, New Delhi, India

Rajeev Chawla
Senior Consultant
Diabetologist and Director
North Delhi Diabetes Centre
Delhi, India

Rajgopal Acharya
Resident
Department of General Surgery
Institute of Medical Sciences
Banaras Hindu University
Varanasi (UP), India

Richik Tripathi
Service Senior Resident
Department of Oral and Maxillofacial Surgery
Faculty of Dental Sciences
Institute of Medical Sciences
Banaras Hindu University
Varanasi (UP), India

RK Singh
Resident
Department of Medicine
Institute of Medical Sciences
Banaras Hindu University
Varanasi (UP), India

Royana Singh
Professor
Department of Anatomy
Institute of Medical Sciences
Banaras Hindu University
Varanasi (UP), India

RP Maurya
Assistant Professor
Department of Ophthalmology
Institute of Medical Sciences
Banaras Hindu University
Varanasi (UP), India

S Singh
Resident
Department of Endocrinology
Institute of Medical Sciences
Banaras Hindu University
Varanasi (UP), India

Samar Banerjee
Professor and Immediate
Past President RSSDI;
President, Association of Clinical Diabetology
Immediate Past President DIPSI;
Editor-in-Chief, Journal of Clinical Diabetology;
International Advisory Board Member,
Davidson's Text Book of Medicine

Sanjay Kalra
Executive Editor
Indian J Endocrinology and Metabolism
Executive Editor
J of Social Health in Diabetes (JoSH Diabetes)
Bharti Hospital and BRIDE
Karnal, Haryana, India

Santosh Kumar Yadav
Research Scholar, Department of Medicine
Institute of Medical Sciences
Banaras Hindu University
Varanasi (UP), India

Sarita Bajaj
Director-Professor and Head
Department of Medicine
MLN Medical College
Allahabad (UP), India

Satvik Khaddar
Resident
Department of Medicine
Institute of Medical Sciences
Banaras Hindu University
Varanasi (UP), India

SC Mohapatra
Professor
Department of Community Medicine
Institute of Medical Sciences
Banaras Hindu University
Varanasi (UP), India

Shivi Jain
Service Senior Resident
Department of Radiodiagnosis and Imaging
Institute of Medical Sciences
Banaras Hindu University
Varanasi (UP), India

SK Singh
Professor
Department of Endocrinology
Institute of Medical Sciences
Banaras Hindu University
Varanasi (UP), India

SS Pandey
Professor, Department of Dermatology
Dean, Faculty of Medicine and
Director, Institute of Medical Sciences
Banaras Hindu University, Varanasi (UP), India

Subhash Kumar Wangnoo
Apollo Centre for Obesity,
Diabetes and Endocrinology
Indraprastha Apollo Hospital
Sarita Vihar, New Delhi, India

Suchi Dwivedi
Consultant Psychiatrist and Medical Officer
CHC, Jamalpur, Mirzapur, India

Sunil M Jain
Total Diabetes Hormone Institute
BCM Health Islands D-44, Scheme 54
Indore (MP), India

Tanushree Chawla
Department of Medicine
MLN Medical College
Allahabad (UP), India

V Balaji
Director and Senior Consultant Diabetologist
Dr V Balaji Diabetes Care Centre
Dr V Seshiah Diabetes Research Institute, Chennai,
Hon. Secretary—Diabetes in Pregnancy Study Group,
India (DIPSI)
Member: WHO Expert Committee for Consultation
on Diagnosis and Screening for GDM, Expert Group
Committee on GDM, Ministry of Health Govt. of India

Vinay Kumar BR
Resident, Department of Medicine
Institute of Medical Sciences
Banaras Hindu University, Varanasi (UP), India

Vipul Garg
Senior Resident, Department of Medicine
Institute of Medical Sciences
Banaras Hindu University, Varanasi (UP), India

Vivek Srivastava
Assistant Professor, Department of General Surgery
Institute of Medical Sciences
Banaras Hindu University
Varanasi (UP), India

VP Singh
Professor, Department of Ophthalmology
Institute of Medical Sciences
Banaras Hindu University,
Varanasi (UP), India

FOREWORD

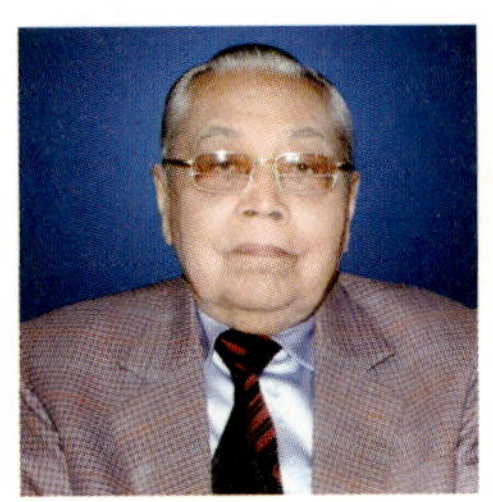

Diabetes, a noncommunicable disease, has acquired a status of epidemic since last two decades surpassing all the barriers of race, ethnicity, poverty and affluency. Though type I diabetes has remained a well understood endocrine disorder, type II diabetes still remains a conglomeration of heterogeneous disorders evolving in different forms of metabolic syndrome in different clinical presentation and genetic polymorphism. Initially thought to be the disease of rich people has shown its presence in the progeny of nutritionally starved mothers and famine-affected population. It has substantially contributed amongst younger population as an etiological factor of premature atherosclerosis, coronary artery disease and stroke. Late marriages, postponement of motherhood and artificial reproductive technique have resulted in higher incidences of gestational diabetes than earlier years. Diabetes is responsible for more than 50% of chronic kidney disease and patients on maintenance hemodialysis program.

Many new antiretroviral drugs, antidepressants and antipsychotics have also contributed in insulin resistance and new onset of diabetes.

Increasing awareness in print and electronic media and self-monitoring of blood glucose have also sensitized the common man, and a large section of population is being recognized as prediabetes which are potential targeted population for diabetes control to prevent the new onset of diabetes or delay its full blown clinical picture.

The present generation of internists, diabetologists and endocrinologists have now too many new drugs as oral antidiabetics, insulin analogs and drugs which restore physiology of insulin secretion. Understanding of glucose metabolism, lipid abnormalities, gene polymorphism, preservation of beta cell and its regeneration with stem cell is now the challenge of the day but equally important is the prevention, and many such efforts have now started showing the result. I hope this book, which deals with fundamental principles of diabetes practice, will be an asset to physicians in day-to-day practice and prevention of diabetes as a national goal.

HS Bajpai
MD FICP
Former
Director, Institute of Medical Sciences
Dean, Faculty of Medicine
Professor and Head of the Department of Medicine
Professor and Head, Division of Endocrinology
Medical Superintendent and Consultant, Sir Sunderlal Hospital
Banaras Hindu University, Varanasi, India

Ex-President, The Association of Physicians of India, UP Chapter, India
Ex-President, Endocrine Society of India, India

FOREWORD

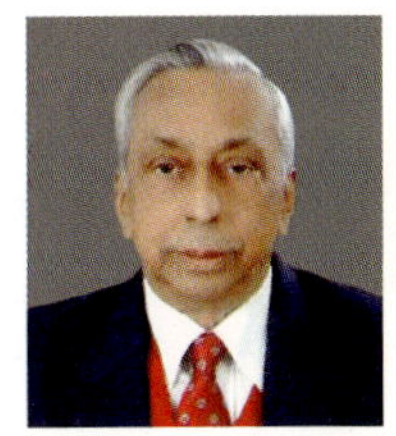

It is a great pleasure for me to write a foreword for this *Fundamentals of Diabetes* to be released during RSSDI-2015 being held at Lucknow. I must congratulate Dr Kamlakar Tripathi who shouldered this responsibility to compile write ups from faculties of national and international repute and edited those to be useful for diabetes practitioners. I am confident this book will be successful in its aim of making easy-to-understand fundamentals of diabetes for all its readers.

I am happy that RSSDI-UP is endeavoring it, on the occasion of 43rd national conference of Research Society for the Study of Diabetes in India (RSSDI) which now has been the largest organization of doctors practicing diabetes. Prof MMS Ahuja, who started the RSSDI in 1972, may never have visualized such a spectacular growth of this organization. I feel it is a very fitting tribute to the great visionary.

In the past ten years, diabetic population has grown fast throughout the world. India is also not remained untouched of this growth impacting adversely health of the nation. It is the need of the hour that every doctor should know the basics of diabetes. I am sure this book *Fundamentals of Diabetes* serves the purpose.

I must congratulate Dr Anuj Maheshwari who conceived this idea with Dr Kamlakar Tripathi and facilitated it to become a reality.

With my best wishes

Prof Amulya Ranjan Sircar
Professor and Ex Head of Department of Medicine
King George's Medical University
Lucknow (UP), India

PREFACE

The idea of writing a book on *Fundamentals of Diabetes* was conceived during the meeting of Executive members of Organizing Committee of Annual Conference of the Research Society for the Study of Diabetes in India (RSSDI) to be held at Lucknow during 2015 and to commemorate the celebration of annual RSSDI to be held for the first time in the state of Uttar Pradesh. The idea was first moved by Prof Anuj Maheshwari, Prof Narsingh Verma, Dr Brij Mohan and subsequently supported by Prof Sarita Bajaj, the Chairperson of Scientific Committee of RSSDI. I was given the privilege to edit the book for which I am obliged to all the members of organizing committee for their trust and faith in me. The editorial board feels obliged to all the authors who readily accepted my invitation and yielded to my request to send their manuscripts in time.

I am thankful to Associate editors Dr Amit Nandan Dwivedi and Dr Richik Tripathi for reviewing the manuscript and Dr Vinay Kumar BR, for his untiring efforts in formatting the text and adding his valuable contribution to some of the chapters on genetics, chronic kidney disease and epidemiology.

The secretarial assistance provided by Dr RK Misra was the most difficult job for transcripting some of the manuscripts and modifying the text to suite the publisher's specification.

In the last, I am indebted to the publishers M/s Jaypee Brothers Medical Publishers (P) Ltd., New Delhi, India for on-time publication and adding a lot of glamour to the book.

Kamlakar Tripathi

CONTENTS

1

CHAPTER

History of Diabetes

Kamlakar Tripathi, Santosh Kumar Yadav

INTRODUCTION

The history of diabetes has its roots in the Vedic literature of Indian medicine in its mythological epics. The first description has been given in Shiv Puran and Shrimad Bhagwat with a reference to the destruction of *"Yagyan"* by the followers and disciples of Lord Shiva. Daksha Prajapati (father-in-law of Lord Shiva) organized a *"Yagyan"* in which he did not invite Lord Shiva. However when his wife "Sati" reached her father's house, she did not find a respectable position in *mandap* for her husband (Shiva) and she felt humiliated and committed suicide. When the followers of Lord Shiva got the news of death of Sati they reached the *"Yagyan"* site and destroyed the *Yagyan,* consumed all the offerings which consisted of "*ghee, sugar, barley, high caloric nuts*", etc.[1,2]

Ever since then the diabetes became a disease of all those people who do not observe ethics, values and consume high caloric fatty diet which is meant for *Yagyan* and do not observe ritual and virtue of any such *Yagyan.*

Charak Samhita (2000 BC conceived and re-published 100 AD) (Fig. 1), the first authentic ayurvedic text, describes diabetes as Prameha which is a urinary disorder and present in different 20 forms. Madhumeha is one of the ultimate complications of the all types of Prameha. Some of these Prameha are in the form of passage of formed elements of blood, chyle, bone marrow, semen, pus and other content which are quite abstract in consistency and do not exist in true clinical form to be separated from each other by the modern physiological and biological description.[3]

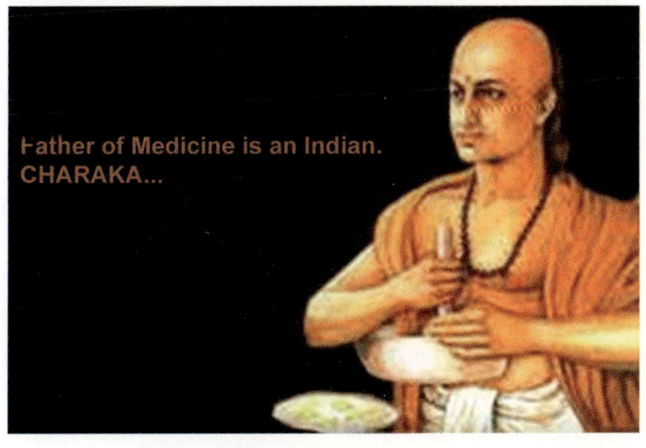

Fig. 1: Father of medicine: Charak

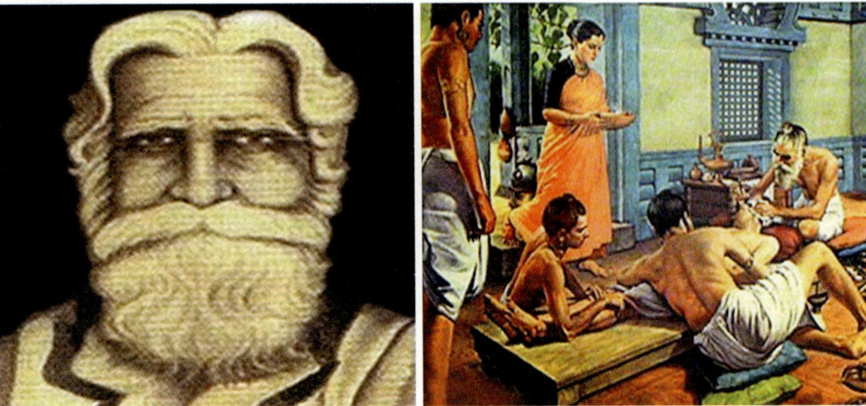

Fig. 2: Sushruta 600 BC practising Ayurveda

Sushruta (Fig. 2) who practiced surgery in the city of Varanasi during 750–500 BC has also given the description about Prameha, which could be due to vitiation of Kapha with different food items which are consumed with altered lifestyle and can lead to Prameha.

The ayurvedic physicians in India were able to treat and manage diabetes with lifestyle modification, observing strict avoidance of high carbohydrate diet, addition of fiber diet to retard the absorption of sugar from intestine and to reduce obesity. During the period of mediaeval history, Vagbhata and Jeevak in association with many Chinese and Tibetan travelers documented many herbs, leaves and fruits having sour taste and many spices which decreased appetite, reduced polyuria and could take care of "Madhumeha".

DIABETES MELLITUS AND THE ISLETS OF LANGERHANS

The Egyptians made the first mention of diabetes around 1500 BC. The Greek physician Aretaeus (130–200 CE) noted a disease with symptoms of constant thirst, excessive urination and loss of weight, and named the condition "diabetes", meaning "flowing through". The first clear reference to diabetes was made by an Arab physician, Avicenna (980–1037 CE), who accurately described in detail the clinical features and complications of the disease and its progress.[4]

It is possible that the sweet taste of the urine in this disease had been noticed by the physician of ancient India, but in modern times this fact was rediscovered by Willis. It may be mentioned that 24 years before Willis observation, there is a reference to the sweet taste of some urine in Moliére's play Le Médecin volant (1650). Reference has been already been made to the differentiation between the urine of diabetes mellitus and that of diabetes insipidus. The proof that the sweet taste of the urine in true diabetes is due to sugar was given in 1776 by Matthew Dobson (1745–1784) of Liverpool, who demonstrated that the residue after evaporation of such urine underwent vinous and acetic fermentation. Dobson made the further important observation that the blood serum in true diabetes also has a sweet taste and he was thus the discoverer of hyperglycemia. That the sugar in diabetic urine is glucose was first shown in 1815 by Michel Eugène Chevreul. Chevreul, one of the great French chemist and a pioneer in the chemistry of the animal fats and vegetable dyes was still as a centenarian carrying out important research; he was also director of the famous Gobelins tapestry works.

Recognition of the association between the pancreas and true diabetes came comparatively late. In 1778 Thomas Cawley, about who practically nothing was known, reported a case of diabetes in which there were numerous calculi in the pancreas. Richard Bright reported morbid changes in the pancreas in such case in 1831, von Recklinghausen described the presence of calculi in 1864 and Frerichs stated in 1884 that 20% of his cases of diabetes showed gross changes in the pancreas. Meanwhile Claude Bernard had been carrying out his important experiments on glycosuria.

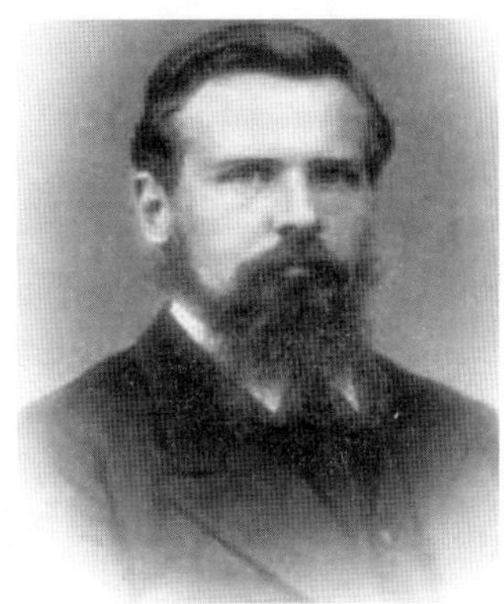
Fig. 3: Paul Langerhans

In an inaugural dissertation published at Berlin in 1869, Paul Langerhans (1847–1988) (Fig. 3) first described the islet of tissue scattered through the pancreas which were histologically distinct form and had no direct connection with the glandular tissue proper. The name of Langerhans was attached to these islet by Gustave Édouard Laguesse (1861–1927) of Lille in 1893, and by this name they have since then been known. Meanwhile, the crucial experiment showing that of diabetes is due to a lesion in the pancreas was made by Joseph von Mering (1849–1908) and Oscar Murkowski, then both at Strasbourg. In 1889 they excised the pancreas in animal and thus produced rapidly fatal diabetes. They also showed that the production of this condition was not due to the loss of the flow of pancreatic juice to the bowel. The conclusion was that the pancreas not only secretes the pancreatic juice, but that some part of it was also closely associated with general metabolism. These experiments were confirmed by Laguesse, who in 1893 suggested that the islets of Langerhans produced an internal secretion. In 1900 Eugene Lindsay Opie, then at Johns Hopkins, but later at St. Louis and the Henry Phipps Institute at Philadelphia, showed that in many cases of diabetes the islet have undergone hyaline degeneration. Other pathological changes in the islet have since been recorded, and a clear statement of the relation between lesion in this tissue and glycosuria was made by WG MacCallum in 1909.[5]

Many attempts were now made to isolate the active principle of the islet, but the difficulties were very great, since the trypsin destroy the internal secretion. It may be said retrospectively that there is no doubt that partial success was achieved in 1908 by Georg Ludwig Zuelzer (1870–1949) of Berlin. Zuelzer succeeded in obtaining a pancreatic extract which was given to eight diabetics with good results. Unfortunately, symptoms later developed which were regarded at the time as toxic, and this important work was abandoned. Eighteen years later, when more was known about the action of the hormone, it was suggested that the supposed "toxic" symptom had really been due to hypoglycemia, resulting from too large or too prolonged doses of a remedy which was successful.

Towards the end of the 19th century, a quantitative blood sugar method was published which used copper reduction and gravimetric measurement. Stanley Benedict devised an improved copper reagent for urine sugar in 1908, and this became, with modifications, the mainstay of urine monitoring of diabetes for over 50 years. Leading specialists in diabetes, notably Elliott Joslin in the USA, advocated a self-management concept relating to diet, exercise and frequent urine testing in an attempt to keep the urine sugar-free. In 1913, Frederick Allen, a leading US diabetologist, identified a clinical need to develop an accurate method for the quantitation of blood sugar for diagnostic purposes. In the first two decades of the 20th century Bang, Folin, Lewis, Benedict, Shaffer and many others pioneered laboratory methods for quantitative blood sugar. Proteins were removed and the reduction of cupric salts, ferricyanide or picrate used with titrimetric or, more often, colorimetric endpoints. Despite continual improvements in reducing sample volume, improving color stability and precision, manual blood sugar estimations in the laboratory were limited and mainly confined to diagnosis and critical care management, rather than for monitoring purposes. A breakthrough in the treatment and improvement in the lives of diabetics came about in 1921 when Frederick G Banting, his assistant, Charles Best, and JR Macleod succeeded in the identification of insulin, the pancreatic hormone deficient in diabetes, which was confirmed in human studies. Large-scale commercial extraction and purification of animal insulin led the way to the treatment for diabetes and to the development of improved testing systems.[6]

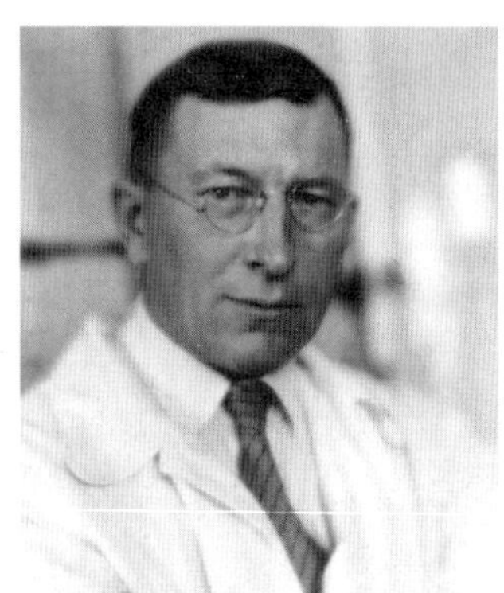
Fig. 4: Frederick Banting

Frederick Grant Banting (Fig. 4) was born on November 14, 1891, at Alliston, Ontario, Canada. He was the youngest of children of William Thompson Banting and Margaret Grant, educated at the Public and High Schools at Alliston, he later went to the University of Toronto to study divinity, but soon transferred to the study of medicine. In 1916 he took his MB degree and joined the Canadian Army Medical Corps, and served, during the First World War in France. In 1918 he was wounded in the Battle of Cambrai, and in 1919 he was awarded the Military Cross for heroism under fire. When the war ended in 1919, Banting returned to Canada and was for a short time a medical practitioner at London, Ontario. He studied orthopedic medicine during the year 1919–1920, Resident Surgeon at the Hospital for Sick Children, Toronto. From 1920 until 1921 he did part-time teaching in orthopedics at the University of Western Ontario at London, Canada, besides his general practice, and from 1921 until 1922 he was Lecturer in Pharmacology at the University of Toronto. In 1922 he was awarded his MD degree, together with a gold medal. Earlier, however, Banting had become deeply interested in diabetes. The work of Naunyn, Minkowski, Opie, Schafer, and others had indicated that diabetes was caused by lack of a protein hormone secreted by the islands of Langerhans in the pancreas. To this hormone, Schafer had given the name insulin, and it was supposed that insulin controls the metabolism of sugar, so that lack of it results in the accumulation of sugar in the blood and the excretion of the excess of sugar in the urine. Attempts to supply the missing insulin by feeding patients with fresh pancreas, or extracts of it, had failed, presumably because the protein insulin in these had been destroyed by the proteolytic enzyme of the pancreas. The problem, therefore, was how to extract insulin from the pancreas before it had been thus destroyed.

While he was considering this problem, Banting read in a medical journal an article by Moses Baron, which pointed out that, when the pancreatic duct was experimentally closed by ligatures, the cells of the pancreas which secrete trypsin degenerate, but that the islands of Langerhans remain intact. This suggested to Banting the idea that ligation of the pancreatic duct would, by destroying the cells which secrete trypsin, avoid the destruction of the insulin, so that, after sufficient time had been allowed for the degeneration of the trypsin-secreting cells, insulin might be extracted from the intact islands of Langerhans. Determined to investigate this possibility, Banting discussed it with various people, among whom was JJR Macleod, Professor of Physiology at the University of Toronto, and Macleod gave him facilities for experimental work upon it. Dr Charles Best (Fig. 5), then a medical student, was appointed as Banting's assistant, and together, Banting and Best started the work which was to lead to the discovery of insulin.

In 1922 Banting had been appointed Senior Demonstrator in Medicine at the University of Toronto, and in 1923 he was elected to the Banting and Best Chair of Medical Research, which had been endowed by the Legislature of the Province of Ontario. He was also appointed Honorary Consulting Physician to the Toronto General Hospital, the Hospital for Sick Children, and the Toronto Western Hospital. In the Banting and Best Institute, Banting dealt with the problems of silicosis, cancer, the mechanism of drowning and how to counteract it. During the Second World War, he became greatly interested in problems connected with flight.

In addition to his medical degree, Banting also obtained, in 1923, the LLD degree (Queens) and the DSc degree (Toronto). Prior to the award of the Nobel Prize in Physiology or Medicine for 1923, which he shared with Macleod, he received the Reeve Prize of the University of Toronto (1922). In 1923, the Canadian Parliament granted him a Life Annuity of $7,500. In 1928 Banting gave the Cameron Lecture in Edinburgh. He was appointed member of numerous medical academies and societies in his country and abroad, including the British and American Physiological Societies, and the American Pharmacological Society. He was knighted in 1934.[7]

DISCOVERY OF INSULIN

Before the discovery of insulin, diabetes was a feared disease that most certainly led to death. Doctors knew that sugar worsened the condition of diabetic patients and that the most effective treatment was to put the patients on very strict diets where sugar intake was kept to a minimum. At best, this treatment could buy patients a few extra years, but it never saved them. In some cases, the harsh diets even caused patients to die of starvation. During the 19th century, observations of patients who died of diabetes often showed that the pancreas was damaged. In 1869, a German medical student, Paul Langerhans, found that within the pancreatic tissue that produces digestive juices there were clusters of cells whose function was unknown. Some of these cells were eventually shown to be the insulin-producing beta cells. Later, in honor of the person who discovered them, the cell clusters were named the islets of Langerhans. In 1889 in Germany, Physiologist Oskar Minkowski and Physician Joseph von Mering, showed that if the pancreas was removed from a dog, the animal got diabetes. But if the duct through which the pancreatic juices flow to the intestine was ligated—surgically tied so the juices could not reach the intestine—the dog developed minor digestive problems but no diabetes. So it seemed that the pancreas must have at least two functions: (1) to produce digestive juices, and (2) "to produce a substance that regulates the sugar glucose this hypothetical internal secretion was the key". If a substance could actually be isolated, the mystery of diabetes would be solved. Progress, however, was slow.[8]

Banting's Idea

In October 1920 in Toronto, Canada, Dr Frederick Banting, an unknown surgeon with a bachelor's degree in medicine, had the idea that the pancreatic digestive juices could be harmful to the secretion of the pancreas produced by the islets of Langerhans. He therefore wanted to ligate the pancreatic ducts in order to stop the flow of nourishment to the pancreas. This would cause the pancreas to degenerate, making it shrink and lose its ability to secrete the digestive juices. The cells thought to produce an antidiabetic secretion could then be extracted from the pancreas without being harmed.

Early in 1921, Banting took his idea to Professor John Macleod at the University of Toronto, who was a leading figure in the study of diabetes in Canada. Macleod did not think much of Banting's theories. Despite this, Banting managed to convince him that his idea was worth trying. Macleod gave Banting a laboratory with a minimum of equipment and ten dogs. Banting also got an assistant, a medical student by the name of Charles Best. The experiment was set to start in the summer of 1921 (Fig. 5).

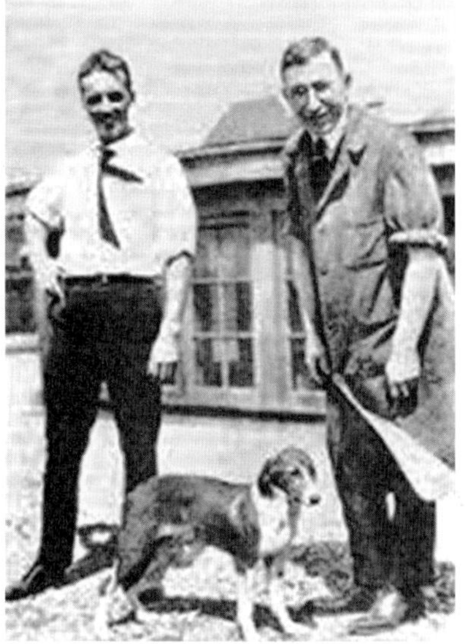

Fig. 5: Banting and Charles Best

Banting and Best began their experiments by removing the pancreas from a dog. This resulted in the following: its blood sugar rose. It became thirsty, drank lots of water, and urinated more often. It became weaker and weaker. The dog had developed diabetes. Experimenting on another dog, Banting and Best surgically ligated the pancreas, stopping the flow of nourishment, so that the pancreas degenerated. After a while, they removed the pancreas, sliced it up, and froze the pieces in a mixture of water and salts.

When the pieces were half frozen, they were ground up and filtered. The isolated substance was named "islet in". The extract was injected into the diabetic dog. Its blood glucose level dropped, and it seemed healthier and stronger. By giving the diabetic dog a few injections a day, Banting and Best could keep it healthy and free of symptoms. Banting and Best showed their result to Macleod, who was impressed, but he wanted more tests to prove that their pancreatic extract really worked.

For the increased testing, Banting and Best realized that they required a larger supply of organs than their dogs could provide, and they started using pancreases from cattle. With this new source, they managed to produce enough extract to keep several diabetic dogs alive. The new results convinced Macleod that they were onto something big. He gave them more funds and moved them to a better laboratory with proper working conditions. He also suggested they should call their extract "insulin". Now, the work proceeded rapidly. In late 1921, a third person, biochemist Bertram Collip, joined the team. Collip was given the task of trying to purify the insulin so that it would be clean enough for testing on humans. During the intensified testing, the team also realized that the process of shrinking the pancreases had been unnecessary. Using whole fresh pancreases from adult animals worked just as well.

Testing on Humans

The team was eager to start testing on humans. But on whom should they test? Banting and Best began by injecting themselves with the extract. They felt weak and dizzy, but they were not harmed. Collip continued his work to purify the insulin. He also experimented with trying to find the correct dosage. He learned how to diminish the effect of an insulin overdose with glucose in different forms. He discovered that the glucose should be as pure as possible. Orange juice and honey are good examples of foods rich in glucose. In January 1922 in Toronto, Canada, a 14-year-old boy, Leonard Thompson, was chosen as the first person with diabetes to receive insulin. The test was a success. Leonard, who before the insulin shots was near death, rapidly regained his strength and appetite. The team now expanded their testing to other volunteer diabetics, who reacted just as positively as Leonard to the insulin extract.

The Nobel Prize

The news of the successful treatment of diabetes with insulin rapidly spread outside of Toronto, and in 1923 the Nobel Committee decided to award Banting and Macleod the Nobel Prize in Physiology or Medicine. The decision of the Nobel Committee made Banting furious. He felt that the prize should have been shared between him and Best, and not between him and Macleod. To give credit to Best, Banting decided to share his cash award with him. Macleod, in turn, shared his cash award with Collip. The Nobel Prize in Physiology or Medicine for insulin has been much debated. It has been questioned why Macleod received the prize instead of Best and Collip. However, Macleod played a central role in the discovery of insulin. It was he who supported the project from the beginning. He supervised the work, and it is also most likely that Macleod's contacts in the scientific world helped the team in getting a speedy recognition of their discovery. Frederick G Banting and John Macleod were awarded the Nobel Prize in Physiology or Medicine in 1923 "for the discovery of insulin".[8]

The Legacy of Insulin; Banting, Macleod, and the rest of the team patented their insulin extract but gave away all their rights to the University of Toronto, which would later use the income from insulin to fund new research. Very soon after the discovery of insulin, the medical firm Eli Lilly started large-scale production of the extract. As soon as 1923, the firm was producing enough insulin to supply the entire North American continent. Although insulin does not cure diabetes, it is one of the biggest discoveries in medicine. When it came, it was like a miracle. People with severe diabetes and only days left to live were saved. And as long as they kept getting their insulin, they could live an almost normal life.

REFERENCES

1. Sri Swami Sivananda. The Bhagavad Gita. Gorakhpur: Geeta Press; 1995.
2. Sharsti JL. The Shiva Puran, vol. 1. New Delhi: Motilal Banarasi Das Publisher; 2008; pp 389-400.
3. Ram Rao B, Sastry JLN. History of Ayurveda (Ayurveda Ka Itihasa): Varanasi: Chaukhambha Orientalia; 2010.
4. Clarke SF, Foster JR. A history of blood glucose meter and their role in self-monitoring of Diabetes mellitus: Br J Biomed Sci. 2012;69(2).
5. Charles Singer, Ashworth E. Underwood, A short History of Medicine: Oxford: Clarendon Press. 1962.
6. Waymouth-Reid E. A method for the estimation of sugar in blood. J Physiol. 1896;20(4-5):316-21.
7. Nobel Lectures, Physiology or Medicine 1922–1941. Amsterdam: Elsevier Publishing Company; 1965.
8. Charles H Best. The Biography.com website. Retrieved. 2015;11:26.

2
CHAPTER

Epidemiology of Diabetes

SC Mohapatra

INTRODUCTION

Diabetes is much beyond the concept of the general population than the "*Sugar Disease*". The Chamber's Dictionary states, "Diabetes is any of several diseases marked by excess discharge of urine". Thus the prevalence of diabetes depends on how it is defined in the study. It is per se a group of diseases where there is "polyuria, polydipsia and polyphagia".

Diabetes is a known disease since 200 years, when Langerhans described the pancreatic islets in 1869 and 20 years after Minkowski experimentally produced diabetes in animal by removing the pancreas. Interestingly, the treatment of insulin for diabetes was discovered by an orthopedic team of Banting and Best in 1921, and by 2119 there will be an estimated diabetic about 387 million. As of 2010, an estimated 285 million people had diabetes, with 90% having type 2 diabetes.[1] International Diabetes Federation (IDF), estimated 381 million people having diabetes by 2013. The incidence is increasing rapidly, and by 2030 the cases will be doubled.[2]

Diabetes mellitus occurs throughout the world, but is more common (especially type 2) in the more developed countries but developing countries like India and China are leading in numbers. The Western European and American incidence study by Guy's Bedford survey was the first of its kind undertaken by glucose tolerance in the community in 1962, which showed the incidence to be 13/1,000 population with 130/1,000 normal population showing blood sugar 120 mg/100 mL of blood after ingestion of 50 g glucose. Recently, the greatest increase in prevalence is, however, expected to occur in Asia and Africa, by 2030. The increase in incidence in developing countries follows the trend of urbanization and lifestyle changes, perhaps most importantly a "Western-style" diet. This has suggested an environmental (i.e. dietary) effect, but there is little understanding of the mechanism(s) at present, though there is much speculation, some of it most compellingly presented. Almost one Chinese adult in ten has diabetes. A 2010 study estimated that more than 92 million Chinese adults have the disease, with another 150 million showing early symptoms. The incidence of the disease is increasing rapidly; a 2009 study found a 30% increase in 7 years.[3]

Box 1: Global burden: Fact sheet
• In 2012, 371 million people had diabetes; the numbers is likely to increase to 552 million by 2030.
• There is a rising incidence of type 2 diabetes globally.
• Approximately 80% of diabetic subjects live in low- and middle-income countries.
• The greatest number of people with diabetes are between 40 years and 59 years of age.
• Almost 50% (183 million) diabetics are undiagnosed.
Although, both type 1 and 2 diabetes contribute to this burden, and prevalence of type 1 diabetes has also increased over the years, type 2 diabetes is the major contributor to the epidemic, contributing more than 90% of all cases of diabetes. About 78,000 children develop type 1 diabetes every year.

In Australia, the age-standardized prevalence of self-reported diabetes in indigenous Australians is almost four times that of non-indigenous Australians.[4] China followed by India has more diabetics than any other country in the world. Every 6 s a person dies. The disease affects more than 62 million Indians, which is more than 7.1% of India's adult population. An estimate shows that nearly 1 million Indians die due to diabetes every year. The average age on onset is 42.5 years. The high incidence is attributed to a combination of genetic susceptibility plus adoption of a high-calorie, low-activity lifestyle by India's growing middle class.[5] A study by the American Diabetes Association reports that India will see the greatest increase in people diagnosed with diabetes by 2030.[6] About 3 million people in the United Kingdom have diabetes mellitus, and they could become high as 6.2 million by 2035 (Box 1).

THE GLOBAL BURDEN

Majority of 382 million people with diabetes, are aged between 40 years and 59 years, and 80% of them live in low- and middle-income countries.[6] The diabetes are on the increase, and more so, type 2 diabetes. Contrast to the other estimates, the IDF states, the number of people with diabetes will increase by 55% by 2035. An additional 21 million cases of high blood glucose in pregnancy are estimated to contribute to the global burden of diabetes. In human as well as financial terms, the burden of diabetes is enormous, provoking 5.1 million deaths and taking up some 548 billion US dollars in health expenditure (11% of the total spent worldwide) in 2013 (Fig. 1). More than 21 million live births were affected by diabetes during pregnancy in 2013. Diabetes UK have also predicted that the National Health Service (NHS) could be spending as much as 16.9 billion pounds on diabetes mellitus by 2035, a figure that means the NHS could be spending as much as 17% of its budget on diabetes treatment by 2035.[7]

The Figure 2 shows the quantum of the increase of the burden from today till 2015 world over, where the African burden will be increasing more than 100%. Diabetes caused 5.1 million deaths in 2013, and it is recorded that every 6 s one person dies of diabetes. Every country is affected by diabetes mellitus today, while exact figure of other kinds of diabetes is not available today. The disease in children as well as the young adults is increasing very fast in most developing countries, probably because of change in lifestyle. This will be leading to the burden on health care needs, cost at the same time flare up in the complications of the disease. It is estimated that Southeast Asia region has 20% of the global diabetic population, and they will be tripled by 2025.[8] During last 20 years, there has been substantial increase in diabetes

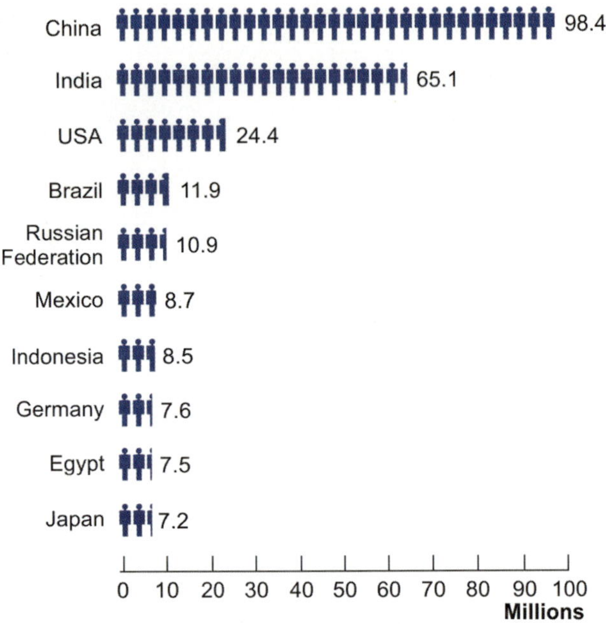

Fig. 1: Global burden of diabetes

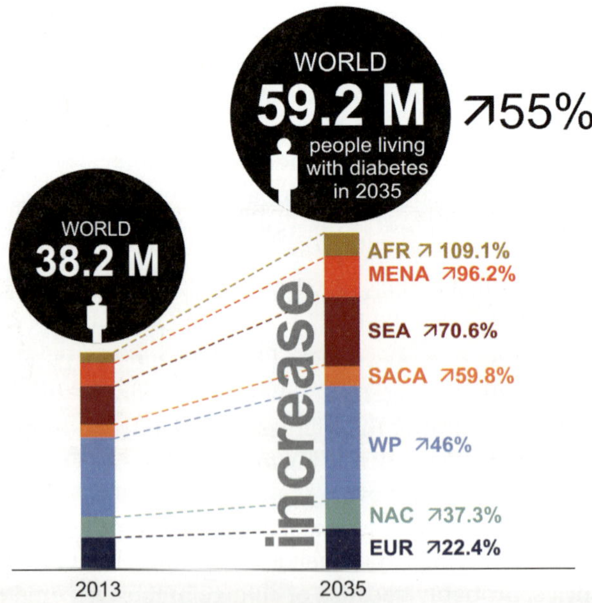

Fig. 2: Expected hike in diabetes

Abbreviations: AFR, Africa; MENA, Middle East and North America; WP, Western Pacific; SACA, South and Central America; SEA, South East Asia; EUR, Europe; NAC, North America and Caribbean

Source: International Diabetes Federation. IDF Diabetes Atlas, 6th edition. Brussels: IDF; 2014.

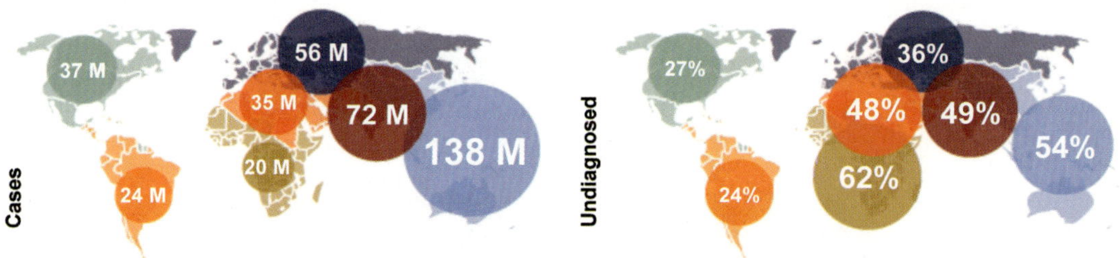

Fig. 3: Cases of diabetes world over
Source: International Diabetes Federation. IDF Diabetes Atlas, 6th edition. Brussels: IDF; 2014.

rates in the North America. In 2010, nearly 26 million people had diabetes; 7 million people remain undiagnosed and 57 million people are estimated to have pre-diabetes in the United States.[9]

The American Diabetes Association cites the 2003 assessment of the National Center for Chronic Disease Prevention and Health Promotion (Centers for Disease Control and Prevention) that one in three Americans born after 2000 will develop diabetes in their lifetimes.[10] Obesity, industrialization, acculturative nutrition and urbanizations have tremendous impact on occurrence of diabetes. The IDF states that indigenous people are especially vulnerable to diabetes. The Figure 3 as presented by IDF is being shown hereunder to highlight the problem as to how serious the problem is the diabetes is a disease of ice-berg where 50% cases remain undiagnosed, since more often than not, diabetes mellitus is diagnosed accidentally than intentionally, particularly in the developing countries where there are no scheduled screening.

EPIDEMIOLOGICAL CONCEPT IN DIABETES

At this juncture, the epidemiological interactions need to be re-defined. In diseases such as diabetes the traditional epidemiological triad does not effectively explain the causation. The host is the poor victim in any way, hence may not be included in the interaction. On the other hand, three other factors affect his health: the agent (particularly in communicable diseases), environment (including lifestyle) and genetic factors (particularly in case of noncommunicable diseases). The gene needs special mention since it could be of the human host or the agent or the vector; in other word, a factor that affects extensively and universally. The Figure 4 depicts the epidemiological quadrate for diabetes mellitus or most noncommunicable diseases, for that matter.

Thus what is essential for health care delivery system is to timely and universally identify the genetic predilection for noncommunicable diseases as primordial prevention measure in order to control disease occurrences. This has been amply proved by Cyprus as to how one nation's culture influences its genes and control disease.

The lives of Cypriots with β-thalassemia have changed over the years. Improved population genetic health care during the past decades has dramatically increased life expectancy for people with two mutations associated with β-thalassemia from 3 or 4 years to almost 30 years

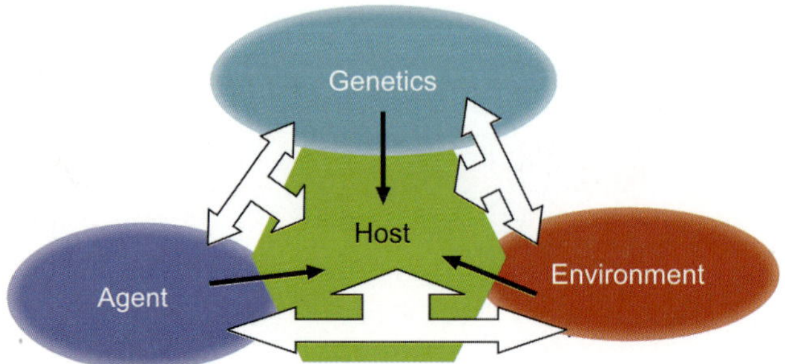

Fig. 4: Concept: epidemiological quadrate

and the prevalence has also reduced.[11] In considering the noncommunicable diseases with the glass of genetics, therefore, the modern epidemiological concept ought to have the next molding of epidemiological quadrate as explained above.

Genetics, the Epidemiological Factor

Non-insulin-dependent diabetes mellitus (NIDDM) shows strong familial aggregation. Twin and family studies have provided firm evidence that the role of the genetic component is relatively strong.[12] NIDDM appears to be the consequence of an interaction between this genetic susceptibility and exposure to environmental factors. In certain populations in which there is evidence of a major genetic component, a "thrifty genotype" has been proposed.[13] By conferring metabolic efficiency, this offers advantages in times of prolonged food deprivation but becomes disadvantageous when food is plentiful. Several genes have been suggested as markers for NIDDM but to date, apart from evidence for abnormalities in the adenosine deaminase[14] and glucokinase genes[15] in some families affected by maturity-onset diabetes of the young, no other consistent abnormalities have yet been found. However, it has become clear today that the gene is the 4th interacting component of diabetes as the epidemiological quadrate for sure. Several environmental factors have been proposed such as physical activity, poverty, nutritional factors, diet, alcoholism, stress, hormonal therapy, body weight and fat distribution, etc. The prevalence increases with age, and particularly in populations undergoing epidemiological transition—a high IGT prevalence may prelude to "epidemic" levels of NIDDM in these communities.[16] In insulin-dependent diabetes mellitus (IDDM) (type 1 diabetes) the concordance was 50%, as against 90% in NIDDM. Thus IDDM is not totally a genetic entity.[17] The IDDM genetic markers are HLA-B8, B15, HLA-DR3 and DR4 and NIDDM is not HLA associated disease.

Other epidemiological determinants include inflammatory or neoplastic pancreatic disorders, cystic fibrosis, synthesis of abnormal insulin, etc. are also partial genetic entities. However viral infections due to rubella, mumps and coxsackie are blamed to be diabetogenic.

Similarly chemical agents such as alloxan and streptozotocin and rodenticides, etc. can also damage the pancreas and produce diabetes. Age-wise, while NIDDM affects the middle aged people nutritional diabetes can be seen in younger age. Sex-wise male and female show equal diabetic load in the developing countries while in India there is male preponderances, which may be due to higher hospital attendance of the males. Obesity, particularly central deposition is accepted as a risk factor for NIDDM, as seen in India and Sri Lanka.

Physical inactivity or sedentary lifestyle is a known risk factor for diabetes. Lack of exercise alters the relationship between insulin and its receptors, and eventually induces NIDDM. Sedentariness also acts indirectly by promoting obesity. On the other hand, low birth weight, premature baby, protein-energy malnutrition, starvation, etc. have a damaging effect on beta cells of pancreas, which impairs carbohydrate metabolism, which may progress to diabetes.

Deficiency of trace elements such as calcium, copper and zinc are suspected to induce diabetes. In some cases, controlled experimental studies have shown dietary fiber have effect in reducing hyperglycemia.[18] High and low level of diabetes has been associated with different social class and groups like many more noncommunicable diseases.

Diagnosis of Diabetes Mellitus

As per WHO,[17] the diagnostic criteria is oral glucose tolerance test (GTT) as given in the Table 1. There has been distinct difference between the type 1 and type 2 diabetes mellitus which has been given in a simplified way in the Table 2.

People of diabetes mellitus not judged clinically not to be in urgent need of insulin to preserve life are classified as non-insulin-dependent. This is classification by exclusion. NIDDM covers a wide spectrum of degrees of glucose intolerance, ranging from the totally asymptomatic to the severely symptomatic. Metabolic status may deteriorate with time or improve with treatment.

Table 1: Diagnosis of diabetes mellitus by oral glucose tolerance test

Diabetes	FPG 2hpp	≥7.0 mmol/L (126 mg/dL) or ≥11.1 mmol/L (200 mg/dL)
Impaired glucose tolerance	FPG	<7.0 mmol/L (120 mg/dL) and ≥ 7.8 and 11.1 mmol/dL
Impaired fasting glucose	2hPP FPG	140 mg/dL and 200 mg/dL 6.1 to 6.9 mmol/L 2hpp <7.8 (110 to 125 mg/dL, (140 mg/dL)

Table 2: Differences between type 1 and 2 diabetes mellitus

Features	*Type 1 diabetes mellitus*	*Type 2 diabetes mellitus*
Pathogenesis	Pancreatic damage	Insulin resistance
Age of onset	Usually <20 years	Usually ≥30 years
Presentation	Sudden	Gradual
Ketoacidosis	Common	Not common
Family trend	<10%	Common
Twin concordance	40%	100%
Acanthosis nigricans	Not seen	Common
Obesity	Not common	Common
HLA association	Common	No association
Insulin requirement	Is a Must	May be needed
Islet cell antibodies	As high as ≥85%	<5%

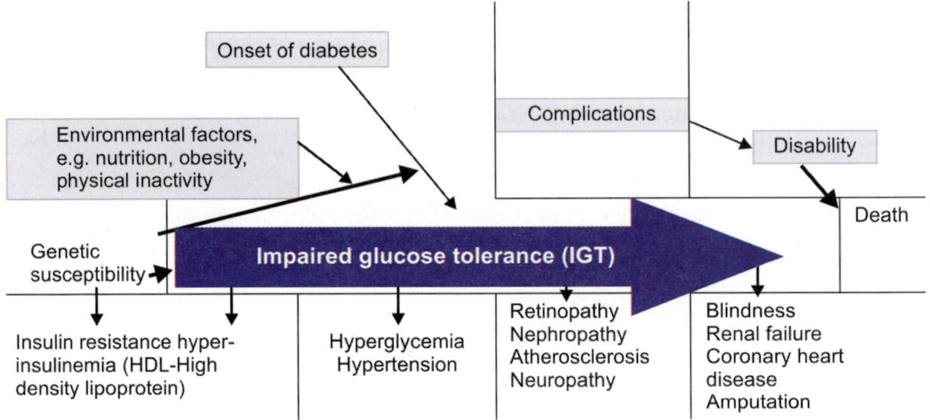

Fig. 5: The natural history of NIDDM

Source: Modified from WHO study group. WHO Technical Report Series; 844. Geneva: WHO; 1994.

The subdivision of NIDDM into obese and non-obese forms is recognized and is included in the 1985 WHO Study Group's classification. As regards Malnutrition-related diabetes mellitus, there is no association between fibrocalculous pancreatic diabetes and gallbladder disease or, in most cases, excessive alcohol intake, and no indication that the characteristic pancreatic fibrosis is postinflammatory in nature.[19] The underlying causative mechanism(s) may relate to the effect of dietary toxins against a background of long-standing malnutrition, as suggested by the association between the global distribution of fibrocalculous pancreatic diabetes and the consumption of dietary toxins in foods such as cassava root (manioc, tapioca). Further investigation is needed of the possible role of cyanogenic glycosides (e.g. linamarin) in initiating cellular injury and causing this form of diabetes when detoxifying mechanisms are inadequate because of insufficient intake of dietary protein rich in sulfur-containing amino acids. Other food toxins may play a similar role. NIDDM and IGT detected only during pregnancy, gestational NIDDM (GDM) and gestational IGT (GIGT) tend "to recur with subsequent pregnancies; GDM carries a very high risk of the ultimate development of permanent NIDDM.

There are at least three major factors of importance: (1) individual or ethnic genetic factors leading to susceptibility; (2) defects in pancreatic beta cell function; and (3) decreased action of insulin in insulin-sensitive tissues (insulin resistance), including skeletal muscle, liver and adipose tissue). The natural history of NIDDM is depicted in the Figure 5. The genetic factors are therefore important epidemiological factors beyond the typical triad, as explained earlier.

Screening for Non-insulin-dependent Diabetes Mellitus

The question of mass community screening for NIDDM remains controversial issue, since covering the whole population is operationally and administratively difficult. Technically, detection of diabetes in asymptomatic or minimally symptomatic individuals will result in effective treatment that may retard its progression and reduce the risk or the severity of complications, thus diminishing premature morbidity and mortality. The sensitivity, specificity and cost-wise diagnostic/screening tools have been depicted in the Table 3, as per WHO.[14]

Table 3: Cost and sensitivity of screening method in diabetes

Diabetes type	*Method*	*Specificity*	*Sensitivity*	*Cost*
NIDDM*	Glycated HbA_{1c} or proteins	+ + +	+/-	+ + +
	Urine glucose	+/-	+/-	+
	Casual blood glucose	+ +	+	+
	Fasting blood glucose	+ + +	+	+
	Oral glucose tolerance test	+ + +	+ +	+ +
IDDM	HLA type	+/-		+ + +
	ICA	+	+	+ + +
	Anti-GAD	+	+	+ + +
	Early insulin secretion	+/-	+	+ +

Keys: -, none; +/-, none or minimal; +, low; + +, intermediate; + + +, high.
* At present screening can be recommended only for high-risk individuals or for epidemiological studies.
Abbreviations: HLA, human leukocyte antigen; ICA, islet cell cytoplasmic antibodies; anti-GAD, antibodies to glutamate decarboxylase.

There can be population screening, which is meant for health care planning, epidemiological research or high prevalence populations. But this is not cost-effective neither cost beneficial. Thus it is recommended to undertake selective screening, taking ethnicity, positive family history, obesity and other factors such as age, previous abnormal GTT, hypertension, macrovascular disease or dyslipoproteinemia, etc. Opportunistic screening is probably one of the most pragmatic way of screening diabetes.[21] Opportunistic screening is highly cost-effective as well as convincing by counseling for the patient. For sure or not, this is the most frequently occurring diagnostic path of diabetes.

PREVENTION AND CONTROL

It cannot be too emphatically said that diabetes can be controlled, but it can definitely be reduced below the public health problem level. Taking a cue from the Western European and American incidence study by Guy's Bedford survey was the cutoff level of public health problem should be set at the incidence to be 13/1,000 population. However there is no set universally accepted cutoff level for diabetes to set as public health problem. It is increasingly accepted that diabetes is a major public health problems. Health care organizations have recognized the enormous personal and public costs of uncontrolled diabetes in terms of complications, patient quality of life and health care system resources. Multilevel systems approach addresses supportive and inhibitory social-environmental factors at multiple levels such as personal, family, health care team, work, neighborhood, community are key areas to be dealt with. The key disciplines contributing to a population-based approach to diabetes include epidemiology, behavioral science, health care services, public health, health economics and quality of life professions. Diabetes is a major public health and economic problem, affecting over 17 million Americans and costing nearly $132 billion a year.[20] The situation over the globe is almost similar with the influential deviation due to lifestyle, nutrition and the health care status.

Primordial Prevention

The carefulness of the health system in a country is inversely proportional to the morbidity status. So is for diabetes. The health programs for prevention of maternal and fetal malnutrition, program for healthy newborn, protection of malnutrition in under-fives and protection of people from starvation are major primordial steps to be included in country's health program. Monthly or annual universal health checkup/screening for abnormalities should be the integral part of health program of all countries. This will prevent risk factors before they appear. No prevention program should be commenced without a properly constituted evaluation component of the health system. Making baseline measurements to establish the prevalence, risk factors including IGT and general and central obesity and to determine levels of physical activity and fitness and of other factors such as insulin resistance, blood lipids and blood pressure, fasting plasma insulin concentration and/or insulin sensitivity should also be assessed periodically, as a part of inbuilt health program of the country. Such step of primordial approach would help preventing many noncommunicable diseases; the component of regular, continuous and timely information collection may be increased depending on the local priority of the country. It is therefore considered as the population strategy of diabetes prevention.

Primary Prevention

This is the important prevention component for both communicable and noncommunicable diseases. As regards diabetes, strict implementation of steps of primordial prevention should be the first step in primary prevention. The other steps of preventive measure includes maintenance of body weight, adoption of healthy diet, including fiber food in daily meals, physical exercise, adopting healthy lifestyle, avoidance of alcohol, restriction on fasting and feasting, etc. The stress should be avoided with escalating spiritual wellbeing by simple Indian habits such as listening religious music, yoga and gardening particularly in the morning. Strict and regular screening of personal health is an integral protection measure of diabetes and many more noncommunicable diseases such as heart disease and cancer. Specific protection measure for type 1 diabetes is genetic counseling, which in south Asian countries, understood as nonpractical. But avoidance of sedentary lifestyle, overnutrition, alcoholism and obesity will help protecting from NIDDM. Persons in risk of diabetes, whether family history is positive, should avoid diabetogenic drugs such as oral contraceptive and chemical agents such as alloxan, streptozotocin and rodenticides, etc. Deficiency of trace elements, such as calcium, copper and zinc, need to be replenished in the subject at risk. These steps are included in the high-risk strategies for diabetes.

Secondary Prevention

It is the key measure of protective strategy in diabetes mellitus which gives emphasis on early diagnosis and adequate effective treatment. The measures include maintenance of blood glucose level close to the normal limits as far as practicable, regulate body weight to normal level, avoidance of feast and fast and adding fiber diets to meal. Regulating blood glucose level with oral hypoglycemic agents or insulin is the only curative-prevention measure. In the meantime, the patient must regularly check the blood and urine sugar, urine for protein and ketone bodies, vision, blood pressure and the kidney function. Glycosylated hemoglobin estimation should be undertaken every 6 months to get the long-term index of glucose control. Personal care of self and responsibility has to be the inbuilt lifestyle of the patient toward avoidance of alcohol and injury, adherence to diet and drug regimen as per medical advice, self-glucose monitoring, understanding hypoglycemia effect and reporting to the consultant timely are the key elements of protective strategy. As per WHO (2011), the Table 4 shows the efficacy of individual protective strategy.[21] Further, the woman found to have glucose intolerance during pregnancy, the high risk of the later development of diabetes[22] offers the important possibility of preventive intervention.

Table 4: The efficacy of individual protective strategy (adapted from WHO)[21]

Individual intervention with evidence of efficacy	*Benefits*
• Lifestyle intervention for preventing type 2 diabetes in high-risk people	• Reduction of 35–58% in incidence
• Metformin for preventing type 2 diabetes in high-risk people	• Reduction of 25–31% in incidence
• Glycemic control in people with HbAlc greater than 9%	• Reduction of 39% in microvascular disease per 1% drop in HbAlc
• Blood pressure control in people having blood pressure higher than 130/80 mm Hg	• Reduction of 359% in macro- and microvascular disease per 10 mm Hg drop in blood pressure
• Annual eye examination	• Reduction of 60–70% in serious vision loss
• Foot care of people with high risk of ulcer	• Reduction of 50–60% in serious foot disease
• Angiotensin converting enzyme inhibitor use in all people with diabetes	• Reduction of 42% in nephropathy and 22% drop in cardiovascular disease

It has been claimed that the vigorous treatment of GDM (gestational diabetes mellitus) with insulin during pregnancy will reduce the risk for the fetus and of overt diabetes later in life in the mother. This requires confirmation by controlled clinical trials. After pregnancy, dietary intervention to prevent obesity and physical exercise (as for prevention of NIDDM) are rational measures, but should also be the subject of planned clinical trials.

All patients of diabetes, irrespective of type 1 or type 2, should carry a personal information card showing the details for treatment, the names of person and physician for contact during any crisis. Education measures for the patient and the family members about care in diabetes are an optimizing measure of prevention and care.

Tertiary Prevention

Tertiary prevention of diabetes aims at the limiting of disability as well as increasing rehabilitation. The aim of this step is to provide capability strategy for the patients to withstand the complications which make the patient disable; such as gangrene of the lower limb, blindness, coronary thrombosis needing instant care, kidney failure or thriving over an insulin coma. The health system needs to develop specialized diabetic clinic and disability skirmishing units. The tertiary health units for diabetes must get involved in regular clinical and epidemiological research as well as public aware measures in form of mass media, print information and senior citizen aware clinics. Establishment of local and national registries have been advocated in this regards.[13] Periodic evaluation and country-wise information dissemination should also be an important national strategy.

REFERENCES

1. Melmed S, Polonsky KS, Larsen PR, Kronenberg HM. Williams Textbook of Endocrinology, 12th edition. Philadelphia: Elsevier/Saunders; 2012. pp 1371-435.
2. Wild S, Roglic G, Green A, Sicree R, King H. Global prevalence of diabetes: Estimates for the year 2000 and projections for 2030. Diabetes Care. 2004;27(5):1047-53.
3. Greens, Kerry (April 4, 2012). Diabetes continuing to spike in China. Reuters. Retrieved 8 June, 2012.
4. Australian Institute for Health and Welfare. Diabetes, an overview. Archived from the original on 2008-06-17.
5. International Diabetes Federation. IDF Diabetes Atlas, 6th edition. Brussels: IDF; 2014.
6. Roglic G, Green A, Sicree R, et al. Global prevalence of diabetes. Diabetes Care. 2004;27:1047-53.
7. http://managingdiabetes.co.uk/articles/diabetesnhsspending.php
8. WHO, Health Situation in South-East Asian Region, 1994-97, SERO, 1999.
9. Washington RE, Andrews RM, Mutter RL. Emergency Department Visits for Adults with Diabetes, 2010. HCUP Statistical Brief No 167. November 2013.
10. Harris MI, Flegal KM, Cowie CC, Eberhardt MS, Goldstein DE, Little RR, Wiedmeyer HM, Byrd-Holt DD. Prevalence of diabetes, impaired fasting glucose, and impaired glucose tolerance in U.S. adults. The Third National Health and Nutrition Examination Survey, 1988–1994. Diabetes Care. 1998;21(4):518-24.
11. Floya Anthias. Cyprus into the New Millennium, Cyprus: How One Nation's Culture Influences Its Genes. Gene letter. 2010;23:44.
12. Bennett PH, Bogardus C, Tuomilehto J, et al. The Epidemiology of NIDDM: obese and non-obese. In: Alberti KGMM, DeFronzo RA, Keen H, et al. (Eds). International Textbook of Diabetes Mellitus. London: John Wiley & Sons Ltd, 1992.
13. Neel JV. Diabetes mellitus: a thrifty genotype rendered detrimental by "progress"? Am J Hum Genet. 1962;14:353-62.
14. Bell GL, Xiang KS, Newman MV, et al. Gene for non-insulin-dependent diabetes mellitus (maturity-onset diabetes of the young subtype) is linked to DNA polymorphism on human chromosome 20q. Pro Natl Acad Sci USA. 1991;88(4):1484-8.
15. Froguel P Vaxillaire M, Sun F, et al. Close linkage of glucokinase locus on chromosomes 7p to early onset NIDDM. Nature. 1992;356(6365):162-4.
16. Virtanen SM, Childhood diabetes in Finland study group. Infant feeding in Finish children <7 years of age with newly diagnosed IDDM. Diabetes Care. 1991;14:415-7.
17. WHO study group. WHO Technical Report Series, 727. Geneva: WHO; 1985.
18. Marshall JA, Hoag S, Shetterly S, et al. Dietary fat predicts conversion from impaired glucose tolerance to NIDDM, Diabetes Care. 1994;17:50-6.
19. WHO study group. WHO Technical Report Series, 844. Geneva: WHO; 1994.
20. Parihar S, Parihar A, Mohapatra A, et al. Can gingival crevicular blood glucometry on dental out-patients be an opportunistic screening innovation for Diabetes Mellitus? Ind J PSM. 2012;43(3):159-64.
21. World Health Organization. WHO global status report on noncommunicable disease, 2010. Geneva: WHO; 2011.
22. O'Sullivan JB. Diabetes mellitus after GDM. Diabetes. 1991;40(Suppl 2):131-5.

3
CHAPTER

Pancreas Islet Cells and Its Development

Royana Singh

INTRODUCTION

The pancreas is an elongated, accessory digestive gland which lies retroperitoneally and transversely across the posterior abdominal wall, posterior to the stomach between the stomach on the right and the spleen on the left—largely in the transpyloric plane. The transverse mesocolon attaches to its anterior margin. The pancreas is both an endocrine and an exocrine gland. Its exocrine secretion, from acinar cells, known as pancreatic juice contains a number of digestive enzymes and is alkaline to neutralize the acidic chyme. The juice enters the duodenum via the main and accessory pancreatic ducts. It also secretes hormones from its endocrine parts, known as the islets of Langerhans. The hormones secreted are insulin and glucagon, which are responsible for maintaining blood glucose homeostasis.

At the midgut junction, the septum transversum generates two pancreatic buds (dorsal and ventral endoderm) which will fuse to form the pancreas. The dorsal bud arises first and generates most of the pancreas. The ventral bud arises beside the bile duct and forms only part of the head and uncinate process of the pancreas (Fig. 1).

In the fetal period, islet cell clusters (ICCs) differentiate from pancreatic bud endoderm. These cell clusters form acini and ducts (exocrine). On the edge of these cell clusters, pancreatic islets (endocrine) are also formed. Pancreatic hormonal function is to secrete insulin and glucagon which together regulate blood glucose levels and also somatostatin.

The pancreas exocrine function begins after birth, while the endocrine function (hormone release) can be measured from 10 weeks to 15 weeks onward. At this stage, it is not clear what the exact roles of these hormones are in regulating fetal growth.[1-3]

- Functions—exocrine (amylase, α-fetoprotein), 99% by volume; endocrine (pancreatic islets), 1% by volume.
- Exocrine function—begins after birth.
- Endocrine function—from 10 weeks to 15 weeks onward hormone release.

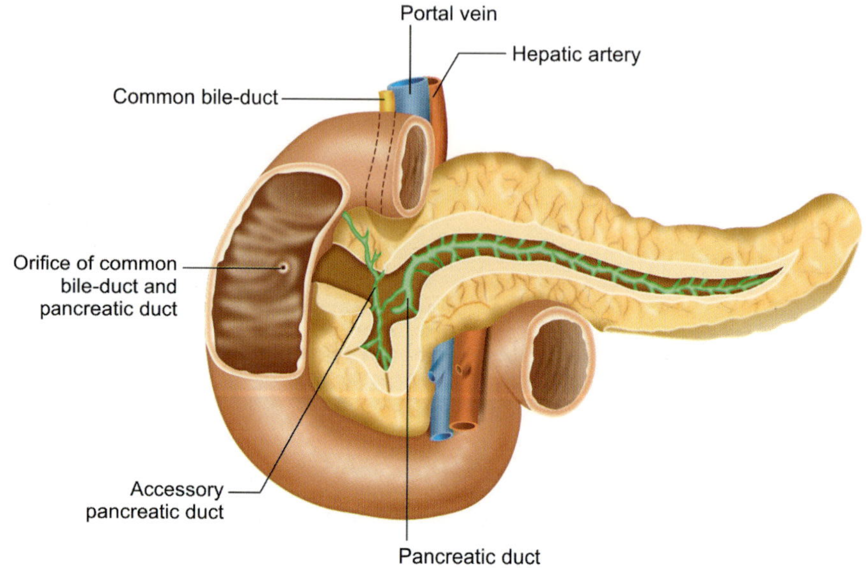

Fig. 1: Adult pancreas (Gray's anatomy)

DEVELOPMENT OF THE PANCREAS

- Pancreatic buds—duodenal level endoderm, splanchnic mesoderm forms dorsal and ventral mesentery, dorsal bud (larger, first), ventral bud (smaller, later).
- Pancreas endoderm—pancreas may be opposite of liver. Heart cells promote/notochord prevents liver formation. Notochord may promote pancreas formation. Heart may block pancreas formation.
- Duodenum growth/rotation—brings ventral and dorsal buds together, leading to fusion of buds.
- Cord of endodermal cells from ducts, from which cells bud off to form islet.
- Pancreatic duct—ventral bud duct and distal part of dorsal bud.

The pancreas develops between the layers of mesentery from the dorsal and ventral pancreatic buds of endodermal cells that arise in the caudal part of the foregut that is developing into proximal duodenum. The dorsal pancreatic bud is in the dorsal mesentery which attaches the developing gut tube to the posterior abdominal wall. The dorsal pancreatic bud is larger than the ventral, and appears first. It grows rapidly between the peritoneal layers of the dorsal mesentery. The ventral pancreatic bud grows between the layers of the ventral mesentery which attaches the developing gut tube to the anterior abdominal wall. It is in close proximity to the gallbladder which develops as a diverticulum. As the duodenum rotates to the right and becomes C-shaped, the ventral pancreatic bud is carried dorsally in a manner similar to the displacement of the entrance of the bile duct. The ventral pancreatic duct comes to lie posterior and inferior to the dorsal pancreatic bud. Later the parenchyma and the duct systems of the dorsal and ventral pancreatic buds fuse. The parenchyma of the pancreas is derived from the endoderm of the pancreatic buds. As the pancreatic buds fuse, their ducts anastomose. The ventral pancreatic duct forms the uncinate process and the inferior part of

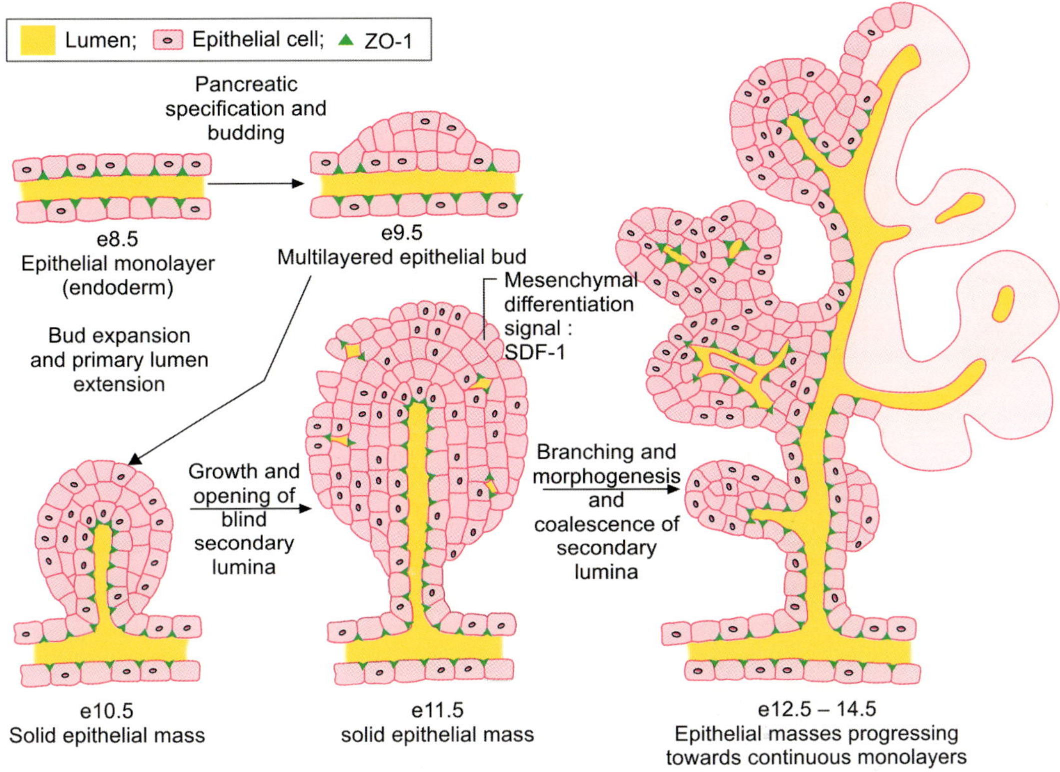

Fig. 2: Development of the exocrine part of the pancreas

the head of the pancreas. The remaining part of the gland is derived from the dorsal pancreatic bud. As the stomach, duodenum and ventral mesentery rotate, the pancreas comes to lie along the dorsal abdominal wall. The main pancreatic duct (duct of Wirsung) forms from the entire duct of the ventral bud and the distal part of the duct of the dorsal bud. The proximal duct of the dorsal bud may persist as the accessory pancreatic duct (duct of Santorini).

The main pancreatic duct and the bile duct enter the duodenum at the site of the major papilla. When present, the site of the accessory duct is at the site of the minor papilla. The pancreas ends up retroperitoneally. The peritoneum of the pancreas fuses with the peritoneum of the posterior body wall to become retroperitoneal. The pancreas is pushed up against the posterior body wall by the transverse colon. In the third month of fetal life, pancreatic islets of Langerhans develop from the parenchymatous tissue and scatter throughout the pancreas.[4-6] This forms the endocrine portions of the pancreas. Insulin secretion begins at approximately the fifth month of fetal life.[7] Glucagon- and somatostatin-secreting cells also develop from the parenchymal cells (Figs 2 and 3).

Pancreatic specification of polarized endodermal cells leads to the formation of a multilayered and then globular mass of epithelial cells with a central duct lumen (pancreatic bud). This lumen, connected to the gut tube lumen, forms extensions within the pancreatic bud, and is surrounded by several layers of cells, linked by adherens junctions (E-cadherin), but lacking tight junctions (ZO-1).

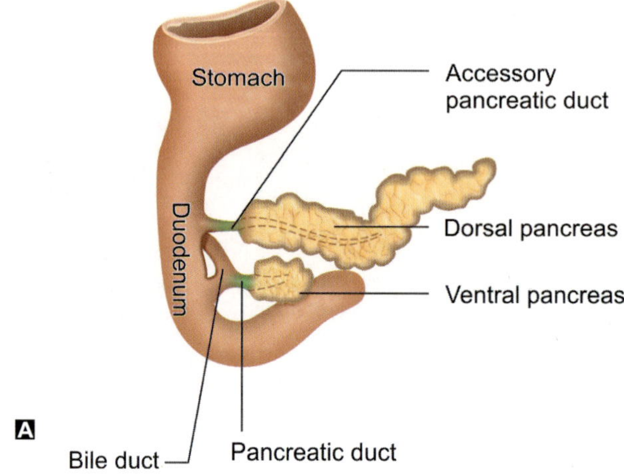

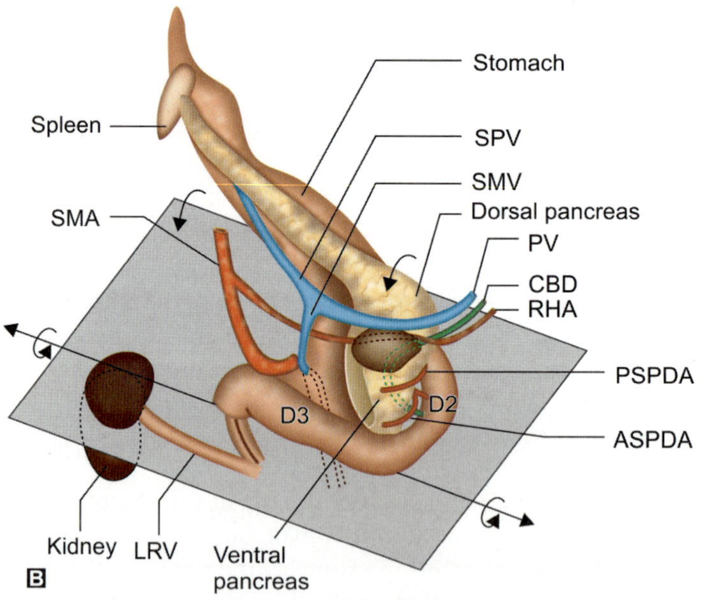

Figs 3A and B: (A) Development of the ventral and the dorsal bud of the pancreas and its rotation for its final position in the abdomen. Fetal pancreas: fetal topographical anatomy of the pancreatic head and duodenum with special reference to courses of the pancreaticoduodenal arteries. (B) A diagram showing joining processes between the dorsal and ventral primordia of the pancreas as well as the hypothetical rotation of the duodenum along a left-right axis. Viewed from the posterosuperior side of the body. A horizontal plane including most parts of the duodenum is shown to emphasize, in contrast to adults, the course of the second portion (Fig. 3B) directing posteriorly rather than inferiorly[10]

DEVELOPMENT OF ENDOCRINE PANCREAS CELLS

There are four main endocrine adult cell types:

1. Alpha-cells secreting glucagon α- and β-cells, δ-cells
2. Beta-cells secreting insulin
3. Delta-cells secreting somatostatin
4. Pancreatic polypeptide (PP) cells secreting pancreatic polypeptide.

Pancreatic G-cells are similar to α-cells in that it is dependent on Arx. Pancreatic G-cells similar to epsilon cells in that both gastrin and ghrelin are frequently coexpressed with glucagon in the embryonic pancreas.[8-10]

Factor Information (Fig. 4)

Factors which help in the differentiation of different protein during development of pancreas.

- Pdx1—pancreas/duodenum homeobox protein 1
  - Transcription (transactivator) factor binds the TAAT element in the promoter region of target genes, mainly those involved in pancreas development.
- Ngn3—neurogenin3
  - Basic helix-loop-helix transcription factor involved in the determination of neural precursor cells in the neuroectoderm.
- NeuroD1—neurogenic differentiation 1
- A basic helix-loop-helix (bHLH) protein that acts as a transcription factor involved in determining cell type during development.

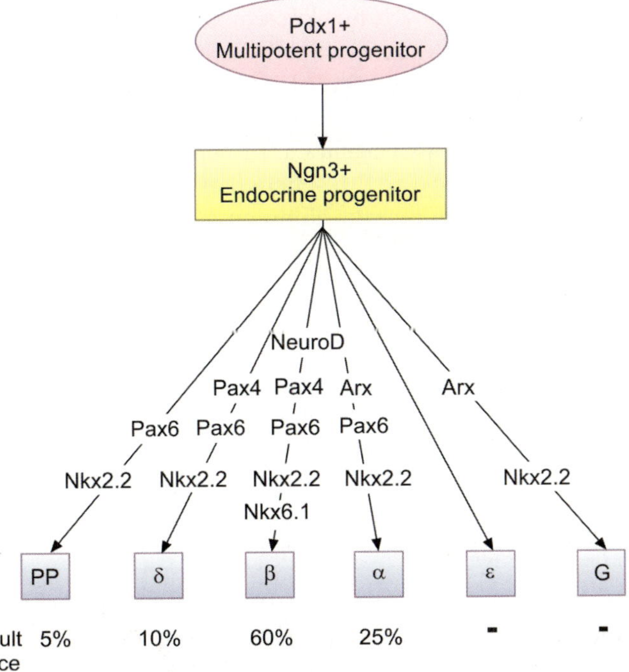

Fig. 4: Progenitors and Pax gene family responsible for the endocrine development of pancreas

- Arx—aristaless-related homeobox, X-link
  - Homeobox protein that belongs to the aristaless-related subset of the paired (Prd) class of homeodomain proteins.
- Pax4—paired box gene 4
  - Transcription factor containing a paired box domain.
- Pax6—paired box gene 6
  - Transcription factor containing a paired box domain.
- Nkx2.2—NK2 homeobox 2
  - Homeobox (Hox) containing transcription factor contains a 60-amino acid evolutionarily conserved DNA-binding homeodomain.
- Nkx6.1—NK2 homeobox 6.1
  - Homeobox (Hox) containing transcription factor contains a 60-amino acid evolutionarily conserved DNA-binding homeodomain required for β-cells development and is completely conserved between rat, mouse and human.

FINDINGS

- Gastrin: a distinct fate of neurogenin3 positive progenitor cells in the embryonic pancreas[3]
  - Neurogenin3(+) [(Ngn3(+)] progenitor cells in the developing pancreas give rise to five endocrine cell types secreting insulin, glucagon, somatostatin, pancreatic polypeptide and ghrelin. Gastrin is a hormone produced primarily by G-cells in the stomach, where it functions to stimulate acid secretion by gastric parietal cells. Gastrin is expressed in the embryonic pancreas and is common in islet cell tumors, but the lineage and regulators of pancreatic gastrin(+) cells are not known. Gastrin is abundantly expressed in the embryonic pancreas and disappears soon after birth.
- Pancreatic mesenchyme regulates epithelial organogenesis throughout development[4]
  - The developing pancreatic epithelium gives rise to all endocrine and exocrine cells of the mature organ. During organogenesis, the epithelial cells receive essential signals from the overlying mesenchyme. Mesenchymal cells regulate pancreatic growth and branching at both early and late developmental stages by supporting proliferation of precursors and differentiated cells, respectively.
- Relative roles of the different Pax6[5]
  - The transcription factor Pax6 functions in the specification and maintenance of the differentiated cell lineages in the endocrine pancreas. It has two DNA-binding domains: (1) the paired domain and (2) the homeodomain, in addition to a C-terminal transactivation domain. The phenotype of Pax6-/- knockout mice suggests nonredundant functions of the transcription factor in the development of glucagon-expressing α-cells as this cell type is absent in the mutants.

MICROSCOPIC FEATURES

Microscopically the pancreas is arranged in 1–10 mm lobules. The parenchyma within the lobules consists almost entirely of the epithelial elements of the pancreas, including the acini, the ducts, and the islets of Langerhans. There is minimal intralobular connective tissue, but fibroconnective tissue containing vessels and nerves separates the lobules.

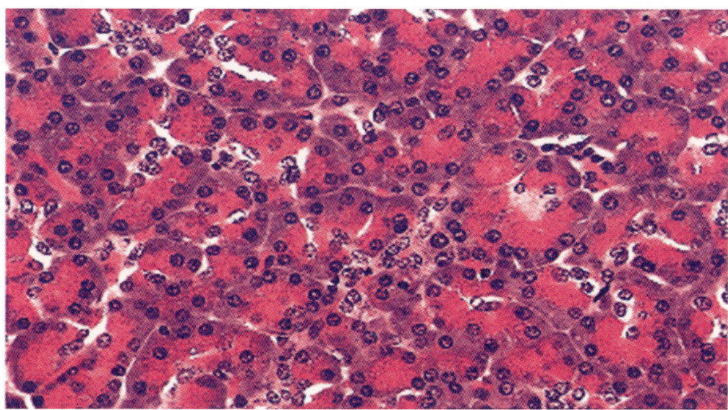

Fig. 5: Acinar cells contain abundant granular eosinophilic cytoplasm in the apical aspect, with basophilic basal cytoplasm. The nuclei are also basally located. Most acini consist of spherically arranged individual acinar cells[8,11]

Acini

Acinar cells make up approximately 85% of the mass of the pancreas and constitute the main exocrine secretory component of the gland. The prototypical architecture of the acinus in routine histologic sections appears to be a single layer of polygonal cells surrounding a minute central lumen, suggesting a spherical configuration; however, the three-dimensional architecture of the pancreatic acini is much more complex.[10] In fact, tubular acini are commonly detected. Also, not all acini are located at the terminal end of ductules. Some acini buds from the sides of the ductules or are situated between two ductules. Anastomosing loops of acini also may be found.[10] Thus, the secretions of a given acinus may pass through a number of different pathways to reach the ductal system.

Individual acinar cells are polarized with basally situated round nuclei and apical granular eosinophilic cytoplasm. The eosinophilia of the apical cytoplasm reflects the accumulation of numerous zymogen granules (Fig. 5), which contrast with the basophilic zymogen granules of salivary serous acini. The zymogen granule content is highly dynamic, depending on the secretory state of the pancreas, which is largely regulated by digestive hormones.[11] The basal cytoplasm of the acinar cells is basophilic due to the high concentration of ribonucleoproteins in the abundant rough endoplasmic reticulum (RER). There may be a clear cytoplasmic zone on the luminal side of the nucleus that contains the Golgi apparatus.

The nuclei are uniform and frequently contain distinct central nucleoli; clumps of chromatin are generally present beneath the nuclear membrane. The acinar cells sit directly upon the basement membrane; in contrast to salivary acini, there are no myoepithelial cells surrounding the pancreatic acini.

Islets of Langerhans

The endocrine component of the pancreas constitutes only 1–2% of the volume of the gland in adults[11,12] but about 10% in the newborn.[13,14] The vast majority of endocrine cells are found in the over one million islets of Langerhans, first described by Paul Langerhans in 1869. Although islets are distributed throughout the pancreas, they are somewhat more numerous in the tail.[15] Apparently random variations in islet concentration may occur from one lobule to the next, resulting in the appearance of plentiful islets in one area and sparse islets in an adjacent region.

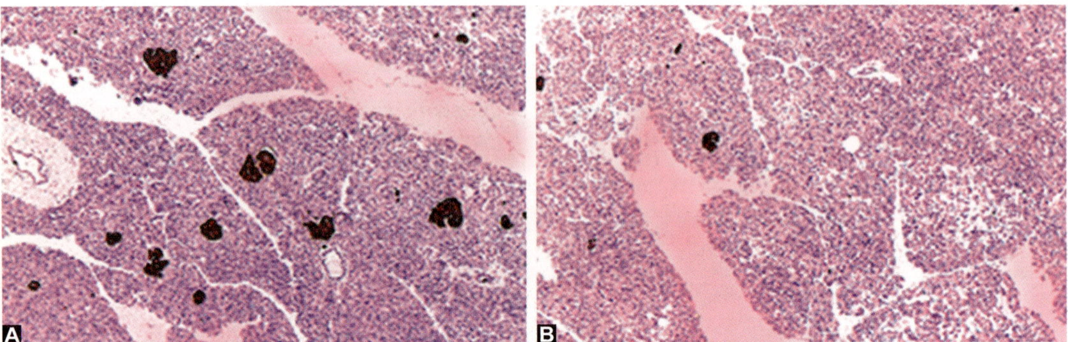

Figs 6A and B: As highlighted by immunohistochemical labeling for chromogranin, the concentration of islets varies considerably from (A) one lobule to (B) the next

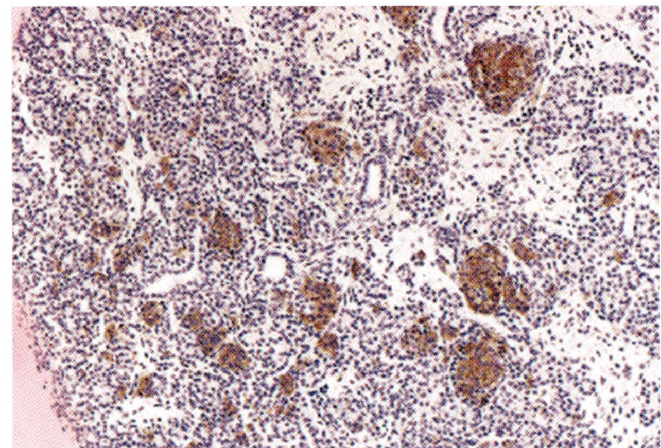

Fig. 7: A fetal pancreas stained immunohistochemically for chromogranin. Note the abundance of endocrine cells relative to acinar cells at this stage of development

The apparent volume of islets observed in histologic sections also varies with the age of the individual and the presence and extent of exocrine atrophy, as commonly occurs in chronic pancreatitis. In the fetus and neonate, the relative volume of endocrine cells far outmeasures that of the adult, especially in the portions derived from the dorsal lobe (Figs 6A and B and 7).[16]

Two types of islets are found. Most (90%) are the compact islets: sharply circumscribed nests usually measuring 75–225 μm, although islets as small as 50 μm or as large as 280 μm also may be found.[17] Compact islets are found predominantly in the body and tail of the gland, with fewer in the head. The second type of islet, the diffuse islet, is essentially restricted to the posteroinferior head of the gland derived from the embryonic ventral lobe.[18,19] These islets are much less numerous than the compact islets and may measure up to 450 μm.

Despite the circumscribed appearance of the compact islets, they are actually composed of interdigitating trabeculae that appear as small lobules in cross section.[17] The cells of the compact islets have uniform round nuclei with coarsely clumped chromatin and inconspicuous nucleoli (Fig. 8). The cytoplasm is pale and amphophilic. Occasional islet cells have nuclei two to four times the size of their neighbors, although no irregularities of shape or chromatin

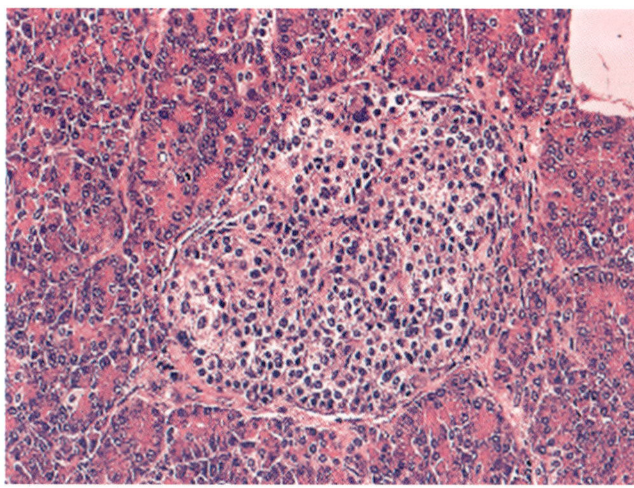

Fig. 8: Compact islets consist of round to oval, generally circumscribed collections of endocrine cells. Small capillaries separate the islet into lobules. The nuclei have a stippled chromatin pattern, and there is moderate amphophilic cytoplasm. Some islet cells contain enlarged nuclei several times the size of those in the neighboring cells

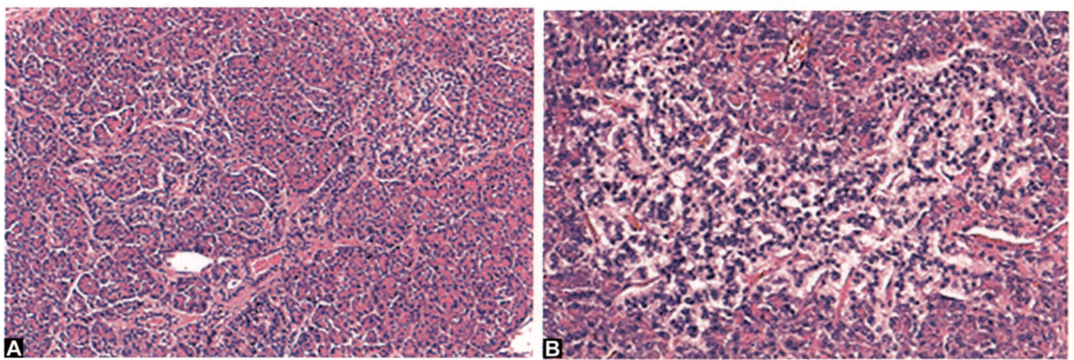

Figs 9A and B: (A) Diffuse islets are composed of trabeculae of endocrine cells interspersed between adjacent acini. (B) The borders of the diffuse islets are ill defined. The cells have somewhat basophilic cytoplasm

pattern are present. These nuclei have a 4n or 8n DNA content and have been shown to occur exclusively in β-cells;[20] they do not have any pathologic significance. Mitotic figures are only rarely encountered in normal islets.[21,22]

The islets contain numerous small vessels, although these capillary-sized vessels are almost in apparent by light microscopy. Essentially all of the islet cells contact the vasculature. In contrast to those supplying the acinar tissue, the capillaries of the islets have a fenestrated endothelium.[11] A thin layer of connective tissue separates the compact islets from the surrounding acinar tissue, but they are not truly encapsulated.

Diffuse islets have a trabecular appearance with winding cords of cells intermingled among acini (Fig. 9A). Because they are less commonly encountered and have a pseudoinfiltrative appearance, they may be mistakenly regarded as neoplastic, an occurrence even more likely in the setting of chronic pancreatitis. In addition to the architectural differences already mentioned, the diffuse islets contain columnar cells within the trabecula. The cytoplasm

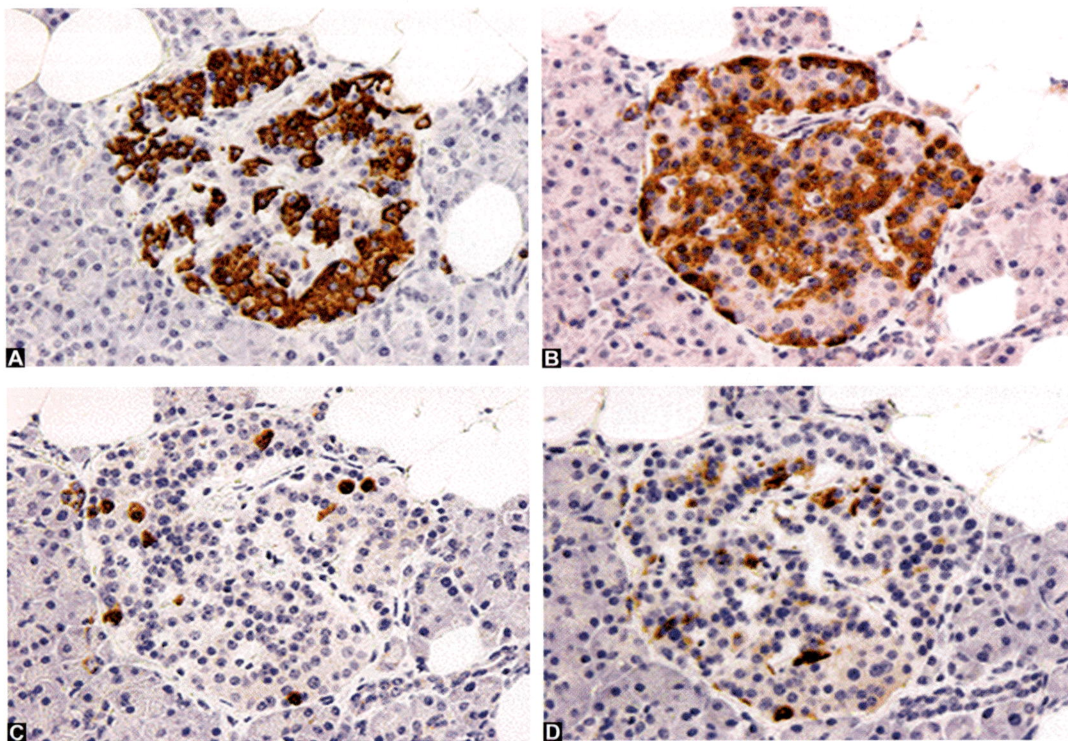

Figs 10A to D: The distribution of the different peptide-producing cells within the islets of Langerhans. (A) Beta-cells (labeled for insulin) are the most numerous and are situated in the central regions of the islet. (B) Alpha-cells (labeled for glucagon) are generally arranged around the periphery. (C) Delta-cells (labeled for somatostatin) and (D) PP cells (labeled for pancreatic polypeptide) are much less numerous and do not display an obvious pattern of arrangement

is basophilic, the nuclei are somewhat hyperchromatic, and there may be more prominent nucleoli than in the compact islets (Fig. 9B).

Each endocrine cell produces only one specific peptide hormone. The four major peptides produced by islet cells are: (1) insulin, (2) glucagon, (3) somatostatin and (4) pancreatic polypeptide.[22] Although some pancreatic endocrine neoplasms produce ectopic peptides such as gastrin or vasoactive intestinal polypeptide, these are not found in normal islet cells. Histochemical staining is used to distinguish the different cell types. Aldehyde-fuchsin stains insulin-secreting β-cells, the Grimelius silver stain labels glucagon-secreting α-cells, and the Hellerstrom-Hellman silver stain identifies somatostatin-secreting δ-cells. Immunohistochemical labeling with antibodies against insulin, glucagon, somatostatin and pancreatic polypeptide provides a more specific method to distinguish the cell types. There is a fairly consistent distribution of the cell types within the compact islets. The β-cells are more centrally located, whereas the α-cells populate the periphery of the islets (Figs 9 and 10). Beta-cells constitute 60–70% and α-cells make up 15–20% of the compact islets, whereas the δ-cells are much less numerous.[17,23,24] Alpha-cells are generally found in close contact with δ-cells,[25] and PP cells are rare in the compact islets, being concentrated in the diffuse islets where they constitute the majority (70%) of the cells (Fig. 11).[25,26] The remaining cells of the diffuse islets

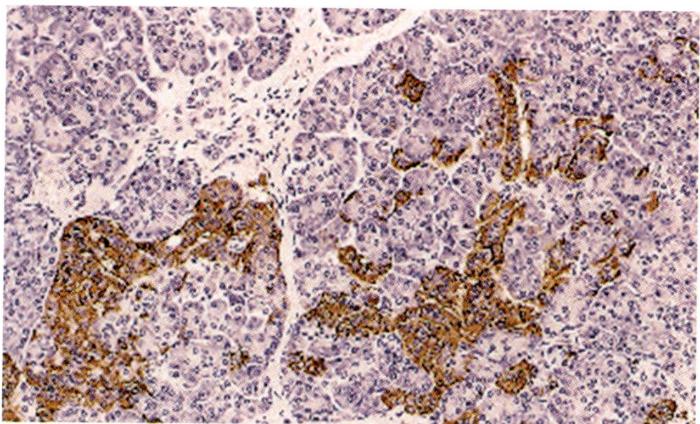

Fig. 11: Immunohistochemistry for pancreatic polypeptide shows positive staining in most of the cells in the diffuse islets

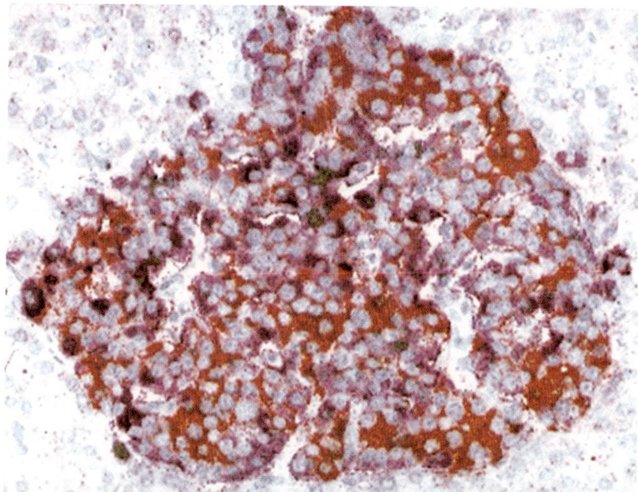

Fig. 12: Triple immunohistochemical labeling of a compact islet for insulin (red-brown reaction product), glucagon (violet reaction product) and somatostatin (green reaction product) shows the characteristic distribution of the different cell types

are largely β-cells (20%), with minor amounts of α- and δ-cells (5% of each). The difference in proportion of cell types between the compact and diffuse islets reflects their different embryologic origins.[18,19] The relative proportion of the different peptide-producing cells also varies with age; for instance, the ratio of β- to δ-cells in the compact islets is many folds higher in adults than in infants, in whom δ-cells constitute one-third of the islet cell population.[14,27] All of the islet cells also express general endocrine markers such as neuron-specific enolase, CD56 (neural cell adhesion molecule), synaptophysin and chromogranin. The last marker is expressed more intensely in α-cells than in β-cells, and the pattern of labeling also reflects the characteristic distribution of the cell types in the compact islets (Fig. 12).

Keratins generally are not detected in islet cells by immunohistochemistry, although there may be some faint labeling with CAM 5.2. Enzymes also are not detectable. Progesterone and CD99 receptors are expressed in normal islets as well as in some pancreatic endocrine neoplasms.[28-30] The homeodomain protein Pdx1, a transcription factor important in pancreatic development, is also expressed in adult islet cells.

Ultrastructural examination of the islets shows polygonal cells joined by tight and gap junctions, suggesting that there may be electronic or metabolic coupling between adjacent cells.[17, 24] Scattered desmosomes are also present. The cytoplasm contains all of the organelles necessary for protein synthesis, including RER, mitochondria, and Golgi apparatus; however, the abundant parallel arrays of RER characteristic of acinar cells are absent (Fig. 13). The granules are also more randomly distributed within the cytoplasm, with some concentration in the basal cytoplasm adjacent to the capillaries into which they are secreted. The granule sizes and morphologies are relatively specific for each cell type.[22,31] Alpha-cell granules measure 200–300 nm and contain an eccentrically located, dense core within a less dense outer region that is separated from the limiting membrane by a thin halo (Fig. 14A). Beta-cells contain 225–375 nm granules with either a finely granular or a crystalline core surrounded by a wide halo underlying the limiting membrane (Fig. 14B). Cytoplasmic lipid inclusions (or ceroid bodies) are often found in β-cells (Fig. 13).[24] Delta-cell granules are slightly smaller (170–220 nm) than α-cell granules and have a uniformly dense core (Fig 14C). Delta-cells have cytoplasmic processes extending toward the α- and β-cells, presumably allowing local paracrine release of somatostatin in addition to systemic release into the bloodstream.[17] The PP cells of the ventrally derived portion of the pancreas have 180–220 nm granules of variable shape and density, whereas the PP cell granules of the remainder of the pancreas are smaller (120–150 nm) and more homogeneous (Fig. 14D).[13] The cells are separated from the fenestrated endothelial cells of the capillaries only by the basement membranes of both cells and minimal interstitial material.[24]

Pancreatic development is also regulated by cell fate determining signals from developmental patterning pathways, such as the Notch and Hedgehog (Hh) signaling pathways. Notch signals are required for epithelial branching and normal exocrine lineage commitment.[33] Of the three Hedgehog genes essential for mammalian embryogenesis [Sonic Hedgehog (Shh), Indian

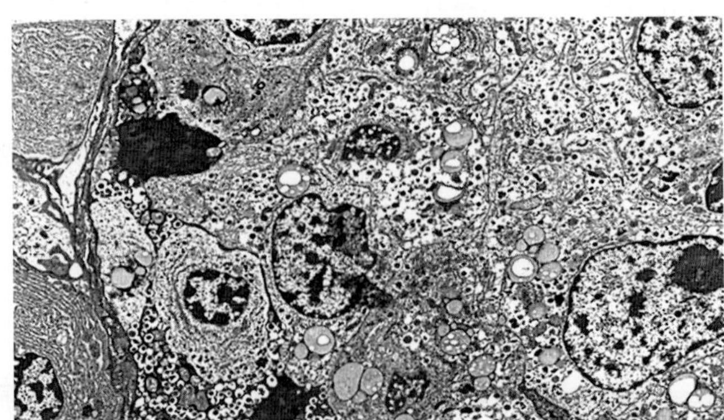

Fig. 13: Ultrastructural appearance of islets of Langerhans. The islets are circumscribed and separated from the adjacent acinar cells (left). The peptide granules are randomly distributed within the cytoplasm. Lipid inclusions (ceroid bodies) are found within the β-cells

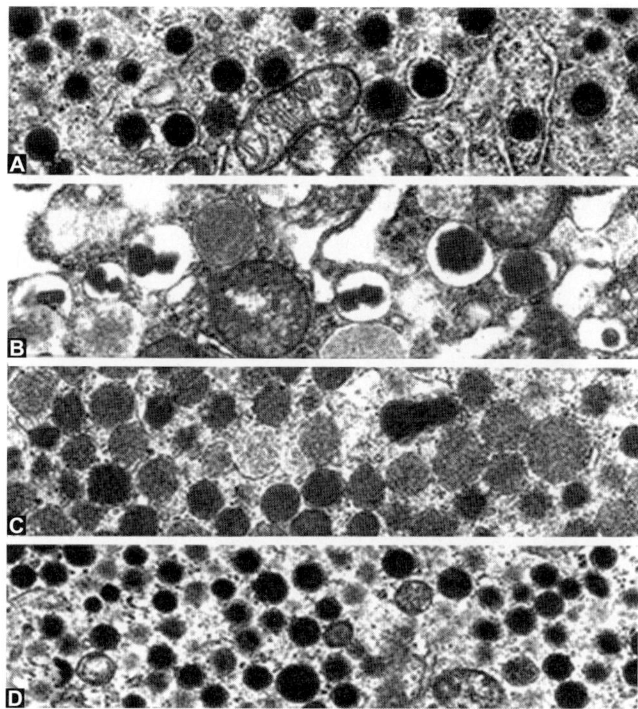

Figs 14A to D: Ultrastructural appearance of islet cell granules. (A) Alpha-cell granules are round and contain an eccentric electron-dense core within a less dense peripheral region. There is a thin halo beneath the limiting membrane. (B) Beta-cell granules are polymorphous and contain crystalline cores with a wide halo beneath the limiting membrane. (C) Delta-cell granules are round with a moderately dense core surrounded by a very thin halo. (D) The granules of PP cells are smaller and have homogeneous hyperdense cores

Source: Reprinted with permission from reference 32.

Hedgehog (Ihh) and Desert Hedgehog (Dhh)], Shh expression in mid-gestational embryos is critical for proper foregut and gastrointestinal development. In contrast, Shh is excluded from the developing pancreas, and repression of Shh permits appropriate transcriptional activation of pancreatic genes.[34]

The developing ducts form solid cellular cords that proliferate into the surrounding mesenchyme. As the ducts branch progressively, luminal spaces are formed. Both acinar and endocrine cells develop from these primitive ducts.[35] The cells at the termini of the branches differentiate into acinar cells during the third month of gestation.[35] The pancreatic lobules are formed by the accumulation of acinar units around ductular branches that are separated by layers of mesenchyme.[36] By the fourth month, the acinar cells contain zymogen granules.[37] The earliest granules identified in acinar cells are elongated and angular, with a fibrillary internal matrix. These granules, along with small spherical granules, may be detected at 15–20 weeks of gestation.[37-39] By 20 weeks, the granules resemble the zymogen granules of the adult pancreas, and the elongate granules disappear. The nature of the elongate granules remains unclear, and enzymes have yet to be detected in them. However, it is interesting that similar "irregular fibrillary granules" have been repeatedly detected in pancreatic neoplasms with acinar differentiation.[39-44]

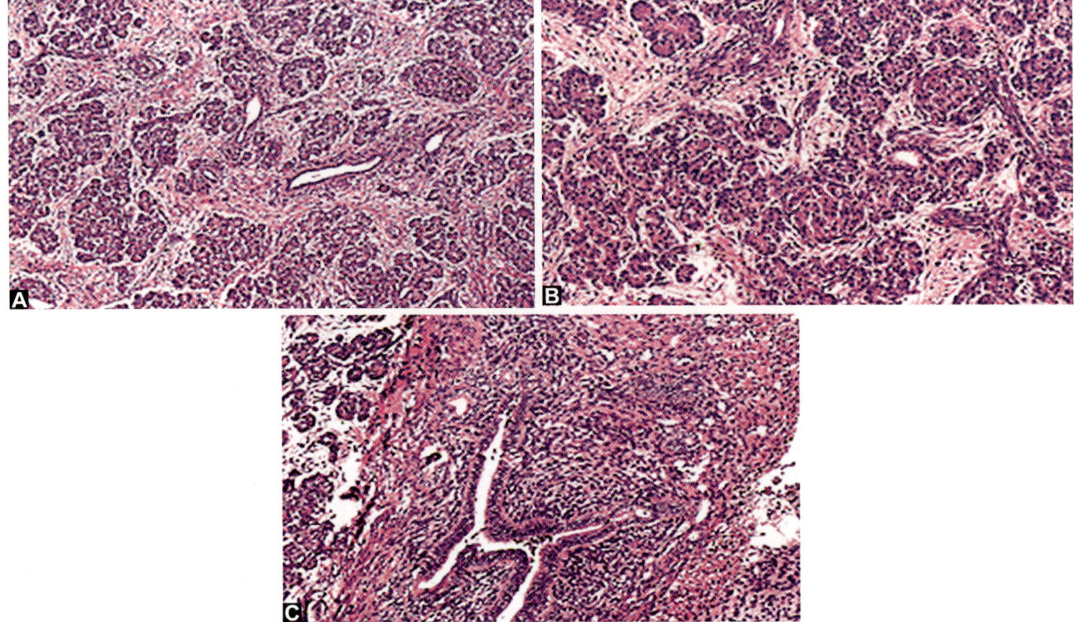

Figs 15A to C: (A) The fetal pancreas at 18–20 weeks of gestation exhibits a well-developed lobular architecture. The loose connective tissue between the lobules is relatively abundant. (B) Both acinar and endocrine elements are well developed and are functioning at this stage. (C) The mesenchyme surrounding the ducts is highly cellular, resembling the so-called ovarian-like stroma of mucinous cystic neoplasms

Islet cells also develop from the ducts at 8–10 weeks of gestation. Most of the islet cells appear to originate from the intralobular and interlobular ducts.[45] In the third month, developing endocrine cell clusters bud off from the ducts and surround capillaries to form discrete islets.[24,46] In even the earliest developing islets, differentiated α- and β-cells can be recognized.[46-48]

At 16 weeks, the α- and β-cells segregate to opposite ends of the islets; these bipolar islets are gradually replaced between 18 weeks and 20 weeks by mantle islets having a central core of β-cells surrounded by a rim of α-cells.[35,46,48] Although the microscopic architecture of the mature adult islets is more complex, the peripheral location of the α-cells found in the mantle islets is roughly maintained.

During the third to fourth months, the pancreatic tissue becomes increasingly organized around the branching ductal structures to form lobules (Figs 15A and B). The characteristics of the ductal lining cells specific to their level within the ductal system become established during this period. The mesenchymal elements of the early pancreas are prominent. The early periductal stroma is highly cellular (Fig. 15C), resembling the ovarian-like stroma that characterizes mucinous cystic neoplasms.[49,50] As the pancreas develops, the mesenchyme becomes increasingly less abundant and less cellular, ultimately constituting a relatively minimal component of the adult gland.

DEVELOPMENTAL ANOMALIES AND HETEROTOPIA

Complete or partial pancreatic agenesis is rare. Complete agenesis is associated with gallbladder agenesis, diaphragmatic hernia and growth retardation. A homozygous deletion in the Pdx1 gene was recently identified in a girl born with complete pancreatic agenesis,[51] interesting because of the role Pdx1 plays in pancreatic development. Most patients with partial pancreatic agenesis survive; but, depending upon the amount of pancreatic tissue that develops, they may have diabetes mellitus. More common than pancreatic agenesis is pancreatic hypoplasia, also referred to as congenital short pancreas. This condition may be part of a congenital syndrome or present as an isolated anomaly. The pancreas appears short and stubby but otherwise retains the normal appearing lobular architecture. Pancreatic hypoplasia typically is not associated with hypofunction.

DEVELOPING PANCREATIC ISLETS

Model of Endocrine Cell and Vessel Organization in Human Islets

1. Alpha-cells (green) and β-cells (red) are organized into a thick folded plate lined at both sides with vessels (blue)[7,8] (Figs 16A and B)
   - Alpha-cells are mostly at the periphery of the plate and in close contact with vessels
   - Beta-cells occupy a more central part of the plate and most of them develop cytoplasmic extension that runs between α-cells and reaches the surface of vessels
2. The plate with adjacent vessels is folded so that it forms an islet.

ADULT PANCREATIC ISLETS

The adult pancreatic islets (islets of Langerhans) contain four distinct endocrine cell types.

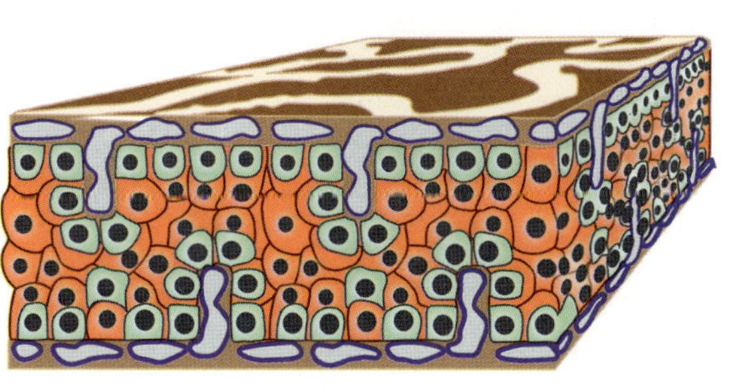

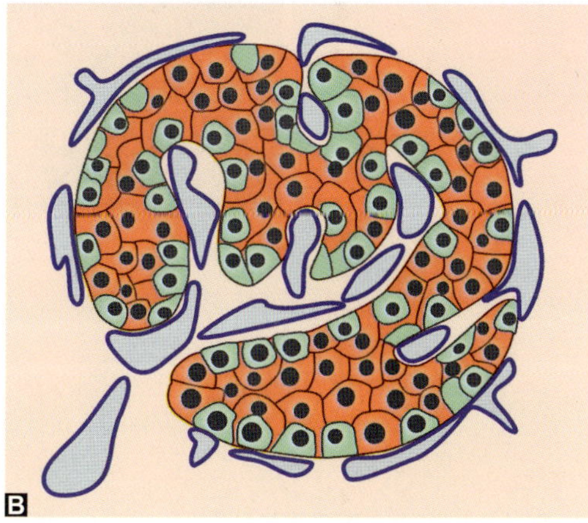

Figs 16A and B: (A and B) Alpha-cells (green) and β-cells (red) are organized into a thick folded plate lined at both sides with vessels (blue)

Alpha-Cells (Fig. 17)

- Glucagon, mobilizes lipid.

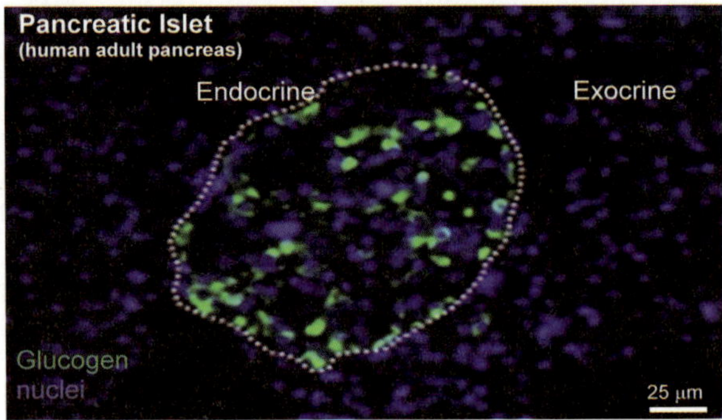

Fig. 17: Alpha-cells

Beta-Cells (Figs 18A to D)

- Insulin, increase glucose uptake
- Stimulate fetal growth, continue to proliferate to postnatal, in infancy most abundant

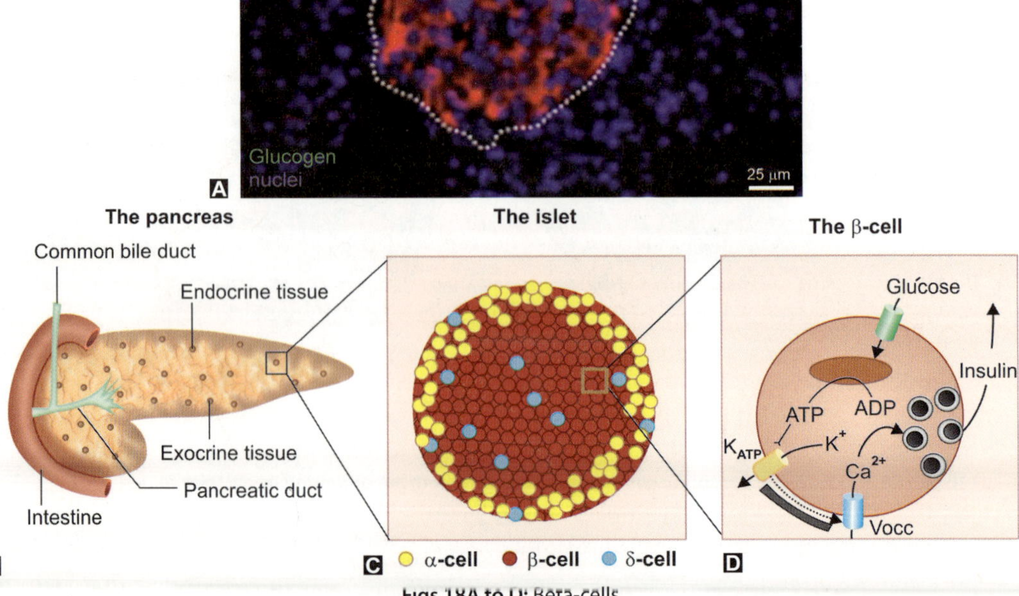

Figs 18A to D: Beta-cells

Molecular—Nkx6.1—NK2 Homeobox 6.1

- Homeobox (Hox) containing transcription factor contains a 60-amino acid evolutionarily conserved DNA-binding homeodomain.
- Required for β-cells development and is completely conserved between rat, mouse and human.

Delta-Cells

- Somatostatin, inhibits glucagon, insulin secretion

F-Cells

- Pancreatic polypeptide

ABNORMALITIES

- Accessory pancreatic tissue—pancreatic tissue located in associated gastrointestinal tract tissues/organs such as the wall of the stomach, duodenum, jejunum or Meckel's diverticulum.
- Annular pancreas—(1 in 7,000 people) pancreas forms as a "ring" of tissue surrounding the duodenum which is subsequently narrowed.
- Diabetes mellitus—maternal diabetes (and hyperglycemia) has been shown to lead to increased fetal islet hyperplasia of the insulin producing β-cells and insulin secretion.
- Intrauterine growth restriction—can lead to a delayed development of the insulin producing β-cells and low insulin secretion.
- Tumors—serous cystadenoma (endocrine tumor), somatostatinoma (tumor of β-cell origin), intraductal papillary-mucinous neoplasm.

REFERENCES

1. Hick AC, van Eyll JM, Cordi S, et al. Mechanism of primitive duct formation in the pancreas and submandibular glands: a role for SDF-1. BMC Dev Biol. 2009;9:66.
2. Scharfmann R, Xiao X, Heimberg H, et al. Beta cells within single human islets originate from multiple progenitors. PLoS One. 2008;3(10):e3559.
3. Suissa Y, Magenheim J, Stolovich-Rain M, et al. Gastrin: a distinct fate of neurogenin3 positive progenitor cells in the embryonic pancreas. PLoS One. 2013;8(8):e70397.
4. Rovira M, Huang W, Yusuff S, et al. Chemical screen identifies FDA-approved drugs and target pathways that induce precocious pancreatic endocrine differentiation. Proc Natl Acad Sci U S A. 2011;108(48):19264-9.
5. Landsman L, Nijagal A, Whitchurch TJ, et al. Pancreatic mesenchyme regulates epithelial organogenesis throughout development. PLoS Biol. 2011;9(9):e1001143.
6. Dames P, Puff R, Weise M, et al. Relative roles of the different Pax6 domains for pancreatic alpha cell development. BMC Dev Biol. 2010;10:39.
7. Jin ZW, Yu HC, Cho BH, et al. Fetal topographical anatomy of the pancreatic head and duodenum with special reference to courses of the pancreaticoduodenal arteries. Yonsei Med J. 2010;51(3): 398-406.

8. Bosco D, Armanet M, Morel P, et al. Unique arrangement of alpha- and beta-cells in human islets of Langerhans. Diabetes. 2010;59(5):1202-10.
9. Cabrera-Vásquez S, Navarro-Tableros V, Sánchez-Soto C, et al. Remodelling sympathetic innervation in rat pancreatic islets ontogeny. BMC Dev Biol. 2009;9:34.
10. Akao S, Bockman DE, Lechene de la Porte P, et al. Three-dimensional pattern of ductuloacinar associations in normal and pathological human pancreas. Gastroenterology. 1986;90:661-8.
11. Fawcett DW. Bloom and Fawcett: A Textbook of Histology, 12th edition. New York: Chapman & Hall; 1994.
12. Williams JA, Goldfine ID. The insulin-acinar relationship. In: Go VL, Brooks FP, DiMagno EP, Gardner J, Lebenthal E, Scheele GA (Eds). The Exocrine Pancreas: Biology, Pathobiology and Diseases. New York: Raven Press; 1986. pp. 347-60.
13. Solcia E, Capella C, Kloppel G. Tumors of the pancreas. In: Rosai J, Sobin LH (Eds). Atlas of Tumor Pathology, 3rd series, fascicle 20. Washington, DC: Armed Forces Institute of Pathology; 1996.
14. Rahier J, Wallon J, Henquin JC. Cell populations in the endocrine pancreas of human neonates and infants. Diabetologia. 1981;20:540-6.
15. Wittingen J, Frey CF. Islet concentration in the head, body, tail and uncinate process of the pancreas. Ann Surg. 1974;179:412-4.
16. Stefan Y, Grasso S, Perrelet A, et al. A quantitative immunofluorescent study of the endocrine cell populations in the developing human pancreas. Diabetes. 1983;32:293-301.
17. Grube D, Bohn R. The microanatomy of human islets of Langerhans, with special reference to somatostatin (D-) cells. Arch Histol Jpn. 1983;46:327-53.
18. Malaisse-Lagae F, Stefan Y, Cox J, et al. Identification of a lobe in the adult human pancreas rich in pancreatic polypeptide. Diabetologia. 1979;17:361-5.
19. Stefan Y, Grasso S, Perrelet A, et al. The pancreatic polypeptide-rich lobe of the human pancreas: definitive identification of its derivation from the ventral pancreatic primordium. Diabetologia. 1982;23:141-2.
20. Ehrie MG, Swartz FJ. Diploid, tetraploid and octaploid beta cells in the islets of Langerhans of the normal human pancreas. Diabetes. 1974;23:583-8.
21. Lecompte PM, Merriam JC Jr. Mitotic figures and enlarged nuclei in the Islands of Langerhans in man. Diabetes. 1962;11:35-9.
22. Pelletier G. Identification of four cell types in the human endocrine pancreas by immunoelectron microscopy. Diabetes. 1977;26:749-56.
23. Bommer G, Friedl U, Heitz PU, et al. Pancreatic PP cell distribution and hyperplasia. Immunocytochemical morphology in the normal human pancreas, in chronic pancreatitis and pancreatic carcinoma. Virchows Arch A Pathol Anat Histol. 1980;387:319-31.
24. Kloppel G, Lenzen S. Anatomy and physiology of the endocrine pancreas. In: Kloppel G, Heitz PU (Eds). Pancreatic Pathology. New York: Churchill Livingstone; 1984. pp. 133-53.
25. Orci L, Baetens D, Ravazzola M, et al. Pancreatic polypeptide and glucagon: non-random distribution in pancreatic islets. Life Sci. 1976;19:1811-5.
26. Orci L, Malaisse-Lagae F, Baetens D, et al. Pancreatic-polypeptide-rich regions in human pancreas. Lancet. 1978;2:1200-1.
27. Orci L, Stefan Y, Malaisse-Lagae F, et al. Instability of pancreatic endocrine cell populations throughout life. Lancet. 1979;1:615-6.

28. Fellinger EJ, Garin-Chesa P, Triche TJ, et al. Immunohistochemical analysis of Ewing's sarcoma cell surface antigen p30/32MIC2. Am J Pathol. 1991;139:317-25.
29. Hochwald SN, Zee S, Conlon KC, et al. Prognostic factors in pancreatic endocrine neoplasms: an analysis of 136 cases with a proposal for low-grade and intermediate-grade groups. J Clin Oncol. 2002;20:2633-42.
30. Weidner N, Tjoe J. Immunohistochemical profile of monoclonal antibody O13: antibody that recognizes glycoprotein p30/32MIC2 and is useful in diagnosing Ewing's sarcoma and peripheral neuroepithelioma. Am J Surg Pathol. 1994;18:486-94.
31. Kloppel G. Endokrines pankreas und diabetes mellitus. In: Doerr W, Seifert G (Eds). Spezielle Pathologische Anatomie. Berlin: Springer; 1981. pp. 523-728.
32. Terada T, Ohta T, Sasaki M, et al. Expression of MUC apomucins in normal pancreas and pancreatic tumours. J Pathol. 1996;180:160-5.
33. Murtaugh LC, Stanger BZ, Kwan KM, et al. Notch signaling controls multiple steps of pancreatic differentiation. Proc Natl Acad Sci U S A. 2003;100:14920-5.
34. Hebrok M. Hedgehog signaling in pancreas development. Mech Dev. 2003;120:45-57.
35. Conklin JL. Cytogenesis of the human fetal pancreas. Am J Anat. 1962;111:181-93.
36. Heitz PU, Beglinger C, Gyr K. Anatomy and physiology of the exocrine pancreas. In: Kloppel G, Heitz PU (Eds). Pancreatic Pathology. New York: Churchill Livingstone; 1984. pp. 3-21.
37. Lebenthal E, Lev R, Lee PC. Prenatal and postnatal development of the human exocrine pancreas. In: Go VL, Brooks FP, DiMagno EP, Gardner J, Lebenthal E, Scheele GA (Eds). The Exocrine Pancreas: Biology, Pathobiology and Diseases. New York: Raven Press; 1986. pp. 33-43.
38. Chong JM, Fukayama M, Shiozawa Y, et al. Fibrillary inclusions in neoplastic and fetal acinar cells of the pancreas. Virchows Arch. 1996;428:261-6.
39. Laitio M, Lev R, Orlic D. The developing human fetal pancreas: an ultrastructural and histochemical study with special reference to exocrine cells. J Anat. 1974;117(Pt 3):619-34.
40. Hassan MO, Gogate PA. Malignant mixed exocrine-endocrine tumor of the pancreas with unusual intracytoplasmic inclusions. Ultrastruct Pathol. 1993;17:483-93.
41. Klimstra DS, Heffess CS, Oertel JE, et al. Acinar cell carcinoma of the pancreas. A clinicopathologic study of 28 cases. Am J Surg Pathol. 1992;16:815-37.
42. Klimstra DS, Rosai J, Heffess CS. Mixed acinar-endocrine carcinomas of the pancreas. Am J Surg Pathol. 1994;18:765-78.
43. Klimstra DS, Wenig BM, Adair CF, et al. Pancreatoblastoma. A clinicopathologic study and review of the literature. Am J Surg Pathol. 1995;19:1371-89.
44. Tucker JA, Shelburne JD, Benning TL, et al. Filamentous inclusions in acinar cell carcinoma of the pancreas. Ultrastruct Pathol. 1994;18:279-86.
45. Cubilla AL, Fitzgerald PJ. Tumors of the exocrine pancreas. In: Hartmann WH, Sobin LH (Eds). Atlas of Tumor Pathology, 2nd series, fascicle 19. Washington, DC: Armed Forces Institute of Pathology; 1984.
46. Robb P. The development of the islets of Langerhans in the human foetus. Q J Exp Physiol Cogn Med Sci. 1961;46:335-43.
47. Clark A, Grant AM. Quantitative morphology of endocrine cells in human fetal pancreas. Diabetologia. 1983;25:31-5.

48. Grasso S, Palumbo G, Fallucca F, et al. The development and function of the endocrine pancreas of fetuses and infants born to normal and diabetic mothers. Acta Endocrinol Suppl (Copenh). 1986;277:130-5.
49. Albores-Saavedra J, Gould EW, Angeles-Angeles A, et al. Cystic tumors of the pancreas. Pathol Annu. 1990;25 Pt 2:19-50.
50. Compagno J, Oertel JE. Mucinous cystic neoplasms of the pancreas with overt and latent malignancy (cystadenocarcinoma and cystadenoma). A clinicopathologic study of 41 cases. Am J Clin Pathol. 1978;69:573-80.
51. Stoffers DA, Zinkin NT, Stanojevic V, et al. Pancreatic agenesis attributable to a single nucleotide deletion in the human IPF1 gene coding sequence. Nat Genet. 1997;15:106-10.

4
CHAPTER

Physiology of Glucose Metabolism, Biochemistry of Cotransporters and Its Clinical Relevance

Narsingh Verma

INTRODUCTION

The main source of energy in most of the Indian diets is carbohydrates which provide 50–80% of daily energy intake.[1] About 80% of this carbohydrate is the plant polysaccharide starch, and most of the remainder consists of the disaccharides sucrose and lactose. Only small amounts of monosaccharides (glucose, fructose) are normally present in the diet. There are two different types of glucose polymers in starch, which is significant because they require different enzymes to digest them fully. About 25% of starch consists of amylose, which is comprised of simple, straight chain polymers of glucose linked by α-1,4-glycosidic bonds. The remainder portion of starch consists of amylopectin, which is similar to amylose; however, in addition to 1,4- linkages there is a 1,6- linkage for every 20–30 glucose units.

Carbohydrate digestion begins in the mouth and continues through to the small intestine. Cellulose and certain other complex polysaccharides found in vegetable matter, referred to as fiber, are not broken down by the enzymes in the digestive tract, and are partially metabolized by bacteria.

DIGESTION OF CARBOHYDRATES: SALIVARY AND PANCREATIC AMYLASE

Food gets mixed with saliva during mastication in the oral cavity and bolus is formed. Saliva contains the digestive enzyme ptyalin (α-amylase), secreted mainly by the parotid glands. This enzyme hydrolyzes starch into the disaccharide maltose and other small polymers of glucose that contain three to nine glucose molecules. Digestion of carbohydrates by salivary α-amylase is of relatively limited importance, as the food remains in the mouth only for a short time, so not more than 5% of all the starches are hydrolyzed, by the time the food is swallowed.

However, the salivary amylase does assume an important role in specific situations. For example, in infants, there is a developmental delay in the production of pancreatic enzymes and so the salivary enzyme assumes a proportionately greater role. Salivary amylase is also an important backup in patients with pancreatic insufficiency, such as in the setting of cystic fibrosis. The optimum pH for the action of α-amylase is 5.6–6.9 and, therefore, it is inactivated in the stomach by gastric juice, which has a pH as low as 1.0. However, it has been demonstrated that amylase activity can be protected if its substrate occupies the active site of the enzyme. Thus, starch digestion sometimes continues in the body and fundus of the stomach for as long as 1 hour before the food becomes mixed with the stomach secretions. On an average 30–40% of the starches can get hydrolyzed, before food and its accompanying saliva become completely mixed with the gastric secretions.

The gastric contents reach the small intestine where the alkaline content of the pancreatic and biliary secretions results in a pH equal to 7.8. Pancreatic secretion like saliva contains a large quantity of α-amylase (94% homologous to salivary amylase) which is almost identical in its function with the salivary amylase but is several times more powerful. It has an optimum pH of about 7.1. Human salivary and pancreatic amylases have optimum activities near neutral pH and are activated by chloride (Cl^-).

Alpha-amylase is an endoenzyme that hydrolyzes internal α-1,4 linkages. α-amylase does not cleave terminal α-1,4 linkages, α-1,6 linkages (i.e. branch points), or α-1,4 linkages that are immediately adjacent to α-1,6 linkages. As a result, starch hydrolysis products are maltose, maltotriose and α-limit dextrin. Maltose is composed of two glucose molecules in α-1,4 linkage, maltotriose consists of three glucose molecules in α-1,4 linkage and α-dextrin has both α-1,6 and α-1,4 links. Because α-amylase has no activity against terminal α-1,4 linkages, glucose is not a product of starch digestion. The intestine cannot absorb these products of amylase digestion of starch, and thus further digestion is required to produce substrates (i.e. monosaccharides) that the small intestine can absorb by specific transport mechanisms (Fig. 1).

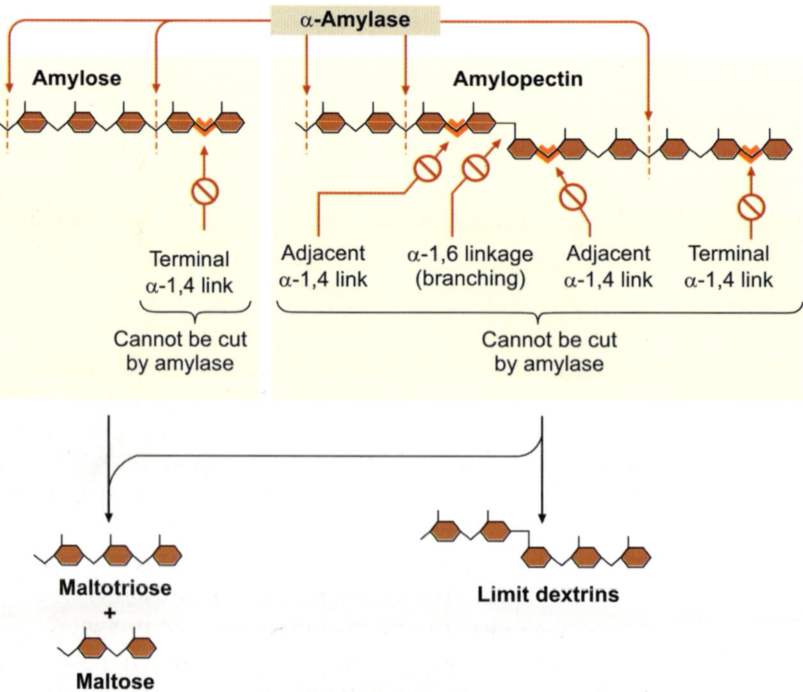

Fig. 1: Digestion of carbohydrates[1]

APPLIED PHYSIOLOGY

Although the action of amylase is rapid, some sources of starch contain proteins and fiber components that may slow the action of this enzyme. This means that the rise in blood glucose that eventually follows the ingestion of starch will have differing kinetics depending on the food in which the starch is contained. Some nutritional supplement manufacturers have tried to take advantage of this by isolating so-called "starch blockers", which they claim can reduce the digestion of starch by inhibiting amylase activity and thereby are useful as aids to weight loss.

However, this is unlikely to be an effective approach, given the marked excess of pancreatic enzymes and the fact that the starch blockers are proteins, and therefore are themselves get digested in gut. Further, any carbohydrate that escapes assimilation in the small intestine is rapidly broken down by bacterial hydrolases in the colon. Although this may carry the price of the generation of gas and bloating, it ultimately allows the caloric content of the starch to be reclaimed.

Disaccharidases

The disaccharidases are located in the brush border cells of the small intestine mucosa. They hydrolyze the disaccharides produced from the action of salivary and pancreatic α-amylase on polysaccharides. In addition, they act on disaccharides that were introduced directly by the diet.

The human small intestine has four brush border oligosaccharidases: (1) lactase, (2) glucoamylase (most often called maltase), (3) sucrase and (4) isomaltase (also known as α-dextrinase or debranching enzyme). Sucrase and isomaltase occur together as a molecular complex, there activities are actually encoded in a single polypeptide chain with two distinct active sites, and thus the complete protein is referred to as sucrase-isomaltase. Lactase has only one substrate; it breaks lactose into glucose and galactose. The other three enzymes have more complicated substrate spectra. All cleave the terminal α-1,4 linkages of maltose, maltotriose and α-limit dextrins. In addition, each of these three enzymes has at least one other activity. Maltase can also degrade the α-1,4 linkages in straight-chain oligosaccharides up to nine monomers in length. The sucrose moiety of sucrase-isomaltase is required to split sucrose into glucose and fructose. The isomaltase moiety of sucrose-isomaltase is the only enzyme that can split the branching α-1,6 linkages of α-limit dextrins. Thus, the only products of sugar digestion are glucose (80%), galactose (10%) and fructose (10%).

They are all water soluble and are absorbed immediately into the portal blood. The activities of the hydrolysis reactions of sucrase-isomaltase and maltase are considerably greater than the rates at which the monosaccharides are absorbed. Thus, uptake, not hydrolysis, is the rate-limiting step. In contrast, lactase activity is considerably less than that of the other oligosaccharidases and is rate limiting for overall lactose digestion-absorption.

The oligosaccharidases have a varying spatial distribution throughout the small intestine. In general, peak oligosaccharidase distribution and activity occur in the proximal jejunum (i.e. at the ligament of Treitz). Considerably less activity is noted in the duodenum and distal ileum, and none is reported in the large intestine. The distribution of oligosaccharides activity parallels that of active glucose transport.

These oligosaccharidases are affected by developmental and dietary factors in different ways. In many nonwhite ethnic groups, as well as in almost all other mammals, lactase activity markedly decreases after weaning in the postnatal period. The regulation of this decreased lactase activity is genetically determined. The other oligosaccharidases do not decrease in the postnatal period. In addition, long-term feeding of sucrose up-regulates sucrase activity. In contrast, sucrase activity is greatly reduced much more by fasting than is lactase activity. In general, lactase activity is both more susceptible to enterocyte injury (e.g. following viral enteritis) and is slower to recover from damage than is other oligosaccharidase activity. Thus, reduced lactase activity (as a consequence of both genetic regulation and environmental effects) has substantial clinical significance in that lactose ingestion may result in a range of symptoms in affected individuals.

Dietary Fiber, although not Digestible, Benefits Gastrointestinal Function

Humans lack enzymes that hydrolyze α-1,4 linkages. Thus, humans are incapable of digesting cellulose, a major constituent of vegetables that consists of glucose residues in α-1,4. Dietary fiber, also known as roughage, consists of nonstarch polysaccharides, such as cellulose, waxes and pectin. Although it is not digestible, consuming dietary fiber offers several advantages to gastrointestinal function. It increases bulk, softens stools and shortens transit time in the intestinal tract—all of which facilitates motility and prevents constipation. For example, many fruits and vegetables are rich in fiber, and their frequent ingestion greatly decreases intestinal transit time. Dietary fiber has also been shown to reduce the incidence of colon cancer by shortening gastrointestinal transit time. A shortened transit time inhibits the formation of carcinogenic bile acids, such as lithocholic acid, as well as reducing the contact time of ingested carcinogens to act on tissue. Another benefit of dietary fiber is the lowering of blood cholesterol. This is accomplished by dietary fiber binding with bile acids, which are formed from cholesterol. Thus, fiber consumption lowers blood cholesterol by promoting excretion.

Absorption of Carbohydrates (Fig. 2)

The three monosaccharide products of carbohydrate digestion, i.e. glucose, galactose and fructose are absorbed by the small intestine in a two-step process involving their uptake across the apical membrane into the epithelial cell and their coordinated exit across the basolateral membrane.

The sodium-glucose transporter 1 (SGLT1) is the membrane protein responsible for glucose and galactose uptake at the apical membrane. Fructose uptake across the apical membrane is mediated by glucose transporter 5 (GLUT5). The exit of all three monosaccharides across the basolateral membrane uses a facilitated sugar transporter (GLUT2).

Glucose uptake across the apical membrane through SGLT1 occurs against the glucose concentration gradient, and is energized by the electrochemical Na^+ gradient, which, in turn, is maintained by the extrusion of Na^+ across the basolateral membrane by the Na^+-K^+ pump. The cotransport of sodium and glucose forms the physiological basis of the treatment of diarrhea, i.e. administration of oral rehydration solutions containing both NaCl and glucose.

The affinity of SGLT1 for glucose is markedly reduced in the absence of Na^+. The varied affinity of SGLT1 for different monosaccharides reflects its preference for specific molecular configurations. SGLT1 has two structural requirements for monosaccharides: (1) a hexose in

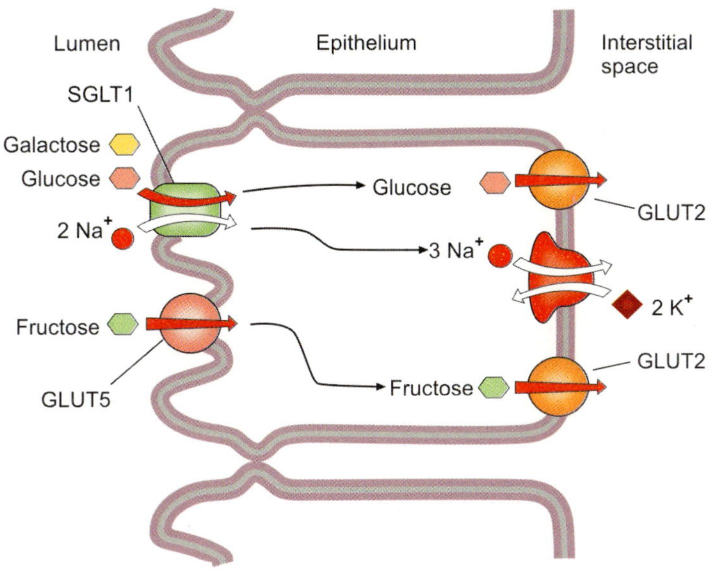

Fig. 2: Absorption of carbohydrates[2,3]

a D-configuration and (2) a hexose that can form a six-membered pyranose ring. SGLT1 does not absorb L-glucose, which has the wrong stereochemistry, and it does not absorb D-fructose, which forms a five-membered ring.

The evolutionary significance of partly luminal and partly surface digestion of carbohydrates is not understood. It may be that the absence of monosaccharides in the intestinal lumen makes bacterial proliferation there more difficult. There may be a kinetic advantage to diffusion of oligosaccharides rather than monosaccharides through the unstirred water layer coating the mucosa. Oligosaccharides are then hydrolyzed at apical membrane promoting their transport.

GLUCOSE-GALACTOSE MALABSORPTION

In patients with glucose-galactose malabsorption (or monosaccharide malabsorption), diarrhea occurs when they ingest dietary sugars that are normally absorbed by SGLT1. Defect in Na^+ coupled monosaccharide absorption results in diarrhea due to the osmotic effects of unabsorbed monosaccharides. Eliminating the monosaccharides (glucose and galactose) as well as the disaccharide lactose (i.e. glucose and galactose) from the diet, it also eliminates the diarrhea. Fructose, which crosses the apical membrane through GLUT5, does not induce diarrhea. Patients with glucose-galactose malabsorption do not have glycosuria (i.e. glucose in the urine), because glucose reabsorption by the proximal tubule normally occurs through both SGLT1 and SGLT2.

Glucose Transport Pathways

Because the lipid bilayer of the eukaryotic plasma membrane is impermeable for hydrophilic molecules, glucose is transported across the plasma membrane by membrane associated carrier proteins, glucose transporters. There are two different types of transporter proteins, which mediate the transfer of glucose and other sugars through the lipid bilayer: (1) sodium-dependent glucose cotransporters (SGLT) and (2) facilitative glucose transporters (GLUT).

SGLT Family

There are twelve members of the human SGLT family in the human genome (gene name SLC5A).[2-4] The SGLT family comprises Na^+-dependent glucose cotransporters (SGLT1 and SGLT2), the glucose sensor SGLT3,[5] the widely distributed inositol and multivitamin transporters SGLT4 and SGLT6, and the thyroid iodide transporter SGLT5.[6]

Sodium-dependent glucose transporters are secondary active cell membrane symporters that transfer sodium down its concentration gradient, usually into the cell, in conjunction with the inward transfer of specific hexose sugars or some other molecules against their concentration gradient. An electrochemical gradient that allows sodium to enter the cell is generated by the active transport of sodium out of the cell at another location within the cell membrane hence the term secondary active.

Genes, substrates and main sites for expression of sodium-glucose cotransporters have been shown in Table 1.

Table 1: Genes, substrates and main sites for expression of sodium-glucose cotransporters[7]

SGLT name	*Substrate*	*Apparent affinity for glucose K0.5 mM*	*Distribution*
SGLT1 (SLC5A1)	Glucose, galactose	0.4	Intestine, trachea, kidney, heart, brain, testes, prostate
SGLT2 (SLC5A2)	Glucose	2	Kidney, brain, liver, thyroid, muscle, heart
SGLT4 (SLC5A9)	Glucose, mannose	2	Intestine, kidney, liver, brain, lung, trachea, pancreas, uterus
SGLT5 (SLC5A10)	Glucose	Not determined	Kidney's cortex
SGLT6 (SLC5A11)	Myo-inositol, glucose	35	Brain, kidney, intestine
SMIT1 (SLC5A3)	Myo-inositol, glucose	> 35	Brain, heart, kidney, lung

The main SGLTs are SGLT1, which is responsible for glucose absorption from the small intestine, and SGLT2, which accounts for reabsorption of most of the glucose filtered by the kidney. SGLT1 is a high-affinity (K0.5 of about 0·4 mM for glucose and about 3·0 mM for sodium), low-capacity glucose transporter with a 2:1 coupling ratio for sodium and glucose. Conversely, SGLT2 is a low-affinity (K0.5 of about 2·0 mM for glucose and about 0·1 mM for sodium), high-capacity glucose transporter with a 1:1 coupling for sodium and glucose.[6,7] SGLT2 inhibitors are called gliflozins and lead to a reduction in blood glucose levels. Therefore, SGLT2 inhibitors have potential use in the treatment of type 2 diabetes. As studied on canagliflozin, a member of this class of drugs, gliflozins enhance glycemic control as well as reduce body weight and systolic and diastolic blood pressure. The gliflozins canagliflozin, dapagliflozin and empagliflozin may lead to ketoacidosis. Other side effects of gliflozins include increased risk of (generally mild) urinary tract infections, candidal vulvovaginitis and hypoglycemia.[7]

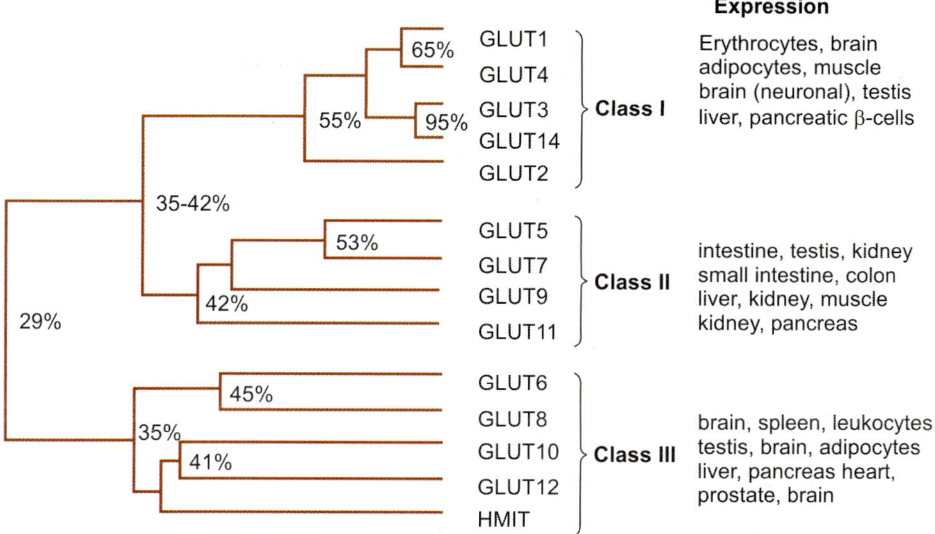

Fig. 3: Dendrogram of the family of human sugar transporter facilitators. Numbers at the branches of the tree indicate percentage of identity[4]

SGLT2 inhibitors represent a novel "glucuretic" therapeutic strategy for the treatment of type 2 diabetes.

The sodium-glucose transporter 3 is expressed in human skeletal muscle and small intestine. Immunofluorescence microscopy indicated that in the small intestine the protein was expressed in cholinergic neurons in the submucosal and myenteric plexuses, but not in enterocytes. Functional studies have shown that human SGLT3 is incapable of sugar transport, leading to the conclusion that SGLT3 is not a Na^+/glucose cotransporter but instead a glucose sensor in the plasma membrane of cholinergic neurons, skeletal muscle and other tissues.[3]

GLUT Family

The human genome contains 14 members of the GLUT family, which can be divided into three subfamilies according to sequence similarities and characteristic elements (Fig. 3).[4]

Among 14 GLUT genes in the human genome, 11 have been shown to catalyze sugar transport.[4,8] The individual isotypes exhibit different substrate specificity, kinetic characteristics and expression profiles, thereby allowing a tissue-specific adaptation of glucose uptake through regulation of their gene expression.[8,9]

Class I Sugar Transport Facilitators

The class I facilitative glucose transporters comprise the thoroughly characterized isoforms GLUT1 to 4 and the recently identified GLUT14.

GLUT1 is expressed in most tissues,[10] though its highest expression levels are in erythrocytes and endothelial cells of the brain. It is responsible for the basic supply of glucose to the cells. GLUT1 is a high-affinity glucose transporter with a Km for glucose of around 3–7 mM.[11]

The Km value for GLUT proteins is the concentration of blood glucose at which transport into the cell takes place at half its maximum rate. A Km of 3–7 mM is below or equal to the average blood glucose concentration of 5–7 mM, enabling tissues to take up glucose at a significant rate, regardless of the amount present in the blood.

GLUT2 is a high-capacity, low-affinity glucose transporter with a Km, around 15–20 mM.[12] Its predominant expression is in pancreatic β-cells, liver, kidney and small intestine (basolateral membrane). In all these tissues, the uptake of glucose is not dependent on the number and activity of the glucose transporters but on the blood glucose concentration;[13] i.e. the amount of incoming glucose in these tissues is proportional to the amount of glucose in the blood. The presence of GLUT2 ensures that glucose is taken up rapidly by the liver only when it is abundant and enables pancreatic β-cells to monitor blood glucose levels directly, and regulate insulin secretion. The presence of GLUT2 in the small intestine and the kidney reflects its role in the transport of glucose across the serosal surface of the epithelial cells which line the intestine and the nephron, after glucose absorption across their luminal surface via the sodium-linked glucose transporter, SLGT1. Thus, transport activity of GLUT2 cannot be saturated by physiologic blood glucose concentrations. In addition to glucose, GLUT2 is able to transport fructose,[14] with higher affinity, glucosamine.[15]

GLUT3 is a high-affinity glucose transporter with a Km for glucose of around 2 mM, much less than the average blood glucose concentration of 5–7 mM, enabling most tissues to take up glucose at a constant rate, regardless of the amount present in the blood. Its predominant expression is in tissues with a high glucose requirement (e.g. brain).[16]

GLUT4 is a high-affinity glucose transporter with a Km around 5 mM. It is expressed in insulin-sensitive tissues (heart, skeletal muscle, adipose tissue).[17] The level of this transporter on the surface of these cells is rapidly regulated by insulin, which stimulates the translocation of GLUT4 from intracellular membranes to the plasma membrane, resulting in an immediate 10- to 20-fold increase in glucose transport.[18-20] In skeletal muscle, translocation of GLUT4 can be induced by muscle contraction and hypoxia.[21,22] GLUT14 is exclusively expressed in testis.

GLUT1, GLUT3 and GLUT4 have also been described to transport dehydroascorbic acid (DHAA). DHAA is a stable oxidation product of ascorbate, which is transported by specific sodium-ascorbic acid cotransporters and mainly stored in skeletal muscle and brain.

Class II Sugar Transport Facilitators

The class II glucose transporters include the fructose-specific transporters GLUT5 and three related proteins, GLUT7, GLUT9 and GLUT11.

GLUT5 mRNA is predominantly expressed in small intestine, testis and kidney. GLUT5 exhibits no glucose transport activity and is responsible for the uptake of fructose.[23]

GLUT7 is a high-affinity transporter for glucose and fructose. GLUT7 mRNA can be detected in small intestine, colon, testis and prostate; within the small intestine, GLUT7 is predominantly expressed in the enterocytes brush border membrane.[24]

GLUT9 exhibits highest expression levels in kidney and liver; lower mRNA levels were detected in small intestine, placenta, lung and leukocytes.[25]

GLUT11 is suggested to be a fructose transporter with low affinity to glucose. GLUT11 is expressed predominantly in pancreas, kidney and placenta, and also moderate expression in heart and skeletal muscle.[26]

Class III Sugar Transport Facilitators

The class III comprises of GLUT6, GLUT8, GLUT10, GLUT12 and H^+-coupled myo-inositol transporter (HMIT).

GLUT6 is a low-affinity glucose transporter, expressed predominantly in brain, spleen and peripheral leukocytes.[27]

GLUT8 is a high-affinity glucose transporter, expressed predominantly in testis, and lower amounts of GLUT8 mRNA were detected in most other tissues, including insulin-sensitive tissues like heart and skeletal muscle.[28] Moreover, GLUT8 was reported to mediate insulin-stimulated glucose uptake in preimplantation embryos.[29] In testis, the protein was associated with the acrosomal region of mature spermatozoa.[30] In addition, GLUT8 may play a role in glucose uptake of adipocytes; its expression was found to be regulated by the metabolism of these cells.[31]

GLUT10 is predominantly expressed in the liver and pancreas.[32]

GLUT12 is predominantly expressed in heart and prostate. GLUT12 seems to sustain the increased glucose consumption in prostate carcinoma and breast cancer.

The HMIT is expressed predominantly in the brain. It specifically transports myo-inositol and related stereoisomers but lacks any sugar transport activity.

GLUCOSE TRANSPORTERS AS COMPONENTS OF THE GLUCOSENSING MACHINERY

A constant monitoring of blood glucose concentrations by specific glucosensing mechanisms is required for the maintenance of the whole-body glucose homeostasis. The best described glucose detection system is that of pancreatic β-cells, which control the insulin secretion. This sensor machinery includes glucose transporters (GLUT2), the enzyme glucokinase and the ATP-sensitive K^+ channel. When the extracellular glucose concentration increases, more glucose enters the β-cell via the low-affinity glucose transporter GLUT2 and is phosphorylated by glucokinase. Glycolytic and oxidative metabolism of glucose raises the ATP-to-ADP ratio, causing ATP to bind to the ATP-sensitive K^+ channel complex. This inactivates the channel and leads to membrane depolarization, influx of calcium and insulin secretion.

REFERENCES

1. ICMR. Nutrient requirements and recommended dietary allowances for Indians: A Report of the Expert Group of the Indian Council of Medical Research. 2009.
2. Wright EM. Renal Na+-glucose cotransporters. Am J Physiol Renal Physiol. 2001;280:F10-8.
3. Hediger MA, Rhoads DB. Molecular physiology of sodium-glucose cotransporters. Physiol Rev. 1994;74:993-1026.
4. Wright EM, Loo DD, Hirayama BA. Biology of human sodium glucose transporters. Physiol Rev. 2011;91:733-94.
5. Berry GT, Mallee JJ, Kwon HM, et al. The human osmoregulatory Na+/myo-inositol cotransporter gene (SLC5A3): molecular cloning and localization to chromosome 21. Genomics. 1995;25:507-13.
6. Balamurugan K, Ortiz A, Said HM. Biotin uptake by human intestinal and liver epithelial cells: role of the SMVT system. Am J Physiol Gastrointest Liver Physiol. 2003;285:G73-7.

7. Tahrani AA, Barnett AH, Bailey CJ. (2013). SGLT inhibitors in management of diabetes. [online] Available from www.thelancet.com/diabetes-endocrinology. [Accessed August, 2015].
8. Gould GW, Holman GD. The glucose transporter family: structure, function and tissue-specific expression. Biochem J. 1993;295:329-41.
9. Zhao FQ, Keating AF. Functional properties and genomics of glucose transporters. Curr Genomics. 2007;8:113-28.
10. Bell GI, Kayano T, Buse JB, et al. Molecular biology of mammalian glucose transporters. Diabetes Care. 1990;13:198-208.
11. Scheepers A, Joost HG, Schürmann A. The glucose transporter families SGLT and GLUT: molecular basis of normal and aberrant function. JPEN J Parenter Enteral Nutr. 2004;28:364-71.
12. Simpson IA, Cushman SW. Hormonal regulation of mammalian glucose transport. Annu Rev Biochem. 1986;55:1059-89.
13. Shepherd PR, Kahn BB. Glucose transporters and insulin action—implications for insulin resistance and diabetes mellitus. N Engl J Med. 1999;341:248-57.
14. Kayano T, Burant CF, Fukumoto H, et al. Human facilitative glucose transporters. Isolation, functional characterization, and gene localization of cDNAs encoding an isoform (GLUT5) expressed in small intestine, kidney, muscle, and adipose tissue and an unusual glucose transporter pseudogene-like sequence (GLUT6). J Biol Chem. 1990;265:13276-82.
15. Mueckler M, Caruso C, Baldwin SA, et al. Sequence and structure of a human glucose transporter. Science. 1985;229:941-5.
16. Burant CF, Bell GI. Mammalian facilitative glucose transporters: evidence for similar substrate recognition sites in functionally monomeric proteins. Biochemistry. 1992;31:10414-20.
17. Fukumoto H, Seino S, Imura H, et al. Sequence, tissue distribution, and chromosomal localization of mRNA encoding a human glucose transporter-like protein. Proc Natl Acad Sci USA. 1988;85: 5434-8.
18. Wood IS, Trayhurn P. Glucose transporters (GLUT and SGLT): expanded families of sugar transport proteins. Br J Nutr. 2003;89:3-9.
19. Uldry M, Ibberson M, Hosokawa M, et al. GLUT2 is a high affinity glucosamine transporter. FEBS Lett. 2002;524:199-203.
20. Kayano T, Fukumoto H, Eddy RL, et al. Evidence for a family of human glucose transporter-like proteins. Sequence and gene localization of a protein expressed in fetal skeletal muscle and other tissues. J Biol Chem. 1988;263:15245-8.
21. Bryant NJ, Govers R, James DE. Regulated transport of the glucose transporter GLUT4. Nat Rev Mol Cell Biol. 2002;3:267-77.
22. Cartee GD, Douen AG, Ramlal T, et al. Stimulation of glucose transport in skeletal muscle by hypoxia. J Appl Physiol. 1991;70:1593-600.
23. Lund S, Holman GD, Schmitz O, et al. Contraction stimulates translocation of glucose transporter GLUT4 in skeletal muscle through a mechanism distinct from that of insulin. Proc Natl Acad Sci. USA. 1995;92:5817-21.
24. Doege H, Bocianski A, Joost HG, et al. Activity and genomic organization of human glucose transporter 9 (GLUT9), a novel member of the family of sugar-transport facilitators predominantly expressed in brain and leucocytes. Biochem J. 2000;350 Pt 3:771-6.
25. Doege H, Schurmann A, Bahrenberg G, et al. GLUT8, a novel member of the sugar transport facilitator family with glucose transport activity. J Biol Chem. 2000;275:16275-80.

26. Carayannopoulos MO, Chi MM, Cui Y, et al. GLUT8 is a glucose transporter responsible for insulin-stimulated glucose uptake in the blastocyst. Proc Natl Acad Sci. USA. 2000;97:7313-8.
27. Schurmann A, Axer H, Scheepers A, et al. The glucose transport facilitator GLUT8 is predominantly associated with the acrosomal region of mature spermatozoa. Cell Tissue Res. 2002;307:237-42.
28. Scheepers A, Doege H, Joost HG, et al. Mouse GLUT8: genomic organization and regulation of expression in 3T3-L1 adipocytes by glucose. Biochem Biophys Res Commun. 2001;288:969-74.
29. McVie-Wylie AJ, Lamson DR, Chen YT. Molecular cloning of a novel member of the GLUT family of transporters, SLC2a10 (GLUT10), localized on chromosome 20q13.1: a candidate gene for NIDDM susceptibility. Genomics. 2001;72:113-7.
30. Macheda ML, Kelly DJ, Best JD, et al. Expression during rat fetal development of GLUT12—a member of the class III hexose transporter family. Anat Embryol (Berl). 2002;205:441-52.
31. Chandler JD, Williams ED, Slavin JL, et al. Expression and localization of GLUT1 and GLUT12 in prostate carcinoma. Cancer. 2003;97:2035-42.
32. Uldry M, Ibberson M, Horisberger JD, et al. Identification of a mammalian H+-myo-inositol symporter expressed predominantly in the brain. EMBO J. 2001;20:4467-77.

5

CHAPTER

Interpretation of Genetics in Diabetes Mellitus

Ashutosh Jain, Vinay Kumar BR, Kamlakar Tripathi

INTRODUCTION

Most cases of diabetes results from the interaction of genetic variation at multiple different chromosomal sites with environmental exposures experienced throughout the lifespan exception being rare monogenic disorders.[1] Varying degrees of insulin resistance and/or dysfunction of the insulin producing beta cells of the pancreas cause diabetes. The disease phenotype is heterogeneous and can be divided into different subtypes depending on the underlying genetic and pathophysiologic cause. Forms of diabetes due to mutations in single genes are rare (2–5% of diabetes cases) have high penetrance and have little influence from environmental factors. In contrast, the common forms of diabetes—type 1 diabetes (T1DM) and type 2 diabetes (T2DM)—are diseases with important genetic underpinnings but with no clear pattern of inheritance.[2] The disease phenotypes result from the interaction of multiple gene variants, each exerting only a modest effect. Recent advances in knowledge of the human genome and molecular approaches to probe the human genome have resulted in dramatic insights into the pathophysiology of several relatively rare monogenic causes of diabetes. Some progress has been made in identifying variants in genes that contribute to the more common polygenic forms of T1DM and T2DM.[3]

CANDIDATE GENES AND LINKAGE STUDIES

A candidate gene approach focuses the search for specific diabetes susceptibility mutations in genes chosen based on their presumed relevance to glucose metabolism. Candidates identified have a greater influence on T1DM risk than that conferred by genes in the human leukocyte antigen (HLA) region of chromosome 6. This region contains several hundred genes known to be involved in immune response similarly new insights into the molecular mechanisms of pancreatic development, insulin signaling, insulin secretion, and body weight regulation have greatly broadened the list of candidate genes for T2DM. Over the last two decades, studies of specific genes have led to the identification of several putative T2DM susceptibility genes.

First degree relatives of Type 1 diabetes mellitus have a higher risk of developing T1DM than unrelated individuals from the general population (approximately 6% vs <1%, respectively).[4] These data suggest that genetic factors are involved with the development of the disease. At present, there is evidence that more than 20 regions of the genome may be involved in genetic susceptibility to T1DM. Those most strongly associated with the disease are the HLA class II genes (i.e. HLA-DR, DQ, DP).

IDDM1

The HLA class II genes, also referred to as IDDM1, contribute approximately 40–50% of the heritable risk for T1DM.[5] When evaluated as haplotypes, DQA1*0501-DQB1*0201 and DQA1*0301-DQB1*0302 are most strongly associated T1DM in Caucasian populations. They are in linkage disequilibrium with DRB1*03 and DRB1*04, respectively. Specific DRB1*04 alleles also modify the risk associated with the DQA1*0301-DQB1*0302 haplotype.

Other reported high-risk haplotypes for T1DM include DRB1*07-DQA1*0301-DQB1*0201 among African-Americans, DRB1*09-DQA1*0301-DQB1*0303 among Japanese, and DRB1*04-DQA1*0401-DQB1*0302 among Chinese. DRB1*15-DQA1*0602-DQB1*0102 is protective and associated with a reduced risk of T1DM in most populations. Recent reports suggest that other genes in the central, class I and extended class I regions may also increase T1DM risk independent of HLA class II genes.[6] Individuals with two high-risk DRB1-DQA1-DQB1 haplotypes have a significantly higher T1DM risk than individuals with no high-risk haplotype. The T1DM risk among those with only one susceptibility haplotype is also increased, but effect is more modest. In addition to IDDM1, two other genes are now known to influence T1DM risk.[7] These include INS and CTLA-4 (Table 1).

Table 1: Several T1DM susceptibility genes

Gene	*Locus*	*Variant*	*Estimated RR*
HLA-DQB1	6p21.3	*0201 and *0302	3–45
INS	11p15.5	Class I	1–2
CTLA-4	2q31-35	Thr17Ala	1–2

INS (Insulin)

The INS gene, located on chromosome 11p15.5, has been designated as IDDM2. Positive associations have been observed with a non-transcribed variable number of tandem repeat (VNTR) in the 5' flanking region.[8] There are two common variants. The shorter class I variant predisposes to T1DM (relative increase: 1–2), whereas the longer class III variant appears to be dominantly protective. The biological plausibility of these associations may relate to the expression of insulin mRNA in the thymus. Class III variants appear to generate higher levels of insulin mRNA than class I variants. Such differences could contribute to a better immune tolerance for class III positive individuals by increasing the likelihood of negative selection for autoreactive T-cell clones. The effect of INS appears to vary by ethnicity, with lesser effects in non-Caucasian populations.[9]

CTLA-4 (Cytotoxic T-lymphocyte-associated 4)

The CTLA-4 gene is located on chromosome 2q31-35 (Anjos and Polychronakos, 2004), where multiple T1DM genes may be located. CTLA-4 variants have been associated with T1DM, as well as other autoimmune disease. CTLA-4 negatively regulates T-cell function. However, impaired activity, which has been associated with the Thr17Ala variant, may increase T1DM risk.

TYPE 2 DIABETES MELLITUS

In contrast to monogenic disorders, where results from single mutations lead to predictable phenotypes, the complex genetic architecture of susceptible and protective alleles in polygenic T2DM is more difficult to discern. Indeed, accumulating data suggest that T2DM is likely a collection of many closely related diseases with varying but often overlapping primary mechanisms that involve both impaired insulin secretion and insulin resistance. Adding to the challenge, T2DM is generally diagnosed later in life as a consequence of significant interactions of lifelong environmental influences with multiple genetic factors. Because of the limited individual impact of single genetic loci, a full understanding of the complex gene–gene and gene–environment interactions in this disease has proven quite challenging.

In the first phase of diabetes gene discovery, investigators used techniques based on linkage analysis to identify potential diabetes-associated genes. This approach, best suited for discovering genes with strong effects within relatively small family-based studies, involves genotyping affected family members for a set of markers to identify regions that are coinherited more commonly in affected family members and therefore potentially point to a genomic region containing a susceptibility locus.

One of the first successes in T2DM genetic research was a study conducted in Icelanders that identified a linkage peak on chromosome arm 5q. Focusing on the various linkage peaks identified in that initial study ultimately led to the association of transcription factor 7-like 2 (TCF7L2) with an increased risk of T2DM.[10] This remains the largest effect size of all known T2DM genes identified to date. The precise mechanisms by which TCF7L2 variants increase risk are not well understood, although various lines of evidence suggest that they involve the enteroinsular axis and impaired insulin secretion and possibly reduced beta cell proliferation.[12] Candidate genes are previously discovered genes that based on their inferred physiologic role, are hypothesized to contribute to the disease of interest if abnormal. In the case of T2DM, genes related to glucose transport, β cell function, and insulin secretion would all be considered reasonable candidates for contributing to the genetic basis of disease. Association studies simply compare the relative frequencies of each variant allele in case and control subjects and determine whether one is overrepresented in disease.

To date, four genes identified using candidate gene association studies have been convincingly associated with T2DM.

PPARG

A proline-to-alanine change in codon 12 (P12A) of the peroxisome proliferator-activated receptor (PPARG) gene was the first genetic variant to be definitively implicated in the common form of T2DM. Since this initial work, the preponderance of evidence has conclusively supported the association of PPARG with T2DM with an odds ratio (OR) of 1.2.

KCNJ11

The potassium inwardly rectifying channel, subfamily J, member 11 (KCNJ11) gene, first described in the context of neonatal diabetes, encodes the beta cell K channel and is functionally closely related to the sulfonylurea receptor, SUR1 encoded by ABCC8. These genes are adjacent to each other on chromosome 11. Work on this locus has confirmed that a less drastic change in a gene implicated in a rare monogenic subtype of diabetes can indeed contribute to its more common form: single nucleotide polymorphism (SNP) E23K of KCNJ11 has now been convincingly associated with T2DM. Subsequent large-scale studies and meta-analyses have consistently associated the lysine variant with T2DM with an OR of 1.15.

WFS1

Another monogenic form of diabetes is Wolfram syndrome, caused by mutations in the Wolfram syndrome 1 (WFS1) gene.

HNF1B

Further research on this maturity-onset diabetes of the young (MODY) gene has produced a conclusive association of an intronic SNP (rs757210) in hepatocyte nuclear factor 1B (HNF1B) (previously known as TCF2) with T2DM.[11]

GWA Studies

Recent dramatic increases in the rate of diabetes gene discovery have occurred with the advent of GWA studies. This new approach has resulted from the confluence of several key scientific achievements: (1) successful sequencing of the entire human genome, leading to (2) identification of the several million SNPs (common variations in a single base pair that explain the vast majority of human heterozygosity), which in turn led to (3) genotyping of 3.8 million SNPs in 270 DNA samples by the International HapMap Project (HapMap) to create a subset of haplotype-tagging SNPs (so-called "tag SNPs" that can serve as efficient proxies for localizing variation within narrow stretches of the genome).

Based on these advances, the following general comments can be made regarding the genetics of T2DM:

- A large number of genes are associated with increased susceptibility to this disease. The approximately 30 genes identified to date are thought to account for a small proportion (estimated at no more than 5–10%) of the total genetic risk for diabetes in the population.
- The genes identified to date individually lead to a modest increase in the risk of diabetes. Persons with these individual polymorphisms have OR between 1.10 and 1.45 when compared with individuals who do not have the at-risk polymorphisms.
- The presence of multiple at-risk polymorphisms in a single individual substantially increases the risk of developing diabetes.

- A significant proportion of the genetic variants associated with increased risk or diabetes appear to do so by inhibiting insulin secretion. Very few appear to increase insulin resistance or obesity.

These advances in our understanding of the human genome proceeded in concert with two additional key steps: (4) the development of affordable, high-throughput genotyping technologies and (5) several large multicenter collections with well-characterized phenotypes assembled and shared through international collaborations. The first GWA scan for T2DM (and all others that followed) was validated by the clear replication of the TCF7L2 association.[11,12]

Whether this is a reflection of the relative importance of the roles of these factors in the pathogenesis of T2DM or whether the design of the genome-wide association study (GWAS) did not allow genetic risk factors for insulin resistance and obesity to be identified is yet to be determined.

CLINICAL APPLICATION OF GENETIC INFORMATION IN DIABETES

By discerning structure in the patterns of gene variation, subtle phenotype differences may be recognized in ways that cannot be achieved with current phenotyping methods. The rapid increase in genome-wide association (GWA)-related publications has fueled expectations that genetic factors can be used to construct susceptibility profiles that will help in the prediction, prevention, and treatment of T1DM and T2DM, thereby ushering in a new era of "personalized medicine." In the following sections, we outline the current knowledge base and potential clinical implications of diabetes genetic testing in four clinical care domains.

Predicting Risk of Developing Diabetes

A major clinical role for genetic testing in medicine has been to predict an individual's risk for developing disease. This works particularly well in monogenic disorders with Mendelian inheritance and reliable penetrance. Examples include testing for the BRCA genes in breast and ovarian cancer and preconception testing for carrier status in parents at risk for cystic fibrosis. Such genetic testing holds two core principles: that the genetic testing improves risk prediction beyond readily available data such as family history, physical examination findings, and basic laboratory tests and that the test results provide "clinically actionable" information. Given the strength of the evidence from landmark studies of diabetes prevention, identifying patients in the prediabetic stage for intensive lifestyle management or metformin therapy has the potential to significantly reduce the incidence and subsequent morbidity and mortality of T2DM. With this potential benefit in mind, researchers have investigated whether genetic testing can improve the identification of high-risk patients. Of the genes confirmed to date, TCF7L2 has the highest OR for predicting diabetes.[12]

Using data from the Framingham Offspring Study, Meigs et al. tested a "genotype score" approach that summed the number of risk-conferring alleles from a panel of the 18 loci known to be associated with T2DM. Genotype score provided only a slightly better prediction of risk than knowledge of common risk factors alone.[13] Other studies using the same 18 genetic loci approach have yielded similar results. While future genetic predication tools may serve a valuable role in identifying particularly high-risk patient subgroups, for current diabetes prevention efforts, individualized genetic information to guide therapy or motivate behavior change may have the most clinical impact among patients who have already been identified as at-risk for diabetes by other methods.

Monogenic Diabetes

Monogenic forms of beta cell diabetes account for approximately 1–2% of all cases of diabetes, yet remain underdiagnosed.[15] Overlapping clinical features with common forms of diabetes, make diagnosis challenging. A genetic diagnosis of monogenic diabetes in many cases alters therapy, affects prognosis, enables genetic counseling and has implications for cascade screening of extended family members.

Neonatal Diabetes

Neonatal diabetes mellitus (NDM) refers to diabetes diagnosed in the first 6 months of life and has an estimated incidence of around 1 in 200,000 live births.[20,21] Historically, patients were treated with insulin as they were assumed to have T1DM, but the discovery in 2004 of the causal role of mutations in the KATP channels in many affected individuals and the successful transfer of these patients from insulin to oral sulfonylurea therapy with improved control and less frequent hypoglycemia has led to the recommendation of genetic testing in all cases of neonatal diabetes.[15]

Neonatal diabetes mellitus may be permanent neonatal diabetes mellitus (PNDM) or transient neonatal diabetes mellitus (TNDM) in which case the diabetes may remit spontaneously within 1–18 months (although relapse to permanent diabetes later in life is common). Fifty percent of cases of PNDM and 20% of TNDM are estimated to result from activating mutations of the KATP channel genes (KCNJ11 or ABCC8) encoding the Kir6.2 and SUR1 subunits respectively.[16] Activating mutations in the KATP channels impair the ability of ATP (generated by pancreatic glucose metabolism) to close the channel, thereby preventing beta cell depolarization and insulin secretion. Consequently, these patients present with diabetic ketoacidosis or marked hyperglycemia, and low levels of circulating endogenous insulin.[1] Orally administered sulfonylurea drugs, commonly used to treat T2DM, close the KATP channel by an ATP independent route and thus increase insulin secretion, although the required dose is frequently considerably higher. Unlike in T2DM however, patients with NDM due to KATP channel mutations who are treated with sulfonylurea therapy have near normalization of glycated hemoglobin (HbA1c) without significant hypoglycemia, suggesting that insulin secretion is well regulated. This phenomenon may be explained by the specific nature of the pathophysiological defect in NDM; unlike T2DM (where multiple factors promote glycemic dysfunction), other physiological regulators of insulin secretion [glucagon-like peptide-1 (GLP-1), etc.] function normally.[28]

In addition to NDM, 20% of patients with KATP channel mutations have associated neurological symptoms including developmental delay, epilepsy, neonatal diabetes "DEND" syndrome, which reflects the presence of extra-pancreatic KATP channels linking cell metabolism to electrical activity in muscle and brain. Glibenclamide therapy (a non-beta cell selective sulfonylurea) in these patients can ameliorate these extra-pancreatic manifestations also.[17,19] Many other genetic etiologies of NDM have been documented; some which are associated with extra-pancreatic manifestations. Insulin therapy is essential for patients with other non-KATP channels forms of NDM.[20]

MONOGENIC DIABETES DETECTED IN ADOLESCENCE OR ADULTHOOD

Glucokinase Monogenic Diabetes

The enzyme glucokinase (GCK), which phosphorylates glucose, functions as a sensor of ambient glucose levels. The effect of a heterozygous inactivating mutation in GCK is mild fasting hyperglycemia (5.5–8.0 mmol/L), minimal or normal post meal time glucose excursions (<3.0 mmol/L glucose during an oral glucose tolerance test), and an HbA1c level within the normal or slightly elevated range (usually 40-60 mmol/L).[18] GCK monogenic diabetes is thought to represent 20–30% of all cases of monogenic diabetes and is inherited in an autosomal dominant pattern.

Since microvascular complications are extremely rare in these patients, the confirmation of GCK mutation allows glucose lowering therapy to be stopped and carries a favorable prognosis without risk of progression of diabetes.[15]

During pregnancy, women with a GCK mutation have a 50% chance of carrying a baby without a GCK mutation, in which case there is an increased risk of macrosomia and its obstetric consequences. Thus, maternal insulin treatment is indicated. Conversely, if the mother carries a baby with a GCK mutation, no treatment is required. Ultrasonographic monitoring of fetal size is currently recommended to decide whether or not to lower maternal glycemia with insulin during pregnancy, although fetal genotyping using maternal blood sampling during early pregnancy may be available in the future.

Hepatocyte Nuclear Factor Monogenic Diabetes

The hepatocyte nuclear factor (HNF) family of proteins are transcription factors, required for the correct functioning of pancreatic beta cells. Three HNF subtype mutations are most commonly associated with monogenic diabetes: HNF1A, HNF4A, HNF1B, with HNF1A mutations being most common. Each heterozygous, loss of function mutation is inherited in an autosomal dominant fashion and results in early and progressive beta cell dysfunction, with diabetes presenting in late childhood or early adulthood. The typical earliest manifestation is postprandial hyperglycemia with fasting normoglycemia, eventually progressing to frank diabetes. HNF4A is also associated with increased birthweight and a tendency to neonatal hypoglycemia, which is thought to reflect fetal hyperinsulinemia and the differential roles for HNF4A in fetal and adult beta cells. The risk of micro- and macrovascular complications is comparable to T1DM and T2DM and correlates with glycemic control.

Early expression of HNF1B is seen in the kidney, liver, genital tract, lung, gut and pancreas. Renal involvement is most consistently described in HNF1B mutation carriers due to abnormal renal development, and includes renal cysts, familial hypoplastic glomerulocystic kidney disease, atypical familiar hyperuricemic nephropathy, single and horseshoe kidney. The penetrance of diabetes in patients with HNF1B mutations is unknown and may present in late adult life. Thus, annual diabetes screening is recommended. Other clinical features include genital tract malformations, abnormal liver function tests, pancreatic atrophy and exocrine insufficiency, gout and hyperuricemia.[22]

Patients with HNF1A and HNF4A frequently demonstrate excellent and durable responses to low dose sulfonylurea therapy, although in some cases higher doses or additional therapy may be required. Thus, insulin therapy can be avoided for many years after diagnosis in most cases, which has clear practical, social, occupational and health cost benefits. Insulin therapy is usually required in those with HNF1B diabetes due to pancreatic atrophy.

Measuring high-sensitivity CRP (hsCRP) may be particularly helpful in discriminating between HNF1A and other forms of diabetes. HNF1A binding sites are located at promoter sites in the gene coding for C-reactive peptide (CRP). Consequently, markedly lower levels of hsCRP are seen in monogenic diabetes as a result of an HNF1A mutation than in other forms of diabetes. The highest discriminatory value of hsCRP is between HNF1A and T2DM, although hsCRP values are also higher among those with HNF4A, GCK, or HNF1B than HNF1A. However, the modest test performance (sensitivity 79%, specificity 70%) requires that additional clinical characteristics are considered in combination.[29] The hsCRP is not useful if elevated (>10 mg/L) as this usually indicates the presence of confounding inflammation, and should be repeated after a few weeks. Insulin resistance is characteristically associated with a reduction in circulating high-density lipoprotein (HDL) levels. Thus, normal or elevated HDL levels indicate that insulin resistance may not be a major component of the disease (i.e. T2DM is less likely). The HDL level displays moderate discrimination when distinguishing between HNF1A carriers and those with T2DM, with a plasma HDL >1.12 mmol/L favoring a diagnosis of monogenic diabetes (75% sensitive and 64% specific). HDL levels are similar between HNF1A, T1DM and healthy controls[6] (Flow chart 1).

Maternally Inherited Diabetes and Deafness

Maternally inherited diabetes and deafness (MIDD) accounts for up to 50% of cases of monogenic diabetes and up to 1% of unselected cases of diabetes. The mt.3243A>G gene mutation is the most common cause of MIDD and affects tRNALeu (UUR) production within the mitochondria.[23,24] Because oocytes (but not spermatozoa) contribute mitochondria to the developing embryo, only females pass mitochondrial mutations to their children (maternal inheritance). Mitochondria are responsible for cellular ATP production, and therefore mutations in its DNA should result in dysfunction within all tissues that are particularly metabolically active. However, it is clear that certain mitochondrial mutations are associated with tissue specific dysfunction (as seen with mt.3243A>G mutations resulting in MIDD) although the mechanisms remain to be fully elucidated.[23] Progressive beta cell failure is seen in those who harbor mutations although the rapidity of insulin production failure is variable. Carriers may also suffer from deafness and macular dystrophy (most commonly) but also strokes and myopathies. Insulin treatment for diabetes is frequently required. Metformin is theoretically contraindicated in MIDD due to concerns about lactic acidosis. Coenzyme Q10 and thiamine replacement is advised to reduce progression of diabetes and hearing loss in the early stages of the disorder.[14]

Status of MODY Genetics in India[27]

India is making rapid advances in the field of molecular genetics, and its application in the field of health and disease. However, few groups of investigators have embarked on the molecular genetic studies in diabetes particularly MODY. The performed studies have been centered on mutations on very few genes which were reported to be relatively common in the Western

Flow chart 1: Diagnostic algorithm for assessment of suspected monogenic diabetes[7]

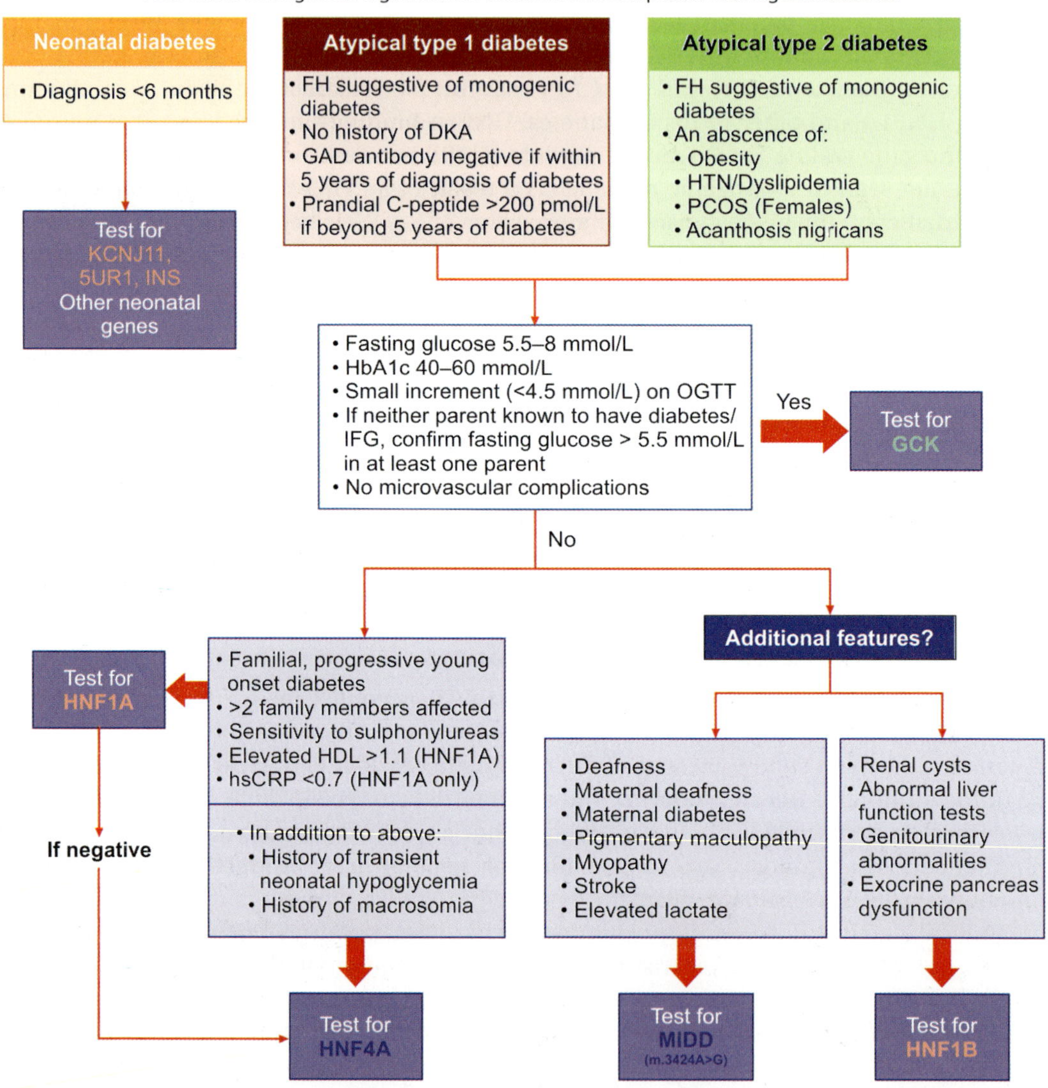

population. Hence, data about MODY in India is basic and preliminary. In 2005, Mohan et al. reported the first SNP in HNF1A gene associated with MODY and early T2DM from India. They identified that frequency of Ala98Val polymorphism in the HNF1A gene is significantly higher in MODY patients. The same polymorphism was associated with earlier age of diabetes onset in T2DM. However, since this study specifically looked at only one polymorphism in HNF1A gene among the several genes involved and there could be several polymorphisms associated with each MODY gene, it cannot be representative of the entire genetic subtypes of MODY.

Another study from Northern India by Sahu et al. showed that A3243G mitochondrial mutation and HNF1A gene mutations were infrequently associated with early-onset T2DM. However, this study attempted to look at the specific etiologies of early-onset type diabetes and was not uniquely focused on the genetic basis of MODY.[25] In 2009 Radha et al. demonstrated that mutations in the HNF1A gene comprise about 9% of clinically diagnosed MODY subjects in southern India. They sequenced the coding and promoter regions of HNF1A gene for mutations in unrelated South Indian subjects, in whom a clinical diagnosis of MODY was made.[26] Nine novel variants comprising seven mutations (one novel mutation-538G>C at promoter region and six novel coding region mutations) and two polymorphisms in the HNF1A gene were identified. They also observed co-segregation with diabetes of the Arg263. His coding region mutation in eight members of one MODY family. In this study, mutations in only one gene that was implicated in MODY was looked for, while there are more than ten genes on the list currently.

In 2011, the first report on HNF4A mutation (MODY1) was published by the same group constituting 3.4% of the clinically diagnosed MODY. They identified three novel mutations in the P2 promoter region of HNF4A. In addition, they also reported SNP of HNF4A that are both susceptible to and protective against MODY and early-onset T2DM.[27]

REFERENCES

1. Permutt MA, Wasson J, Cox N. Genetic epidemiology of diabetes. J Clin Invest. 2005;115(6):1431-39.
2. American Diabetes Association. Diagnosis and classification of diabetes mellitus. Diabetes Care.2012;35(1):S64-S71.
3. Horenstein RB, Shuldiner AR. Genetics of diabetes. Rev Endocr Metab Disord. 2004;5(1):25-36.
4. Dorman JS, Bunker CH. HLA-DQ locus of the human leukocyte antigen complex and type 1 diabetes mellitus: a HuGE review. Epidemiol Rev. 2000;22(2):218-27.
5. Hirschhorn JN. Genetic epidemiology of type 1 diabetes. Pediatr Diabetes. 2003;4(2):87-100.
6. Nejentsev S, Reijonen H, Adojaan B, et. al. The effect of HLA-B allele on the IDDM risk defined by DRB1*04 subtypes and DQB1*0302. Diabetes. 1997;46(11):1888-92.
7. Anjos S, Polychronakos, C. Mechanisms of genetic susceptibility to type 1 diabetes: beyond HLA. Mol Genet Metab. 2004;81(3): 187-95.
8. Bennett ST, Wilson AJ, Esposito L, et al. Insulin VNTR allele-specific effect in type 1 diabetes depends on identity of untransmitted paternal allele. The IMDIAB Group. Nat Genet. 1997; 17(3):350-2.
9. Undlien DE, Hamaguchi K, Kimura A, et al. IDDM susceptibility associated with polymorphisms in the insulin gene region. A study of Blacks, Caucasians, and Orientals. Diabetologia. 1994;37(80:745-9.
10. Grant SF, Thorleifsson G, Reynisdottir I, et al. Variant of transcription factor 7-like 2 (TCF7L2) gene confers risk of type 2 diabetes. Nat Genet. 2006;38(3):320-3.
11. Grant RW, Moore AF, Florez JC. Genetic architecture of type 2 diabetes: recent progress and clinical implications. Diabetes Care. 2009;32(6):1107-14.
12. Florez JC, Jablonski KA, Bayley N, et al. TCF7L2 polymorphisms and progression to diabetes in the Diabetes Prevention Program. N Engl J Med. 2006;355(3):241-50
13. Meigs JB, Shrader P, Sullivan LM, et al. Genotype score in addition to common risk factors for prediction of type 2 diabetes. N Engl J Med. 2008;359(21):2208-19.
14. Carroll RW, Murphy R. Monogenic diabetes: a diagnostic algorithm for clinicians. Genes (Basel). 2013;4(4):522-35.
15. Murphy R, Ellard S, Hattersley AT. Clinical implications of a molecular genetic classification of monogenic beta-cell diabetes. Nat Clin Pract Endocrinol Metab. 2008;4(4): 200-13.

16. Shields BM, Hicks S, Shepherd MH, et al. Maturity-onset diabetes of the young (MODY): how many cases are we missing? Diabetologia. 2010;53(12):2504-8.
17. Hattersley A, Bruining J, Shield J, et al. The diagnosis and management of monogenic diabetes in children and adolescents. Pediatr Diabetes. 2009;10(12):33-42.
18. Ellard S, Bellanne-Chantelot C, Hattersley AT, et al. Best practice guidelines for the molecular genetic diagnosis of maturity-onset diabetes of the young. Diabetologia. 2008;51(4):546-53.
19. Vaxillaire M, Bonnefond A, Froguel P. The lessons of early-onset monogenic diabetes for the understanding of diabetes pathogenesis. Clin Pract Endocrinol Metab. 2012;26(2):171-87.
20. Temple IK, Gardner RJ, Mackay DJ, et al. Transient neonatal diabetes: widening the understanding of the etiopathogenesis of diabetes. Diabetes. 2000;49(8):1359-66.
21. Slingerland AS, Shields BM, Flanagan SE, et al. Referral rates for diagnostic testing support an incidence of permanent neonatal diabetes in three European countries of at least 1 in 260,000 live births. Diabetologia. 2009; 52(8):1683-5.
22. Maestro MA, Cardalda C, Boj SF, et al. Distinct roles of HNF1beta, HNF1alpha, and HNF4alpha in regulating pancreas development, beta-cell function and growth. Endocr Dev. 2007;12:33-45.
23. Murphy R, Turnbull DM, Walker M, et al. Clinical features, diagnosis and management of maternally inherited diabetes and deafness (MIDD) associated with the 3243A>G mitochondrial point mutation. Diabet Med. 2008;25(4):383-99.
24. Maassen JA, Janssen GM, 'tHart LM. Molecular mechanisms of mitochondrial diabetes (MIDD). Ann Med. 2005;37(3):213-21.
25. Sahu RP, Aggarwal A, Zaidi G, et al. Etiology of early-onset type 2 diabetes in Indians: islet autoimmunity and mutations in hepatocyte nuclear factor-1alpha and mitochondrial gene. J Clin Endocrinol Metab. 2007;92(7):2462–7.
26. Radha V, Ek J, Anuradha S, et al. Identification of novel variants in hepatocyte nuclear factor-1alpha gene in South Indian patients with maturity onset diabetes of young. J Clin Endocrinol Metab. 2009;94(6):1959-65.
27. Anuradha S, Radha V, Mohan V. Association of novel variants in the hepatocyte nuclear factor 4A gene with maturity onset diabetes of the young and early onset type 2 diabetes. Clin Genet. 2011;80(6):541-9.
28. Pearson ER, Flechtner I, Njølstad PR, et al. Switching from insulin to oral sulfonylureas in patients with diabetes due to Kir6.2 mutations. N Engl J Med. 2006;355(5):467-77.
29. McDonald TJ, Shields BM, Lawry J, et al. High-sensitivity CRP discriminates HNF1A-MODY from other subtypes of diabetes. Diabetes Care. 2011;34(8):1860-2.

6
CHAPTER

Classification and Diagnosis of Diabetes

Radhika Jindal, Asim Siddiqui, Subhash Kumar Wangnoo

INTRODUCTION

Diabetes mellitus is a group of metabolic diseases of multiple etiologies characterized by hyperglycemia together with disturbances of carbohydrate, fat and protein metabolism resulting from defects in insulin secretion, insulin action, or both. The chronic hyperglycemia of diabetes is associated with microvascular damage affecting, particularly, eyes, kidneys, nerves and heart, together with an increased risk of macrovascular disease.[1]

HISTORY OF DIABETES CLASSIFICATION

A major requirement for epidemiological and clinical research and for the clinical management of diabetes is an appropriate system of classification that provides a framework within which to identify and differentiate its various forms and stages.

In 1964, the World Health Organization (WHO) Expert Committee, made the first real attempt to classify diabetes.[2] It resorted to a symptomatic classification on one hand, and age of onset on the other. Thus, it described "asymptomatic" diabetes and "clinical" diabetes, with diagnostic criteria based on the oral glucose tolerance test (OGTT); it also had "potential" diabetes and "latent" diabetes. Its age categorization of diabetes comprised: infantile or childhood diabetes (0–14 year old), young diabetes (15–24 years old), adult diabetes (25–64 years old) and elderly diabetes (65+ years old). In addition, the classification "juvenile" diabetes was confusingly retained for anyone requiring insulin and showing ketosis. It also had "brittle" diabetes, "gestational" diabetes, "pancreatic" diabetes and "endocrine" diabetes. This was a start and more information became available in the succeeding years.

In 1979, the National Diabetes Data Group (NDDG) in the USA, and in 1980, the second report of the WHO Expert Committee on Diabetes Mellitus offered a classification that was accepted internationally.[3,4] Two main classes of diabetes were suggested: insulin dependent diabetes mellitus (IDDM) (type 1) and noninsulin dependent diabetes mellitus (NIDDM) (type 2). "Other types" and "gestational diabetes mellitus (GDM)" completed the list. Two risk classes—previous abnormality of glucose tolerance and potential abnormality of glucose tolerance—were also introduced and replaced categories such as prediabetes and potential diabetes. "Borderline" diabetes was replaced by impaired glucose tolerance (IGT). In 1985, the WHO Study Group also added malnutrition-related diabetes mellitus, and the terms "type 1" and "type 2" diabetes were dropped.[5]

Based on increasing knowledge, WHO revisited the classification in 1999[6] as did the American Diabetes Association (ADA) in 1997.[7] It was recognized that the terms IDDM and NIDDM, although superficially appealing, were often confusing and unhelpful—as in patients with insulin treated type-2 diabetes mellitus (T2DM). The new classification attempted to encompass both etiology and clinical stages of the disease as well as being useful clinically. This was based on the suggestion of Kuzuya and Matsuda.[8] This acknowledges that diabetes may progress through several clinical stages (e.g. from normoglycemia to ketoacidosis) while having a single etiologic process such as autoimmune attack on the beta cells. Similarly, it is possible that someone with type-2 diabetes can move from insulin requirement to no pharmaceutical intervention through modification of lifestyle. The main classes are type-1 diabetes mellitus (T1DM), T2DM, other specific types and gestational diabetes. It should be noted that T2DM is largely categorization by exclusion. As new causes are discovered, they will be included under "other specific types" as has occurred for maturity-onset diabetes of the young (MODY). WHO re-examined the classification in 2006, when no changes were recommended,[9] and again in 2009, when some updating was done, but there were no fundamental changes.[1]

CURRENT CLASSIFICATION OF DIABETES

The currently used classification is an etiologic classification (Box 1).[10] Diabetes can be classified into four clinical categories:

1. Type 1 diabetes (due to β-cell destruction, usually leading to absolute insulin deficiency) (Table 1).
2. Type 2 diabetes (due to a progressive insulin secretory defect on the background of insulin resistance) (Table 1).
3. Other specific types of diabetes due to other causes, e.g. genetic defects in β-cell function, genetic defects in insulin action, diseases of the exocrine pancreas (such as cystic fibrosis), and drug- or chemical-induced (such as in the treatment of HIV/AIDS or after organ transplantation).
4. Gestational diabetes mellitus (diabetes diagnosed during pregnancy that is not clearly overt diabetes).

Box 1: Etiologic classification of diabetes mellitus

1. Type 1 diabetes (β-cell destruction, usually leading to absolute insulin deficiency)
   A. Immune mediated
   B. Idiopathic

2. Type 2 diabetes (may range from predominantly insulin resistance with relative insulin deficiency to a predominantly secretory defect with insulin resistance)

3. Other specific types:
   A. Genetic defects of β-cell function
      i. Maturity-onset diabetes of the young (MODY) 3 [Chromosome 12, hepatocyte nuclear factor (HNF)-1α]
      ii. MODY 1 (Chromosome 20, HNF-4α)
      iii. MODY 2 (Chromosome 7, glucokinase)
      iv. Other very rare forms of MODY (e.g. MODY 4: Chromosome 13, insulin promoter factor-1; MODY 5: HNF-1β; MODY 6: Chromosome 2, NeuroD1; MODY 7: Chromosome 9, carboxyl ester lipase)
      v. Transient neonatal diabetes (most commonly ZAC/HY AMI imprinting defect on 6q24)
      vi. Permanent neonatal diabetes (most commonly KCNJ11 gene coding Kir6.2 subunit of β-cell KATP channel)
      vii. Mitochondrial DNA
      viii. Others
   B. Genetic defects in insulin action: Type A insulin resistance/Leprechaunism/Rabson-Mendenhall syndrome/Lipoatrophic diabetes/Others
   C. Diseases of the exocrine pancreas: Pancreatitis/Trauma/Pancreatectomy/Neoplasia/Cystic fibrosis/Hemochromatosis/Fibrocalculous pancreatopathy/Others
   D. Endocrinopathies: Acromegaly/Cushing's syndrome/Glucagonoma/Pheochromocytoma/Hyperthyroidism/Somatostatinoma/Aldosteronoma/Others
   E. Drug or chemical induced: Vacor/Pentamidine/Nicotinic acid/Glucocorticoids/Thyroid hormone/Diazoxide/β-Adrenergic agonists/Thiazides/Dilantin/Gamma-interferon/Others
   F. Infections: Congenital rubella/Cytomegalovirus/Others
   G. Uncommon forms of immune-mediated diabetes: Stiff-man syndrome/Anti-insulin receptor antibodies/Others
   H. Other genetic syndromes sometimes associated with diabetes: Down syndrome/Klinefelter syndrome/Turner syndrome/Wolfram syndrome/Friedreich ataxia/Huntington chorea/Laurence-Moon-Biedel syndrome/Myotonic dystrophy/Porphyria/Prader-Willi syndrome/Others

4. Gestational diabetes mellitus

Table 1: Differences between Type 1 and Type 2 diabetes mellitus[5]

Features	*Type 1 diabetes mellitus*	*Type 2 diabetes mellitus*
Pathogenesis	Pancreatic damage	Insulin resistance
Age of onset	Usually <20 years	Usually ≥30 years
Presentation	Sudden	Gradual
Ketoacidosis	Common	Not common
Family trend	<10%	Common
Twin concordance	40%	100%
Acanthosis nigricans	Not seen	Common
Obesity	Not common	Common
HLA association	Common	No association
Insulin requirement	Is a must	May be needed
Islet cell antibodies	As high as ≥85%	<5%

Abbreviation: HLA, human leukocyte antigen

Type 1 Diabetes (β-Cell Destruction, Usually Leading to Absolute Insulin Deficiency)

Immune-mediated Diabetes

Previously known as insulin-dependent diabetes or juvenile-onset diabetes, it results from a cellular-mediated autoimmune destruction of the β-cells of the pancreas. The rate of β-cell destruction is quite variable, being rapid in some individuals (mainly infants and children) and slow in others (mainly adults). The disease has strong human leukocyte antigen (HLA) associations. It commonly occurs in childhood and adolescence, but it can occur at any age, even in the 8th and 9th decades of life. Markers of the immune destruction of the β-cell include islet cell autoantibodies, autoantibodies to insulin, autoantibodies to glutamic acid decarboxylase (GAD65), and autoantibodies to the tyrosine phosphatases IA-2 and IA-2b. When fasting hyperglycemia is initially detected, one and usually more of these autoantibodies are present in 85–90% of individuals.

Idiopathic Diabetes

Some forms of type 1 diabetes have no known etiologies. Individuals with this form of diabetes suffer from episodic ketoacidosis and exhibit varying degrees of insulin deficiency in between the episodes. There is absence of β-cell autoimmunity, and it is not HLA associated. An absolute requirement for insulin therapy in affected patients may come and go.

Type 2 Diabetes (Ranging from Predominantly Insulin Resistance with Relative Insulin Deficiency to Predominantly Insulin Secretory Defect with Insulin Resistance)

Previously known as noninsulin-dependent diabetes, type 2 diabetes, or adult-onset diabetes; this is the most common form of diabetes. It encompasses individuals who have insulin resistance and usually have relative (rather than absolute) insulin deficiency. At least initially, and often throughout their lifetime, these individuals may not need insulin treatment for their survival. Autoimmune destruction of β-cells does not occur.

Most patients with this form of diabetes are obese, and obesity itself causes some degree of insulin resistance. Even those who are not obese may have an increased percentage of body fat distributed predominantly in the abdominal region. The increased visceral fat and the associated insulin resistance predisposes to type 2 diabetes. Since the hyperglycemia develops gradually, and at earlier stages it is often not severe enough for the patient to notice any of the classic symptoms of diabetes, it frequently goes undiagnosed for many years. But still, the patients are at increased risk of developing macrovascular and microvascular complications. Patients with this form of diabetes may have insulin levels that appear normal or elevated; the higher blood glucose levels in these diabetic patients would be expected to result in even higher insulin values had their β-cell function been normal. Thus, insulin secretion is defective in these patients and insufficient to compensate for insulin resistance. Ketoacidosis seldom occurs spontaneously in this type of diabetes; when seen, it usually arises in association with the stress of another illness such as infection. The risk of developing this form of diabetes increases with age, obesity, lack of physical activity, prior GDM, presence of hypertension or dyslipidemia, and its frequency varies in different racial/ethnic subgroups. It is often associated with a strong genetic predisposition; however, the genetics of this form of diabetes are complex and not fully defined. Insulin resistance may improve with weight reduction and/or pharmacological treatment of hyperglycemia but is seldom restored to normal.

Other Specific Types of Diabetes

Genetic Defects of the β-Cell

Several forms of diabetes are associated with monogenetic defects in β-cell function. Known as MODY, these are characterized by impaired insulin secretion with minimal or no defects in insulin action. The onset of hyperglycemia characteristically occurs at an early age (generally before age 25 years). They are inherited in an autosomal dominant pattern. Abnormalities have been identified at different genetic loci on different chromosomes.

Diabetes diagnosed in the first 6 months of life is known as neonatal diabetes. It can either be transient or permanent. It is not autoimmune mediated. The most common genetic defect causing transient disease is a defect on ZAC/HYAMI imprinting, whereas permanent neonatal diabetes is most commonly due to a defect in the gene encoding the Kir6.2 subunit of the β-cell KATP channel. Diagnosing the latter has implications, since such children can be well managed with sulfonylureas.

Genetic Defects in Insulin Action

There are unusual causes of diabetes that result from genetically determined abnormalities of insulin action. The metabolic abnormalities associated with mutations of the insulin receptor may range from hyperinsulinemia and modest hyperglycemia to severe diabetes. Patients may have features of insulin resistance in the form of acanthosis nigricans; women may be virilized and have enlarged, cystic ovaries. In the past, this syndrome was termed type A insulin resistance. Leprechaunism and the Rabson-Mendenhall syndrome are two pediatric syndromes that have mutations in the insulin receptor gene with subsequent alterations in insulin receptor function and extreme insulin resistance. The former has characteristic facial features and is usually fatal in infancy, while the latter is associated with abnormalities of teeth and nails and pineal gland hyperplasia.

Diseases of the Exocrine Pancreas

Any process that diffusely injures the pancreas can cause diabetes such as pancreatitis, trauma, infection, pancreatectomy and pancreatic carcinoma. Damage to the pancreas must be extensive for diabetes to occur except that caused by cancer; adenocarcinomas that involve only a small portion of the pancreas have been associated with diabetes. This implies a mechanism other than simple reduction in β-cell mass. If extensive enough, cystic fibrosis and hemochromatosis will also damage β-cells and impair insulin secretion. Fibrocalculous pancreatopathy may be accompanied by abdominal pain radiating to the back and pancreatic calcifications identified on X-ray examination.

Endocrinopathies

Several hormones (e.g. growth hormone, cortisol, glucagon and epinephrine) antagonize insulin action. Excess amount of these hormones (e.g. acromegaly, Cushing's syndrome, glucagonoma, pheochromocytoma, respectively) can cause diabetes. This generally occurs in individuals with pre-existing defects in insulin secretion, and hyperglycemia typically resolves when the hormone excess is resolved.

Endocrine disorders which induce hypokalemia—somatostatinomas and aldosteronoma—can cause diabetes, at least in part, by inhibiting insulin secretion. Hyperglycemia generally resolves after successful removal of the tumor.

Drug and Chemical-induced Diabetes

Insulin secretion can be impaired by many drugs. These drugs may not cause diabetes by themselves, but they may precipitate diabetes in individuals with insulin resistance. In such cases, the classification is unclear because the sequence or relative importance of β-cell dysfunction and insulin resistance is unknown. Certain toxins such as Vacor (a rat poison) and intravenous pentamidine can permanently destroy pancreatic β-cells. There are also many drugs and hormones that can impair insulin action, thus leading to insulin resistance. Examples include nicotinic acid and glucocorticoids. Patients receiving α-interferon have been reported to develop diabetes associated with islet cell antibodies and, in certain instances, severe insulin deficiency.

Infections

Certain viruses have been associated with β-cell destruction. Diabetes occurs in patients with congenital rubella, although most of these patients have HLA and immune markers characteristic of type 1 diabetes. In addition, coxsackievirus B, cytomegalovirus, adenovirus, and mumps have been implicated in inducing certain cases of the disease.

Uncommon Forms of Immune-mediated Diabetes

The stiff-man syndrome is an autoimmune disorder of the central nervous system characterized by stiffness of the axial muscles with painful spasms. It is associated with high titers of the GAD autoantibodies, and about one-third patients develop diabetes.

Anti-insulin receptor antibodies can cause diabetes by binding to the insulin receptor, thereby blocking the binding of insulin to its receptor in target tissues. However, in some cases, these antibodies can act as an insulin agonist after binding to the receptor and can thus cause hypoglycemia. Anti-insulin receptor antibodies are occasionally found in patients with systemic lupus erythematosus and other autoimmune diseases. As in other states of extreme insulin resistance, patients with anti-insulin receptor antibodies often have acanthosis nigricans. Previously this syndrome was termed type B insulin resistance.

Other Genetic Syndromes sometimes Associated with Diabetes

Many genetic syndromes are accompanied by an increased incidence of diabetes. These include the chromosomal abnormalities of Down syndrome, Klinefelter syndrome and Turner syndrome. Wolfram syndrome is an autosomal recessive disorder characterized by insulin-deficient diabetes and the absence of β-cells at autopsy. Additional manifestations include diabetes insipidus, hypogonadism, optic atrophy and neural deafness.

Gestational Diabetes Mellitus

Gestational diabetes mellitus has been defined as any degree of glucose intolerance with onset or first recognition during pregnancy. Although most cases resolve with delivery, the definition applied whether or not the condition persisted after pregnancy and did not exclude the possibility that unrecognized glucose intolerance may have antedated or begun concomitantly with the pregnancy.

DIAGNOSIS OF DIABETES

In the presence of classical symptoms like thirst, polyuria, weight loss and recurrent infections, a casual venous plasma glucose level of 200 mg/dL (11.1 mmol/L) or more is sufficient for a definite diagnosis of diabetes. But in an asymptomatic person with moderate hyperglycemia, a second confirmatory test is essential.

Diagnostic Tests

Glycosuria was earlier used as the major diagnostic test in the 19th century. In the 20th century, with the availability of measurement of blood glucose, it came into use as the main diagnostic test and has remained so. The initial tests for the measurement of blood glucose were laborious and were not very specific. Gradually over the years, blood glucose measurement became relatively easy and rapid to perform. With the introduction of enzymatic assays, the results became specific. The OGTT was first devised in the early years of the 20th century and slowly came into use for diagnosis. There was no universal agreement on precisely which tests should be performed and what concentrations of glucose were diagnostic for diabetes. Glycosuria continued to be used for diagnosis until the 1960s.

In 1964, the first WHO Expert Committee scrapped the use of glycosuria as a diagnostic test, and suggested that only the 50-g and the 100-g OGTTs should be used.[2] The fasting glucose criterion was set at 130 mg/dL (7.2 mmol/L); but this was venous whole blood, so, for plasma, it would be about 150 mg/dL (8.3 mmol/L). However, nonspecific tests for glucose were used at that time, so a true plasma glucose would have been between 130 mg/dL (7.2 mmol/L) and 140 mg/dL (7.8 mmol/L). The WHO Committee was also the first to suggest that the 2-hr value alone after an oral glucose load was sufficient, and that the intervening values were unhelpful. It suggested 130 mg/dL for venous whole blood—independent of the size of the glucose load. It also introduced the category of "borderline diabetes"—the forerunner of IGT. Also it was the first one to suggest that people should be carbohydrate loaded for at least 3 days before the OGTT—an advice that still holds today, but to which adherence is rare. But despite the efforts, there was little standardization of testing.

In 1979, the NDDG in the USA, and in 1980, the second WHO Expert Committee set the thresholds for the venous fasting plasma glucose at 140 mg/dL (7.8 mmol/L) and 144 mg/dL (8.0 mmol/L) respectively.[3,4] It was agreed that only a 75 g oral glucose (anhydrous) should be used for the OGTT, and in children, a weight-related dose of 1.75 g/kg was recommended. The 2-hr post load thresholds for venous plasma glucose were 198 mg/dL (11.0 mmol/L) for WHO, and 200 mg/dL (11.1 mmol/L) for NDDG. These values were based on the bimodality in certain high prevalence populations like the Pima Indians. They also emphasized the need for two separate abnormal tests for diagnosing diabetes in an asymptomatic individual. However, a casual venous plasma glucose level of 200 mg/dL (11.1 mmol/L) or more in the presence of symptoms was sufficient to make the diagnosis. "Borderline diabetes" was replaced by IGT, which was defined as fasting glucose below the diagnostic value for diabetes, and the 2-hr value between 140 mg/dL and the threshold for diabetes.

In 1985, the WHO group met again and adjusted the fasting and 2-hr values to be consistent with the NDDG criteria.[5] Thus, universally, the fasting threshold was 140 mg/dL (7.8 mmol/l) and the 2-hr value 200 mg/dL (11.1 mmol/L).

Subsequently, in 1997 and 1999, an ADA Expert Committee[7] and a WHO Consultation[6] agreed that the threshold for the fasting plasma glucose was too high. They lowered it to 126 mg/dL (7 mmol/L), partly based on the cross-sectional relationship between the fasting plasma glucose and retinopathy. However, the 2-hr value remained unchanged. Impaired Fasting Glucose (IFG) was introduced as a new category to cover the levels of glucose that were not diagnostic of diabetes, but were clearly above normal, and carried an increased risk of subsequently developing diabetes. ADA recommended the use of FPG alone for the diagnosis of diabetes, but WHO did not support this view. This was because, even if the FPG is normal, a significant number of people will have diabetic values 2-hr after a glucose load. Thus, WHO recommended that if IFG is detected, a complete 75 g, 2-hr OGTT should be done; except in epidemiological studies, where OGTT may not be practicable.

In 2003, another ADA Expert Committee changed the lower threshold for the diagnosis of IFG to 100 mg/dL (5.6 mmol/L). The range for IFG now became 100 mg/dL to 125 mg/dL (5.6 mmol/L to 6.9 mmol/L).[11]

Current Diagnostic Criteria

The diagnostic criteria were further considered by both ADA and WHO in 2010.[1,12] Only the venous plasma glucose values should be used for definitive diagnosis, as all the evidence on which the diagnostic thresholds are based is for the venous plasma glucose. The plasma glucose criteria remain the same for diagnosis (Table 2).

Table 2: Current diagnostic criteria of diabetes mellitus[1,12]

Type of diabetes	*Glucose mm/dL*			
	Whole blood		*Plasma*	
	Venous	*Capillary*	*Venous*	*Capillary*
Diabetes mellitus				
a. Fasting	≥120	≥120	≥140	≥140
b. 2 hours after glucose load	≥180	≥200	≥200	≥200
Impaired glucose tolerance test				
a. Fasting	<120	<140	<140	<140
b. 2 hours after glucose load	120–180	140–180	140–180	140–180

Diabetes Mellitus

- Fasting plasma glucose level of ≥126 mg/dL (7 mmol/L)
- 2-hr post glucose load plasma glucose of ≥200 mg/dL (11.1 mmol/L).

Impaired Glucose Tolerance

- Fasting plasma glucose level of <100 mg/dL
- 2-hr post glucose load plasma glucose of ≥140 mg/dL (7.8 mmol/L) to <200 mg/dL.

Impaired Fasting Glucose

- Fasting plasma glucose level of ≥100 mg/dL (5.6 mmol/L) to <126 mg/dL (7 mmol/L)
- 2-hr post glucose load plasma glucose of <140 mg/dL (7.8 mmol/L).

Due to the day-to-day variability of blood glucose measurements, it is important that the diagnosis of diabetes be made only when two abnormal values have been found on separate days—except in the presence of symptoms and signs. The ADA continues to use fasting glucose alone as a definitive diagnostic test, while the WHO advocates the OGTT if IFG is present. However, the WHO accepts the use of fasting plasma glucose as a screening test.

Use of HbA1c as a Diagnostic Test for Diabetes

In 2010, the ADA accepted the use of HbA1c for the diagnosis of diabetes.[12] The A1C test should be performed using a method that is certified by the National Glycohemoglobin Standardization Program and standardized or traceable to the Diabetes Control and Complications Trial reference assay. Epidemiological data show a similar relationship of A1C with the risk of retinopathy as seen with FPG and 2-hr post glucose. The A1C has several advantages to the FPG and OGTT, including stability, low assay variability, reproducibility day to day, convenience (in that no special preparation of the patient is needed and it can be done any time of the day), the sample is stable at room temperature, and it is not affected by acute illness. It also reflects a period of hyperglycemia, rather than just a single point of time. The disadvantages are the cost, lack of availability worldwide, lack of standardization in many places, and problems in countries where there is a high prevalence of hemoglobinopathies or high red cell turnover rates.

A cut off HbA1c of 6.5% (48 mmol/mol) or more is used for the diagnosis of diabetes. In addition, the range of 5.7% (39 mmol/mol) to 6.4% (46 mmol/mol) is considered as a high risk range—equivalent to IFG and IGT. National Health and Nutrition Examination Survey data indicate that the A1C cut point of ≥6.5% identifies one-third fewer cases of undiagnosed diabetes than a fasting glucose cut point of ≥126 mg/dL (7.0 mmol/L).[13] Numerous studies have confirmed that, at these cut points, the 2-hr OGTT value diagnoses more screened people with diabetes.[14] In reality, a large portion of the diabetic population remains undiagnosed. Of note, the lower sensitivity of A1C at the designated cut point may be offset by the test's ability to facilitate the diagnosis (Table 3).

Table 3: Cost and sensitivity of screening method in diabetes[7]

Diabetes type	*Method*	*Specificity*	*Sensitivity*	*Cost*
NIDDM	Glycated HbA_{10} or proteins	+++	+/-	+++
	Urine glucose	+/-	+/-	+
	Casual blood glucose	++	+	+
	Fasting blood glucose	+++	+	+
	Oral glucose tolerance test	+++	++	++
IDDM	HLA type	+/-		+++
	ICA	+	+	+++
	Anti-GAD	+	+	+++
	Early insulin secretion	+/-	+	++

Abbreviations: NIDDM, noninsulin dependent diabetes mellitus; IDDM insulin dependent diabetes mellitus; HLA, human leukocyte antigen; ICA, islet cell antibodies; GAD, glutamic acid decarboxylase.

Diagnosis of Gestational Diabetes Mellitus

Gestational diabetes mellitus has been defined as any degree of glucose intolerance with onset or first recognition during pregnancy. Over the years, various diagnostic criteria with different cutoffs have been used for the diagnosis of GDM. The WHO recommended the 75-g OGTT for the diagnosis of GDM (Box 2).[15] The cut offs used were: fasting plasma glucose 126 mg/dL, and a 2-hr plasma glucose 140 mg/dL.

Box 2: Diagnosis of gestational diabetes mellitus

First prenatal visit:

- Measure FPG (Fasting plasma glucose), A1C, or random plasma glucose on all or only high risk women[#]
- If results indicate overt diabetes, treatment and follow-up as for pre-existing diabetes*
- If results not diagnostic of overt diabetes and FPG ≥5.1 mmol/L (92 mg/dL) but ≤7 mmol/L (126 mg/dL), diagnosed as gestational diabetes mellitus (GDM); and FPG ≤5.1 mmol/L (92 mg/dL), test for GDM from 24 weeks to 28 weeks gestation with a 75 g oral glucose tolerance test (OGTT)**
- 24–28 weeks gestation: Diagnosis of GDM
- 2-hr 75-g OGTT: Perform after overnight fast on all women not previously found overt diabetes or GDM during testing earlier in this pregnancy
- Overt diabetes, if FPG ≥7 mmol/L (126 mg/dL)
- GDM, if one or more values equal(s) or exceed(s) thresholds [FPG >92 mg/dL (5.1 mmol/L), 1-hr post glucose >180 mg/dL (10.0 mmol/L), 2-hr post glucose >153 mg/dL (8.5 mmol/L)]
- Normal, if all values on OGTT less than thresholds

Decision to perform for evaluation of glycemia on all pregnant women or only on women with characteristics indicating a high risk for diabetes is to be made on the basis of the background frequency of abnormal glucose metabolism in the population and on local circumstances.

* To be applied to women without known diabetes antedating pregnancy. Postpartum glucose testing should be performed for all women diagnosed with overt diabetes during pregnancy or GDM.

** The panel concluded that there have been insufficient studies performed to know whether there is a benefit of generalized testing to diagnosis and treat GDM before the usual window of 24–28 weeks gestation.

International Association of Diabetes and Pregnancy Study Groups (IADPSG) reviewed published results of the Hyperglycemia and Adverse Pregnancy Outcomes (HAPO) study, additional unpublished HAPO study findings, and the results of other works that examined associations of maternal glycemia with perinatal and long-term outcomes in offspring.[16] They then recommended the following steps given in Box 3.[16]

In 2011, the ADA Professional Practice Committee recommended the use of the IADPSG criteria for the diagnosis of GDM.[17] However, in 2014, the ADA recommends that GDM screening can be accomplished with either of two strategies: the "one-step" 2-hr 75-g OGTT or the "two-step" approach with a 1-hr 50-g (nonfasting) screen followed by a 3-hr 100-g OGTT for those who screen positive (Box 3):

Box 3: Strategy for the detection and diagnosis of hyperglycemic disorders in pregnancy (IADPSG)[10]

- "One-step" (IADPSG consensus): Perform a 75-g OGTT, with plasma glucose measurement fasting and at 1 and 2 hr, at 24–28 weeks of gestation in women not previously diagnosed with overt diabetes. The OGTT should be performed in the morning after an overnight fast of at least 8 hr. The diagnosis of GDM is made when any of the following plasma glucose values are exceeded:
  - Fasting: ≥92 mg/dL (5.1 mmol/L)
  - 1 hr: ≥180 mg/dL (10.0 mmol/L)
  - 2 hr: ≥153 mg/dL (8.5 mmol/L)
- "Two-step" (National Institutes of Health consensus): Perform a 50-g glucose loading test (nonfasting), with plasma glucose measurement at 1 hr (Step 1), at 24–28 weeks of gestation in women not previously diagnosed with overt diabetes. If the plasma glucose level measured 1 hr after the load is ≥140 mg/dL* (10.0 mmol/L), proceed to 100-g OGTT (Step 2). The 100-g OGTT should be performed when the patient is fasting.

The diagnosis of GDM is made when the plasma glucose level measured 3 hr after the test is ≥140 mg/dL (7.8 mmol/L).

*The American College of Obstetricians and Gynecologists recommends a lower threshold of 135 mg/dL in high-risk ethnic minorities with higher prevalence of GDM.

The Diabetes in Pregnancy Study Group India (DIPSI) reported practice guidelines for GDM in the Indian environment.[18] They recommend that due to high prevalence, screening is essential for all Indian pregnant women. As a pregnant woman walks into the antenatal clinic in the fasting state, she has to be given a 75 g oral glucose load without regard to the time of the last meal and at 2 hrs a venous blood sample is to be collected for estimating plasma glucose. GDM is diagnosed, if 2-hr plasma glucose is >140 mg/dL.

CONCLUSION

The diagnosis of diabetes should be made with certainty and caution. This is because once diagnosed, an individual is labeled to be having this chronic ailment for a lifetime. The management of diabetes requires continuous care on part of the patient, his family and care givers. Defining/classifying the type of diabetes is also important as it affects the management and prognosis. Diagnosing diabetes in a symptomatic individual is not difficult. However, in an asymptomatic patient with moderate hyperglycemia, a second confirmatory test is essential.

REFERENCES

1. World Health Organization. Consultation on the definition, diagnosis and classification of diabetes mellitus. Geneva: World Health Organization; 2011.
2. World Health Organization. Diabetes Mellitus. Report of a WHO Expert Committee. Geneva, 24–30 November 1964. World Health Organization Technical Report Series No. 310. Geneva: World Health Organization; 1965.
3. National Diabetes Data Group. Classification and diagnosis of diabetes mellitus and other categories of glucose intolerance. Diabetes. 1979;28(12):1039-57.
4. World Health Organization. WHO Expert Committee on Diabetes Mellitus. Second Report. Geneva, 26 September–1 October 1979. World Health Organization Technical Report Series No. 646. Geneva: World Health Organization; 1980.
5. World Health Organization. Diabetes Mellitus: Report of a WHO Study Group. Geneva, 11–16 February 1985. World Health Organization Technical Report Series 727. Geneva, World Health Organization; 1985.
6. World Health Organization. Report of a WHO Consultation. Definition, diagnosis, and classification of diabetes mellitus and its complications. 1. Diagnosis and classification of diabetes mellitus. WHO/NCD/NCS/99.2. Geneva: World Health Organization; 1999.
7. Expert Committee on the Diagnosis and Classification of Diabetes Mellitus. Report of the Expert Committee on the Diagnosis and Classification of Diabetes Mellitus. Diabetes Care. 1997;20(7):1183-97.
8. Kuzuya T, Matsuda A. Classification of diabetes on the basis of aetiologies versus degree of insulin deficiency. Diabetes Care. 1997;20:219-20.
9. World Health Organization and International Diabetes Federation Technical Advisory Group. Definition and diagnosis of diabetes mellitus and intermediate hyperglycemia. Report of a World Health Organization/International Diabetes Federation Consultation. Geneva: World Health Organization; 2006.
10. American Diabetes Association. Diagnosis and classification of diabetes mellitus. Diabetes Care. 2014;37(Suppl.1):S81-90.
11. The Expert Committee on the Diagnosis and Classification of Diabetes Mellitus. Follow up report on the diagnosis of diabetes mellitus. Diabetes Care. 2003;26(11):3160-7.
12. American Diabetes Association. Diagnosis and classification of diabetes mellitus. Diabetes Care. 2010;33(Suppl.1):S62-9.
13. Cowie CC, Rust KF, Byrd-Holt DD, et al. Prevalence of diabetes and high risk for diabetes using A1C criteria in the U.S. population in 1988–2006. Diabetes Care. 2010;33(3):562-8.
14. Picón MJ, Murri M, Muñoz A, et al. Hemoglobin A1c versus oral glucose tolerance test in postpartum diabetes screening. Diabetes Care. 2012;35(8):1648-53.
15. Alberti KG, Zimmet PZ. Definition, diagnosis and classification of diabetes mellitus and its complications. Part 1: diagnosis and classification of diabetes mellitus provisional report of a WHO consultation. Diabet Med. 1998;15(7):539-53.

16. Metzger BE, Gabbe SG, Persson B, et al; International Association of Diabetes and Pregnancy Study Groups Consensus Panel. International Association of Diabetes and Pregnancy Study Groups recommendations on the diagnosis and classification of hyperglycemia in pregnancy. Diabetes Care. 2010;33(3):676-82.
17. American Diabetes Association. Diagnosis and classification of diabetes mellitus. 2011;34 (Suppl 1): S62-9.
18. Seshiah V, Das AK, Balaji V, et al. Gestational diabetes mellitus--guidelines. J Assoc Physicians India. 2006;54:622-8.

7

CHAPTER

Management of Type 1 Diabetes

Jamal Ahmad

INTRODUCTION

Diabetes mellitus is one of the most common endocrine and metabolic diseases of childhood. Type 1 diabetes is a chronic autoimmune disease in the vast majority and accounts for over 90% of childhood and adolescent diabetes. It results from the destruction of the glucose responsive insulin-secreting beta cells of the pancreatic islets. In general, beta-cell damage is immune mediated and other clinical features occur related to other autoimmune processes. Its principal clinical features reflect significant insulin deficiency. It is likely that the clinical symptoms only manifest when 90% or more of the beta cells are lost. The effects of insulin deficiency are further enhanced at the time of insulin resistance such as infections or illness and stress. This may explain the link between clinical onset of type 1 diabetes and acute stresses.

Till recently diabetes in children (defined as onset below 12 years) and adolescents (defined as onset between 12 and 19 years) was almost exclusively type 1 diabetes, but this has changed, as there is increased recognition of a number of different forms of non-type 1 diabetes in the young. This includes type 2 diabetes, maturity onset diabetes of young, fibrocalculous pancreatic diabetes and diabetes due to genetic disorders. Fifty percent of individuals with type 1 diabetes are diagnosed before the age of 16 years. The rate of beta-cell loss in type 1 diabetes is highly variable. It is probable that type 1 diabetes presenting in prepubertal childhood may reflect a more aggressive destructive process, while, at the other extreme, type 1 diabetes present in adult life with a slow evolution to an absolute need for insulin replacement. The later is called as "latent adult onset diabetes" (LADA), and confounds the clinical definition of type 1 diabetes.

The diagnosis of type 1A diabetes may be made by finding evidence of autoimmunity [the presence of anti-islets-cell antibodies-antiglutamic acid decarboxylase (GAD), anti-islet-associated protein 2 (IA-2) antibodies in the blood]. Absence of such antibodies does not mean the diagnosis is not type 1, as the antibodies tends to disappear but their presence is usual in type 1 diabetes where there is at least some residual insulin-secretory capacity. However, there is recognition that type 1 diabetes may be heterogenous, as in some patients, evidence of autoimmunity is lacking (type 1 B).

EPIDEMIOLOGY

Epidemiological incidence studies define the onset of type 1 diabetes by the date of first insulin injection because of the variable time between the onset of symptoms and diagnosis shows an annual incidence rates for childhood type 1 diabetes (0–14 years age group) comparing different countries of the world.[1] Type 1 diabetes is a disorder that arises following the autoimmune destruction of insulin producing pancreatic beta cells. The disease is most often diagnosed in children and adolescents, usually presenting with a classic triad of symptoms, i.e. polydypsia, polyphasia, polyuria and with severe hyperglycemia, necessitating the need for exogenous insulin replacement on a lifelong basis. Type 1 diabetes probably accounts for 50% of all diagnosed cases of diabetes. About 40–60% of persons with type 1 diabetes are younger than 20 years of age at onset. The worldwide prevalence of type 1 diabetes is 0.1–0.3% with 78,000 new cases every year, especially among young individuals (<5 years). Some 79,100 children under 15 years are estimated to develop type 1 diabetes annually worldwide.[2] According to the reports of SEARCH group,[3] the incidence of type 1 diabetes peaks around the age of 10 years and is highest among non-Hispanic Whites followed by non-Hispanic Blacks, Hispanics, Asia and Pacific Islanders and American Indian/Alaskan Natives. The South-East-Asia Region (SEAR) has a high prevalence of type 1 diabetes in children, with an estimated 77,900 children affected. In 2013, alone an estimated 12,600 children under the age of 15 in SEAR developed type 1 diabetes.[2]

India accounts for most of the children with type 1 diabetes in the SEAR and its incidence rate was frequently used in extrapolation for other countries in the region, and therefore, the estimates in India are of great significance. In the 1990s, Menon et al.[4] reported the prevalence that ranged from 0.8% to 3.61% during the period from 1964–1989. In a population-based study conducted in South India for a period of 1991–1994, the incidence for the 4 year period was 10.5/100,000/year (CI 5.0) for children up to 15 years of age.[5] Similarly a study from Karnal district in 2008, showed a prevalence of 18.3/100,000 in the 0–14 years of age group.[6] Clinic-based data show that more than 60% of type 1 diabetes patients registered were childhood and adolescent onset type 1 diabetic patients.

ETIOLOGY AND PATHOGENESIS OF TYPE 1 DIABETES

The prevalence of type 1 diabetes is unknown but there are number of possible contributory factors and some of them are discussed below:

Genetic Factors

Type 1 diabetes is a chronic T-cell mediated disease in which there is selective autoimmune destruction of beta cells of the pancreas. Type 1 diabetes occurs as a result of complex interactions between multiple genes[7-9] and environmental influences, which may both promote and protect against disease. The disease clusters in some families, but with no distinct pattern of inheritance. The concordance rates in monozygotic twins for type 1 diabetes can reach 50% compared to 6% for dizygotic twins. The sibling recurrence risk ratio (risk to siblings + risk to general population value for type 1 diabetes) value for type 1 diabetes is 15 (6.0 + 0.4 or 6% to 0.4%), and twin studies suggest that 80–85% of familial aggregation is accounted for by genes (Table 1). Type 1 diabetes has been noted to coexist with other autoimmune diseases—notably, Graves' disease and coeliac disease—in certain families, implying the involvement of common autoimmune pathways.

Table 1: Approximately frequency of islet autoantibodies (Ab+) and development of diabetes mellitus for initially nondiabetic relatives

Relationship	*% DM*	*%Ab+ (GAD), 512, or Insulin*	*Comments*
Monozygotic twin	50%	50%	Almost all Ab+ progress to DM
Dizygotic twin	6%	10%	Risk similar to sibling
Sibling	3.2%	7.4%	—
Offspring father	4.6%	6.5%	Diabetes risk greater than offspring of diabetic mother
Offspring mother	3%	5%	Lower risk relative to offspring of diabetic father
Parent	1%	4.1%	Many parents with single Ab+
DR3/4, DQ8 sibling	>25%	>50%	Highest risk for non-twin relatives

Abbreviations: DM, diabetes mellitus; GAD, glutamic acid decarboxylase.
Source: Adapted from In: C Ronald Kahn, Gordon Weir, George King, Alan Jacobson, Robert Smith, Alan Moses (Eds). Joslin's Diabetes Mellitus, 14th edition, Chapter 42. Philadelphia: Lippincott Williams & Wilkins. pp. 729.

Improved understanding of the "allelic structure" and biological pathways involved in type 1 diabetes is expected to facilitate the identification of new therapeutic targets for the development of new treatments. DNA biomarkers could also assist the risk production at a population level. This is clinically relevant since individuals can survive with only 20% intact beta-cell mass and the time to reach this level of destruction can be delayed in some individuals.

Genes belonging to the human leukocyte antigen (HLA) system on chromosome constitute the most important risk factor.[10,11] The chromosomal locations of these "diabetes genes are called inherited susceptibility loci. There are now at least 18-insulin-dependent diabetes mellitus susceptible loci (IDDM1 to IDDM18).[12] HLA make up the human major histocompatibility complex (MHC), which presents antigens to immune system, but now more than 40 additional loci are known to significantly affect type 1 diabetes risk.

Identifying Susceptibility Genes in Type 1 Diabetes

The indirect association studies generally exploit linkage disequilibrium, i.e. nonrandom association of alleles, between single nucleotide polymorphisms (SNPs) to assist in the identification of casual gene variants. These were aimed to determine if the frequencies of gene variants, usually SNPs, in plausible biological candidate were significantly over represented or under-represented in cases with type 1 diabetes versus unaffected healthy controls. In contrast, direct association studies involve the screening of potentially functional SNPs for association. In addition, family-based association studies have also been used, which can implement case-controlled studies. The transmission disequilibrium test is the most popular family-based method and employs parent-offspring trios. The test assesses distortion in transmission frequency from the expected 50:50 transmission of a gene variant from heterozygous parents to an affected offspring across a large number of families, and, unlike case-control studies, is not subjected to potential bias caused by population stratification.

Recently genome wide association studies (GWAS) have been used to identify genome loci associated type 1 diabetes. In contrast to the traditional methods of using a candidate gene approach, GWAS scans the whole genome for SNPs that occur more frequently in people suffering from type 1 diabetes. The associated SNPs that are used to mark the susceptibility loci. By using the SNP typing technology, a number of additional susceptibility loci were discovered from type 1 diabetes namely: CLEC16A, CHQTNFα, UBASH 3A, CD226, PTPN2,CTSH, SH2B3, ERBBB, PRKCQ, TAGAP, interleukin (IL)-2RA, TNFA1P3, BACH2, IL-7R, IL-2, CCRS, IFIHI, IL-IRAP, RGSI, IL-10, IL-19, IL-20, GLIS3, CD69 and IL-27.[13-15]

More than 30 years ago, the biological candidate gene approach revealed strong associations between type 1 diabetes and allelic variants at the HLA loci on chromosome 6p21. Linkage studies have also consistently demonstrated linkage to HLA region in type 1 diabetes.16,17 The association studies in European populations have demonstrated significant risk to type 1 diabetes at the HLA-DQB1 locus. Increased susceptibility is observed for the DQBI*-O3-O2 and DQBI020 alleles whereas DQBI0602 is dominantly protective. The greater risk of type 1 diabetes occurs in those individuals who are heterozygous for DRBI*04-DQBI* 0302/DRBI* 03DQBI*0201, and the risk is even greater in sibling has type 1 diabetes. Recently studies under the direction of the type 1 diabetes Genetics Consortium (https://www.t1dgc.org/home) have identified susceptibility and protective DR-DQ haplotypes for type 1 diabetes.

Genetic association studies have largely replaced linkage studies, since association studies have greater power to detect common alleles with modest effect on risk. Furthermore, linked genomic intervals may be quite large and, potentially, contain hundreds of genes, whereas, in genomic association studies, linkage disequilibrium generally extends only up to hundreds of kilobases.

Viral Infections and Toxins

Epidemics of enteroviral infections in the autumn and winter months are associated with an increase in the incidence of type 1 diabetes. Several viruses (e.g. Coxsackie B, enteroviruses, rubella, mumps and cytomegalovirus) have been implicated in the etiology of type 1 diabetes. Also, T cells target the envelope proteins (VP1, VP2 and VP3) of Coxsackievirus B4, but the T cell proliferative response was reduced markedly in type 1 diabetic patients compared with control subjects, which eventually results in destruction of beta cells. Ingestion of the rodenticide Vacor is also known to be associated with development of type 1 diabetes.

Environmental Factors

Exposure to antigenic substances early in life is thought to contribute to type 1 diabetes. Undissolved gluten causes subclinical inflammation of intestinal mucosa, which raises the proportion of aggressive T cells. The functional state of beta cells also plays a role in the pathogenesis of type 1 diabetes, and food intake with a high glycemic index increases the insulin demand and forces the beta cell to produce more insulin, which accelerates its destruction.

Nutrition and Dietary Factors

Breastfeeding appears to provide protection against the risk of developing type 1 diabetes. The benefits have been attributed to bioactive substances, which promote the maturation of the immune system, reduce insulin resistance and prevent excessive weight gain during childhood. Early introduction of cow's milk appears to be a risk factor for the development of type 1 diabetes. Some of the patients of type 1 diabetes have IgG antibodies to bovine serum albumin, a protein in the cow's milk with similarities to the islet cell antigen. This protein may stimulate autoantibody production leading to islet cell destruction as a result of molecular mimicry.

C-peptide Assay for Assessment of Pancreatic Beta-cell Reserve

At the time of diagnosis of type 1 diabetes, 80–90% of pancreatic beta cells are destroyed. C-peptide determination has gained lot of interest and is used to understand the course of type 1 diabetes. Very young children especially those with onset after infections tend to have loss C-peptide. The heterogeneity of diabetes at clinical onset along with the increasing incidence in children and adolescent makes it if interest to test of C-Peptide may improve the classification of newly diagnosed children. Kartz et al.[18] reported testing c-peptide levels of 0.38±0.37 ng/mL can distinguish type 1 diabetes from type 2 diabetes with 83%.

Immune-mediated Destruction of Pancreatic Beta Cells

Type 1 diabetes is an immune-mediated organ specific disease. The disease is induced by an environmental event or events operating in a genetically susceptible individual. Many genes are implicated in the genetic susceptibility of type 1 diabetes as discussed above, the most important are in the HLA region of chromosome 6. The risk of developing childhood onset type 1 diabetes is about 1:400 in the general population but 1:2 in an identical twin of a young diabetic twin, 1:10 in an identical twin of an adult diabetic twin, and 1:17 in a sibling of a subject with type 1 diabetes; the risk is only 1:5 if the sibling is HLA-identical to the effected sibling. The risk of developing diabetes by age of 20 years is greater with a type 1 diabetic father (8%) then with a type 1 diabetic mother (2%).

Whatever the nature of the environmental effect, the interaction of environmental and genetic factors at different stages leads to induction of immune changes, including the activation of T lymphocytes and B lymphocytes, with the latter producing autoantibodies. The destructive immune response targets the pancreatic islets and the destruction can be mediated directly by cellular processes or indirectly through the release of cytokines and chemokines.

The younger is the onset of the disease, the more severe is the destructive immune process. Several autoantibodies have been identified in newly diagnosed cases of type 1 diabetes. Currently, four major antibodies namely, the 65 kDa form of glutamic acid decarboxylase (GAD65), insulinoma antigen 2 (IA 2), insulin autoantibodies (IAA) and zinc transporter 8 (Zn T8) have been shown to be found in type 1 diabetes and approximately 94% of all type 1 diabetes patients have at least one of these antibodies at clinical onset.[19] Monitoring these autoantibodies is currently the most reliable biomarker in the prodromal phase of type 1 diabetes since their appearance typically precedes overt type 1 diabetes onset for years or even decades.[20] The prevalence of multiple types of autoantibodies identifies individuals with the highest risk of progression to clinical disease in those in the prediabetes stage of type 1 diabetes (Fig. 1).

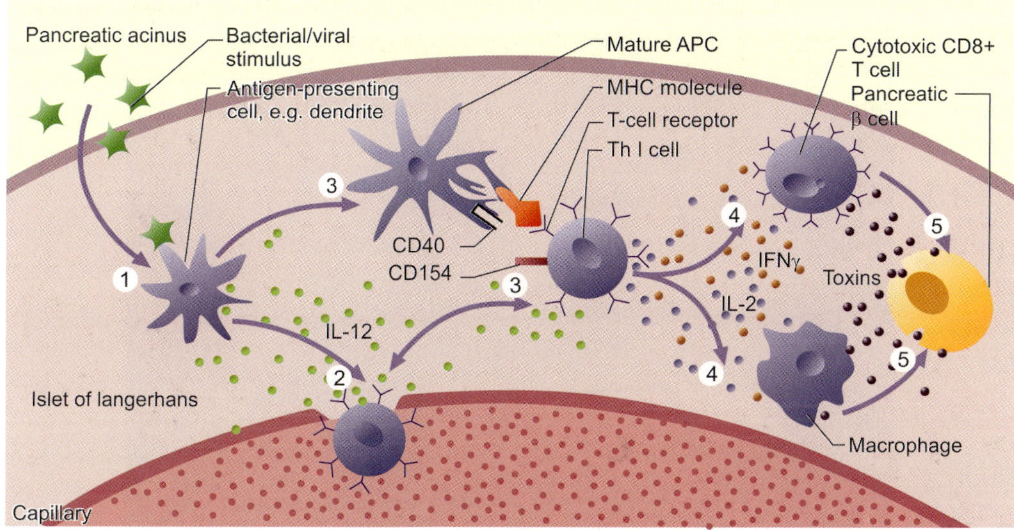

Fig. 1: Immune-mediated destruction of β-cells. Upon activation (1), antigen-presenting cells (APCs), such as dendritic cells, produce interleukin (IL)-2 cytokines that stimulates the production of Th1 lymphocytes (2). T cell receptor (TCR) and CD154 molecules on the surface of the Th1 cell bind to the MHC and CD40 molecules on the surface of the APC (3). The lymphocytes also produce large amount of interferon-gamma (IFN-γ) which, together with IL-2 cytokines, induces macrophages to become cytotoxic, and also stimulates cytotoxic CD8=+ cells (4). Both of these release mediators that are toxic to pancreatic islet cells (5).

Abbreviation: MHC: Major Histocompatibility complex.

Source: Adapted from Diabetes Clinician's Desk Reference, special Pharma edition 2014. CRC Press Taylor & Francis Group: Boca Raton; 2014. pp. 39.

The Pathogenesis of Type 1 Diabetes

There is a continuous spectrum of loss of insulin secretory capacity associated with autoimmune diabetes.

Stage 1: There must be some form of "original sin" in relation to allowing T-lymphocytes with the potential to recognize beta-cell autoantigens to emerge from the thymus. This allows the peripheral immune system to be populated from birth with adaptive immune cells with the capability of attacking beta cells. The HLA genes that confer disease susceptibility could operate through ineffective thymus function.

Stage 2: It requires a focus of islet inflammation that involves damage to beta cells. Beta cell autoantigens are released and taken up by tissue resident dendritic cells that are induced to mature by inflammatory stimuli that pertain. Dendritic cells migrate to the pancreatic lymph nodes and in the presence of incomplete thymic tolerance, presentation of islets proteins to naïve beta cell-specific CD4 and CD-8 lymphocytes with relevant T-cell receptor ensues.

Stage 3: There is a relative imbalance in immune regulation that allows the beta cell specific T lymphocytes to undergo activation and maturation to a proinflammatory phenotype. It is likely that genes that are relevant could subtly lower the threshold at which autoreactive T-lymphocyte activation takes place, or they could negatively influence pathways of immune regulation.

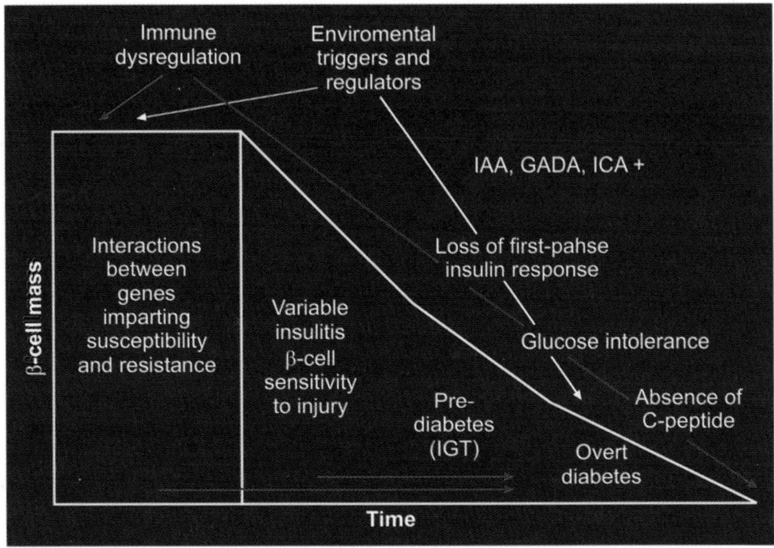

Fig. 2: Pathogenesis of type 1 diabetes

Abbreviations: IAA: Insulin autoantibodies; GADA, Glutamic acid decarboxylase antibodies; ICA, Islet cell antibodies; IGT, Impaired glucose tolerance.

Source: Adapted from Lancet. 2001;258:221.

Stage 4: In this stage, the migration of autoreactive T-lymphocytes to the inflamed islets occurs, leading to perpetuation of the inflammation and further damage to beta cells in a highly targeted fashion. The autoantibodies may contribute to the inflammatory process via immune complex formation and islets becomes devoid of beta cells.

Stage 5: The inflammatory process becomes chronic, perhaps with a lapsing and remitting rhythm. It could be speculated that the relapses and remissions are now being influenced by events irrelevant to the original insult, and, again virus infections may play a role. Beta-cell destruction spreads through lobules until the full metabolic disease emerges (Fig. 2).

PHASES OF TYPE 1 DIABETES

Type 1 diabetes is characterized by:

- Preclinical diabetes
- Presentation of diabetes
- Partial remission or honeymoon phase
- Chronic phase of life-long dependency on administered insulin.

RECOMMENDED CARE

Preclinical Diabetes

It refers to the months or years preceding the clinician presentation of type 1 diabetes when islets antibodies can be detected as markers of beta cell autoimmunity. In addition to this, the

risk of type 1 diabetes can further be determined by genetic markers. The parameters currently helping to define the preclinical phase include:
- Islets cell autoantibodies
- Glutamic acid decarboxylase autoantibodies (65 kDa GAD isoform)
- IA2 (also known as ICA 512 or tyrosine phosphatase) autoantibodies
- Insulin autoantibodies
- HLA typing.

Risks of Progression to Diabetes

- HLA-DR3-DQAI*0501-DQBI*0201 (susceptible genotype)
- HLA DR4-DQAI*0301-DQBI*0302 (susceptible genotype)
- HLADR2-DQAI*0102-DQBI*0602 (protective genotype)

Islets autoimmunity can be transient and one raised islet antibody alone has little prognostic value. If an individual is under 45 years and does not have HLADR2-DQAI*0102-DQBI*0602 then:
1. Impaired first phase insulin release on intravenous glucose tolerance testing confers a 60% risk over the next 5 years
2. Two or more islets antibodies raised without impaired first phase insulin release confers a 25–50% risk over the next 5 years. Neither screening of any population nor intervention in the preclinical phase should occur outside the context of defined clinical studies.

Presentation of Type 1 Diabetes

- Clinical presentation of diabetes can vary from nonemergency presentations (e.g. polyuria, polydipsia, weight loss and enuresis) to severe dehydration, shock and diabetic ketoacidosis.
- Prospective follow-up of high risk subjects shows that diagnosis of type 1 diabetes can be made in asymptomatic individuals in majority of the cases.
- Some individuals have a rapid onset of symptoms and present within days in diabetic ketoacidosis; other have a slow onset over several months.
- A blood glucose measurement (plasma glucose ≥200 mg/dL confirms the diagnosis. The blood glucose measurement should be laboratory estimation rather than a home glucose monitor or bed side reading. Hands should be washed since glucose from sweets or fruit can give a false reading.

Nonemergency Presentations

- Recent onset of enuresis in a previously toilet-trained child, which may be misdiagnosed as a urinary tract infection or the result of excessive fluid ingestion.
- Vaginal candidiasis, especially in prepubertal girls
- Chronic weight loss or failure to gain weight in a growing child
- Irritability or decreasing school performance
- Recurrent skin infections.

Emergency Presentations

- Severe dehydration

- Frequent vomiting
- Continuing polyuria despite the presence of dehydration
- Weight loss due to fluid loss and loss of muscle and fat
- Vomiting and abdominal pain, which may be misdiagnosed as gastroenteritis
- Flushed cheeks due to ketoacidosis
- Acetone detected in breath
- Hyperventilation of diabetic ketoacidosis (Kussmaul Respiration) is characterized by a high respiratory rate and large tidal volume of each breath which gives it a sighing quality
- Disordered sensorium (disoriented, semicomatose or rarely comatose)
- Decreased peripheral circulation with rapid pulse rate
- Hypotension or shock with peripheral cyanosis (a late sign and rare in children with diabetic ketoacidosis).

Diagnostic Difficulties Leading to Late Diagnosis

- Very young children may present in severe ketoacidosis because of more rapid onset of severe insulin deficiency and because the diagnosis was not considered early.
- Hyperventilation of ketoacidosis may be misdiagnosed as pneumonia or asthma (cough and breathlessness distinguish these conditions from diabetic ketoacidosis).
- Abdominal pain associated with ketoacidosis may stimulate an acute abdomen.
- Polyuria and enuresis may be misdiagnosed as urinary tract infection.
- Polydipsia may be thought to be psychogenic.
- Vomiting may be diagnosed as gastroenteritis or sepsis.
- Severe ketoacidosis if untreated is fatal. Therapy is urgent and referral to specialized services is essential.

Partial Remission or Honeymoon Phase in Type 1 Diabetes

- In many children and adolescents, insulin requirements decrease transiently following initiation of insulin treatment. This has been strictly defined as insulin requirements of less than 0.5 units per kg of body weight per day with an HbA1c ≤7%.
- The partial remission phase commences within days or weeks of this start of insulin therapy and may last for weeks to months. During this phase, blood sugar levels remain fairly stable within the normal range, despite fluctuations in diet and exercise.
- Ketoacidosis at presentation and young age reduce the likelihood of a remission phase.
- The families to be advised of the transient nature of the partial remission phase. They should be advised that as the child comes out of this phase an increasing amount of insulin is needed.

Chronic Phase of Lifelong Dependence on Insulin

The progression from the partial remission phase into the chronic phase of lifelong dependence on insulin is usually a gradual decrease in residual beta function but may be accelerated by an intercurrent illness. At present, exogenous insulin replacement remains the only form of replacement therapy for children with type 1 diabetes.

MANAGEMENT OF TYPE 1 DIABETES

Almost 95 years after the discovery of insulin, people with type 1 diabetes still use subcutaneous insulin to manage their condition. Insulin treatment is mandatory and lifesaving. It relieves osmotic symptoms, reverses most of the pathophysiological changes within a few weeks of starting treatment. It also prevents early death from diabetic ketoacidosis. People with diabetes still die prematurely from long-term complications and the quality of most of the patients is shattered by poor vision, lower limb amputations, recurrent hypoglycemia and renal replacement therapy. The DCCT/EDIC trial in type 1 diabetes has clearly shown that tight glycemic control can delay or postpone both micro- and macrovascular complications, however, the limitation of current treatment prevent most of type 1 diabetic patients from achieving tight glycemic control. The recent progress in the treatment in the form of cell therapy or closed looped technology will help us in achieving tight glycemic control and improve quality of life.

Aims of Diabetes Management

The immediate aims of treatment are:

- To relieve the symptoms
- To restore the abnormal physiology as closely to normal as possible
- To prevent the onset of diabetic ketoacidosis
- Optimal psychosocial adjustment
- Normal growth and development
- An individualized plan of diabetes care incorporating the particular needs of a child or adolescent and the family.

In the long term, the main principle of treatment is to encourage patients to maintain sufficiently tight metabolic control without side effects to minimize the chances of developing the microvascular complications of diabetes. It is clearly the responsibility of healthcare team to try and ensure that each of the patients achieve the best possible level of metabolic control of which they are capable and which they wish to achieve. One should also keep in mind the limitations of current therapy and quality of life. Therefore, the glycemic targets will differ according to the overall aims of treatment for that particular individual, and setting them should incorporate the patient's own views.

The best approach for treatment of type 1 diabetes involves multiple daily insulin injections (regular insulin before each meal and intermediate/long-acting insulin twice a day or at bed time) which are medically recommended. This approach is helpful in achieving not only the flexibility in lifestyle but also in maintaining good glycemic control.

Hospital versus Ambulatory Stabilization

At diagnosis the decision should be made between hospital admission and ambulatory initiation of treatment. In appropriately chosen patients, there are no disadvantages of ambulatory management compared to inpatient management of children and adolescents who develop diabetes but are not dehydrated or acidosis may be successfully managed out of hospital if expert diabetes support teams are available.

Relative Contraindications to Ambulatory Initiation of Insulin Therapy include

- Very young age (under 2 years)
- Ketoacidosis
- Dehydration (moderate to severe)
- Profound grief reaction in the family
- Significant psychosocial/psychiatric problems in family
- Geographic isolation/lack of communication facilities.

The basic elements of type 1 diabetes management are:

- Insulin administration
- Nutrition management
- Physical activity
- Self-monitoring of blood glucose
- The avoidance of hypoglycemia.

INSULIN THERAPY

Insulin was discovered in 1921 and transformed the management of type 1 diabetes, until then a fatal disorder. Until the 1980s, insulin was obtained by extraction and purification from pancreas of cows and pigs (bovine and porcine insulins). Recombinant DNA technology enabled large-scale production of human insulin. More recently, the amino acid sequence of insulin has been altered to produce analogues of insulin, which differ in the rate of absorption from the site of injection.

The duration of action of short-acting, unmodified insulin ("soluble" or "regular" insulin), which is clear solution, can be extended by the addition of protamine and zinc at neutral pH [isophane or NPH (neutral protamine Hagedorn) insulin] or excess zinc ions (lente insulins). Those modified depot insulins are cloudy preparations. Premixed formulations containing short-acting and isophane insulin in various proportions are available. The pharmacokinetics of these various insulins is shown in Figure 3.

Rapid-acting Insulin

Insulin has a tendency to aggregate into dimers and hexamers which retard the absorption and biological availability. Therefore, human soluble insulin for therapeutic use has important limitations, largely due to the tendency of its single molecule to aggregate at high concentration into hexamers.

This property is presumably important to its physiological packaging as insulin granules within the beta cells, but, when prepared for therapeutic use, the aggregation slows the rate of absorption of insulin from subcutaneous depots into the blood stream. The relative delay in the action of soluble human insulin contributes to the immediate postprandial rise in blood glucose during treatment, and explains the desirability of injecting 30 minute or more before eating this properly has driven the development of insulin analogues, which have more favorable pharmacokinetics profiles following subcutaneous injections.

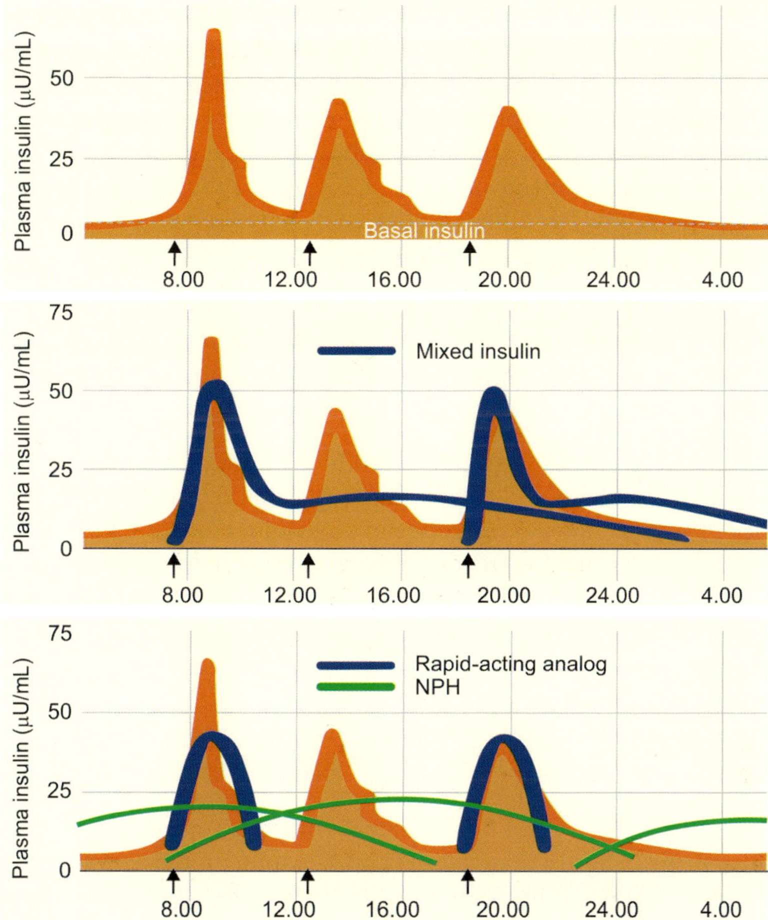

Fig. 3: Insulin regimens: The pattern of physiological basal-bolus insulin secretion (top), with peak action at mealtime (arrow), can be mimicked by therapy schedules. These can use both rapid-acting and long-acting [neutral protamine Hagedorn (NPH)] insulin or mixed (rapid/longer-acting) insulin or a single injection of long-acting insulin with rapid-acting insulin at mealtimes.
Source: Adapted from Diabetes Clinician's Desk Reference, special Pharma edition 2014. CRC Press Taylor & Francis Group: Boca Raton; 2014. p. 159.

Three rapid acting-insulin analogues have been developed, exploiting structural homology with insulin like growth factor (IGF-1), a hormone with less tendency to self-association. Insulin lispro is produced by substituting a proline with a lysine amino-acid residue; insulin aspart (switching a proline residue by aspartic acid). Insulin glulisine by exchange of asparagine and glutamic acid with two lysine residues. All three rapid-acting insulin analogues exhibit similar pharmacokinetic properties. They dissociate more readily than conventional human insulin, producing free insulin profiles following subcutaneous injections that are faster in onset, rise to a higher peak, and have shorter duration. This will match more closely to an endogenous meal insulin profile. HbA1c is slightly better and there are reductions in symptomatic night hypoglycemic.

Immediate-acting Insulin

The duration of action of insulin of human or animal structure can be prolonged by creating suspensions with either protamine (NPH insulins) or Zn (lente insulins). In recent years, NPH insulins have increasingly replaced lente preparations, as they can be combined with soluble insulin to create premixed biphasic insulin. Since the duration of action is generally up to 12–14 hours, they are best given twice a day (first thing in the morning and at bed time). The absorption profile has a marked peak at 6–8 hours, which can increase the risk of hypoglycemia, especially at night. Rate of absorption is also variable; thus a bolus may enter the blood stream at a relatively rapid rate on one day and then more slowly the next; variability calculated according to changes in fasting glucose values can be as high as 50%.

Long-acting Insulin Analogues

Long-acting insulin analogues have been developed in an attempt to replace basal insulin secretion more effectively. Insulin glargine is produced by adding two basic arginine amino-acid residues on to the β-chain and substituting a glycine for an asparagines residue on the alpha chain. These substitutions have produced an insulin that is suitable at a relatively acid pH, and then becomes crystalline at the more alkaline environment of the subcutaneous tissue. Insulin glargine has both a flatter insulin profile than NPH and a longer duration of action; in most individuals, this is around 18–20 hrs. One injection a day is thought to provide adequate basal insulin replacement for many individuals with type 1 diabetes, although others need glargine given twice a day.

Insulin detemir is manufactured by adding a myristic acid moiety to the β-chain of the human insulin molecule, increasing its affinity for albumin binding and delaying its absorption from subcutaneous tissue. This prolongs its duration of action to around 16–18 hrs; some individuals can replace basal insulin adequately with one injection a day, although many requires two. It appears to have a mare marked peak insulin profile and slightly less variability than insulin glargine in some individuals.

Insulin degludec (rDNA origin) is an ultra-long-acting basal insulin analogue, produced by coupling Des B30 threonine insulin to fatty acid side chain, developed by Novo Nordisk, under the brand name Tresiba, is available and administered by subcutaneous injection once daily (noninferiority with glargine). Daily administration of degludec has glucose-lowering benefits not different from glargine, with purportedly less hypoglycemia.

Biphasic or Premixed Insulins

There are numbers of biphasic or premixed insulins available that are usually given twice a day; before breakfast and before the evening meal. The biphasic insulin that is most widely consists of 25–30% quick-acting insulin (either human soluble or insulin analogue) with 70–75% NPH (neither long-acting insulin analogue) can be mixed with soluble insulin in the same syringe.

Combination of a Basal Insulin with an Ultra-long Duration of Action and a Mealtime Insulin

The first combination of a basal insulin with an ultra-long duration of action and a mealtime insulin is one pen (Ryzodeg) has been developed by Novo and is now available. 1 mL solution contains 100 units insulin degludec/insulin aspart in the ratio of 70/30. Ryzodeg can be administered once or twice daily with meal. There is no clinical experience with the use of Ryzodeg in pregnancy and in those who are breastfeeding.

STORAGE CONDITIONS

The following storage conditions should be recognized:

- Insulin is stable at room temperature for several weeks provided there are no extremes of temperature.
- Unused vials should be refrigerated (stored at 4–8°C) but never frozen.
- Insulin may lose its potency after opening the vial or when exposed to high temperatures.
- Insulin vials should be discarded after 3 months of opening if kept refrigerated and after 1 month at room temperature.
- Penfill cartridges and disposable insulin pen should be discarded after 21–28 days at room temperature. The manufacturer's expiry date should be adhered to.

INSULIN REGIMEN AND DELIVERY

The ultimate aim of insulin therapy is to provide physiological insulin replacement. However, commonly used insulins and delivery methods have approximated this very poorly. The availability of new (and future) insulin analogues and alternate delivery methods (insulin pumps) offers the potential more closely to approximate normal physiology in suitable subjects. The choice of insulin types and insulin regimen has to be guided by a variety of factors:

- Age of patient
- Lifestyle factor
- Patient and family preference and management skills
- Metabolic targets
- Duration of diabetes
- Experience of healthcare team
- Affordability and sustainability
- Association complications, including hypoglycemia.

Any insulin regimen has to be considered in the wider context of a total diabetes management packages, which must include dietary management, exercise, blood glucose monitoring, initial and ongoing education, regular medical follow-up, and psychological care.

Insulin Regimens

The insulin regimens need to aim to:

- Provide appropriate basal insulin requirements to cover the need across 24 hours.
- Provide sufficient insulin levels when needed to cover food intake.
- Have adequate provision for adjustment and correction when needed.
- Minimize blood glucose fluctuation and risk of hypoglycemia and hyperglycemia.
- Achieve short-term and long-term metabolic targets.
- Many regimens are in common use; children and adolescent will often evolve from one regimen to another in order to meet the goals of therapy.

One injection daily: Either intermediate-acting insulin or short/rapid-acting plus intermediate-acting insulin. Such a regimen is rarely appropriate for children and adolescent with type 1 diabetes.

Two injections daily: A mixture of short/rapid-acting and intermediate-acting insulin given before breakfast and before the main-evening meal. Historically it was common to initiate patient-administered subcutaneous insulin therapy as simply as possible, in terms of frequency of insulin injections, using twice-daily premix insulin, often at a starting dose of 10 units twice daily. This can work reasonably well, particularly in the early days, when the patients regain some residual endogenous insulin secretion after the control of the presenting hyperglycemia (the so called honeymoon phase).

The twice-daily mixed insulin regimen might be a combination of soluble insulin or a rapid-acting insulin analogue (aspart or lispro) together with an isophane. The relative proportion of the quick-acting and medium-acting insulin varies in different commercially available preparations, but the most common combination is 25–30% quick acting and 70–75% isophane. A range of premixed insulins containing other proportions, like 50:50 preparations are also available with this regimens, some units prefer to give two-thirds of the total dose in the morning and one-third in the evening.

While the above approach has the merit of apparent simplicity there are risks to starting individuals with type 1 diabetes on twice-daily premixed insulin. Such a regimen may control blood sugar reasonably tightly over the first few months, or even years, particularly of that person enters a strong "honeymoon phase" as the preserved endogenous insulin will smooth out the deficiencies in the exogenous regimen. However, once endogenous insulin secretion begins to decline, then twice-daily premixed insulin is, by its nature, inflexible, since adjusting the dose will affect both the quick-acting insulin and the long-acting component.

In a conventional twice-daily insulin regimen, the long-acting, the long-acting insulin component of the morning dose provides the insulin to cover the mid-day meal as well as the background requirement for the day time, but, clearly, longer-acting insulin will be unable to provide the rapid rise in insulin concentration needed to respond to eating. This can lead to marked increases in blood glucose immediately after the mid-day meal and during the early part of the afternoon. The evening dose of a twice-daily regimen is usually taken before evening meal, between 17:00 and 20:00, or later. For this injection, the 30% quick-acting component will increase insulin concentration to cover the evening meal, and the 70% longer-acting component is intended to provide background cover through night. However, the latter will have its greatest effect around 8–10 hrs after injection. This often translates into a clock-time of around 2:00 to 3:00, depending upon the dose, which can lead to nocturnal hypoglycemia. Because, the insulin action wanes thereafter, any regimen that administers a medium-acting insulin before a fairly early evening meal, are relatively ineffective in controlling the fasting (prebreakfast) blood glucose.

The other limitation of premixed insulin is another consequence of a formulation that covers both basal and meal requirements. This means that increasing the dose to deal with a larger meal, or reducing the insulin dose, when someone is not hungry, may cause the glucose to fall or rise at other times.

The limitations of premixed insulin may not be manifested in the early stages of type 1 diabetes, since continued secretion of endogenous insulin will mask their inflexibility, particularly in controlling blood glucose overnight. However, attempts to move patients from two injections a day to multiple doses, injecting four or five injections a day, are resisted for obvious reasons. Once individuals are used to twice-daily insulin, the suggestion to switch to an intensive five injections each day, splitting the meal and basal insulin in combination with frequent glucose monitoring, will not be treated enthusiastically.

The modern approach to insulin therapy in type 1 diabetes encourages active participation in diabetes self-management; this may be more acceptable if newly diagnosed individuals are encouraged to self-manage their diabetes actively from the day of diagnosis. The aim is to use insulin "physiologically" allowing the patients to maintain a flexible eating pattern, eating different amount at different times. If such an approach is planned, patients are initially started on quick-acting insulin before meals with background insulin added, if necessary, on the basis of fasting blood glucose measurements. Some units prefer to start both premeal and background insulin from the start, believing that limiting initial prescriptions to premeal fast-acting insulin may be insufficient to switch off hepatic ketone production and, therefore, potentially dangerous. There is evidence that tightly controlling blood sugar from the beginning of therapy prolongs the preservation of residual insulin secretion, which would support such an approach.

TOTAL DAILY INSULIN DOSAGE AND DISTRIBUTION

Factors affecting insulin doses are age, weight, stage of puberty, duration of diabetes, food intake and distribution, exercise pattern, daily routines, results of monitoring and intercurrent illness. As a general guide, total daily insulin doses are as follows:

- Partial remission phase (any age): <0.5 units/kg/day
- Preadolescent children (beyond remission phase): 0.7–1 unit/kg/day
- During puberty (beyond remission phase): 1.2–1.5 units/kg/day or higher.

The distribution of total daily insulin dose varies greatly between individuals and requires individual titration. Twice-daily insulin injection regimens: approximately 60–75% of the total daily insulin dose is given in the morning and 25–40% at night with approximately 30% of each dose being short-acting insulin. Basal bolus regimens: typically 40–60% of the total daily insulin dose is given as intermediate-acting or long-acting insulin before bed, with the remainder divided up into premeal bolus. Insulin pump therapy: typically 45–60% (lower end of this range in young children and higher end of this range often in adolescents) of the total insulin given as basal insulin and the remainder is provided by premeal boluses.

Basal insulin requirements are considerably reduced (around 20%) when using physiological regimens involving glargine or insulin pumps.

INSULIN ADMINISTRATION

Insulin Absorption

The rate of absorption of insulin is affected by many factors as follows:

- Insulin type
- Insulin site.

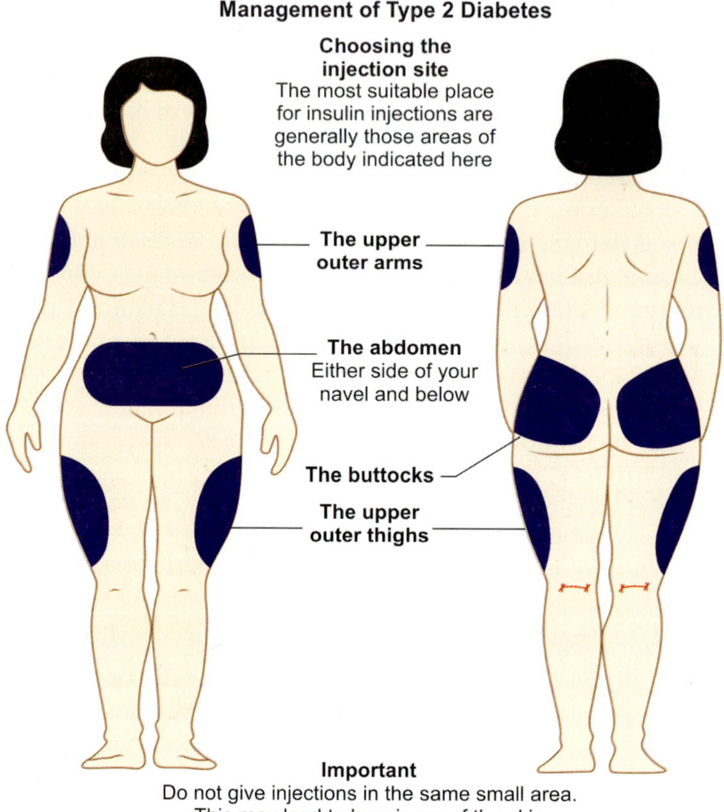

Fig. 4: Recommended insulin injection sites

Soluble insulin is absorbed more slowly and consistently from the subcutaneous site compared to intramuscular injections. There is less difference with rapid-acting analogous. Thus subcutaneous injections are preferred. Insulin is also absorbed at different rates from different anatomical locations. Absorptions are quickest from the abdomen, followed by buttock and slowest from the thigh (nonexercising). However, these differences are less pronounced with both rapid-acting and long-acting analogous. Thus it is recommended that short/rapid-acting insulin or mixed doses of insulin be injected in the abdomen. It is recommended that evening doses of intermediate-acting insulin be given in the (nonexercising) thigh to optimize the overnight profile of action. The upper arm is used by some for injecting however, this is generally not recommended in younger children because the thin the layer of subcutaneous tissues at this stage and the increased risk of intramuscular injections.

Rotation between different anatomical sites from day to day is not recommended since this has been shown to be associated with higher and more variable blood glucose levels (Fig. 4).

- Injection depth (Table 2).

Table 2: Mean cutis/subcutis thickness

Mean cutis/subcutis thickness (mm) (measured by ultrasound without compression)		
Site	***Male child***	***Female child***
Abdomen	9	15
• Thigh anterolateral	10	14
• Thigh anterior	10	13
Buttock	19	26

Source: Adapted from Birkebaek NH, Johansen A, Solvig J. Cutis/subcutis thickness at insulin injection sites and localization of simulated insulin boluses in children with type 1 diabetes mellitus: need for individualization of injection technique? Diabetic Med. 1998;15(11):965-71.

In assessing the suitability of different infection sites, studies have examined subcutaneous tissues thickness and site of deposition of injection.[21] There is a significant risk of intramuscular injection (and hence more rapid absorption) which is increased in lean individual, especially boys. This can be minimized by using a two-finger pinch technique and an injection angle of 45°. Shorter needles reduce the risk of intramuscular injection. In general, most children and adolescents should use 8 mm needle with a pinch-technique and 45° angle and if lean and using pens, 5 or 6 mm needle may be appropriate.

Intramuscular injection of insulin can increase absorption from the thigh by up to 50%, but it has been reported that there is no difference between subcutaneous and intramuscular absorption from the abdomen.

- *Insulin dose*: Insulin has dose-dependent absorption kinetics: small doses are absorbed more quickly than large doses.
- *Temperature*: Insulin absorption is increased with increased ambient and body temperature, related to increased subcutaneous blood flow. Therefore, care should be taken in hot weather and warm bath after insulin injection.
- *Exercise*: Exercise causes increased insulin absorption, again predominantly related to increased subcutaneous blood flow. For this reason, the thigh is not recommended prior to exercise.
- *Age of child and fat mass*: Large fat mass is associated with increased subcutaneous tissue thickness and therefore, slower absorption. Since younger children are often leaner, insulin absorption is often faster.
- *Presence of lipohypertrophy or lipoatrophy*: Adverse changes at the injection site can considerably affect absorption. Lipohypertrophy is a common problem in diabetes management and absorption of insulin from those sites is delayed and erratic. This can be avoided by moving the injection site from day to day within the same anatomical area of the body, or periodically moving to another anatomical site. Prevalence of lipohypertrophy has been estimated at 20–30% in patients with type 1 diabetes. Other factors associated with lipohypertrophy are presence of insulin antibodies.

Insulin Delivery Devices

Insulin Syringes and Pens

Insulin syringes are disposable plastic syringes designed for single use only and are available in a range of sizes [40 units (0.4 mL); 50 units (0.5 mL) and 100 units (1 mL)] and needles length (6 mm and 12.7 mm).

Insulin pens are also available which contains prefilled cartridges (3 mL) of insulin. Cartridges are available for the rapid-acting analogous, short acting and isophane insulins but not for lente and ultralente insulins which are not stable in pen systems. Needle length available are 5, 8 and 12.7 mm. Families should know how to use an insulin syringe even if the delivery device is primarily a pen in case of unexpected failure of the pen. Disposable pens are also available for some insulin types.

Practical Aspects of Insulin Administration

Disinfection of the skin is not necessary prior to insulin injections. However, injections should be given through clearly healthy skin. Some patients inject through clothing at times for reasons of convenience and no significant problems have been reported with the practice.

The age at which children can reliably draw up and administer the insulin injection or use an insulin pen varies markedly between children. Many children assist in the insulin injection routine from 9 years to 10 years of age and many can easily use an insulin pen from that age. White insulin syringes and needles are recommended for single use only; surveys indicate that some patients reuse syringes and needles and that this is not associated with increased infections or other adverse events. Insulin syringes and pen needles need to dispose of in a safe and hygienic way.

Insulin Adjustment

Appropriate adjustment of insulin is critical if goals of therapy are to be achieved. Patients on insulin injection therapy are advised to make adjustment to the appropriate dose in approximately 10% increments and observe the effects of this over several days before making further changes.

Side Effects of Insulin Therapy

- Hypoglycemia
- Weight gain
- Peripheral edema (insulin treatment causes salt and water retention in the short term)
- Insulin antibodies (animal insulin)
- Local allergy (rare)
- Lipodystrophy at injection sites.

The most common side effect is hypoglycemia. A common problem is fasting hyperglycemia (the dawn phenomenon) associated with normal circadian rhythm and causing release of counter-regulatory hormones during the later part of night, which antagonize insulin action before wakening.

Alternative Insulin Therapies

"Open loop" systems are battery powered portable pumps providing subcutaneous or intravenous infusion of insulin without reference to the blood glucose concentration. The rate of insulin infusion is variable and can be preprogrammed to match diurnal variation in requirements and manually boosted at meal times. In practice, the "loop" is closed by the patient performing blood glucose estimations and the use of these devices requires a high degree of patient motivation. These increasingly sophisticated systems can achieve excellent glycemic control but widespread therapeutic use is limited by cost.

Glycemic Control

Intensive diabetes management: The Diabetes Control and Complication Trial (DCCT) confirmed the benefit of maintaining near normoglycemia in reducing the development and progression of diabetic microvascular complications in adolescents and adults. Long follow-up of patients after the completion of DCCT, in the EDIC (Epidemiology of Diabetes Interventions and Complications) study, showed increasing reduction of microvascular and macrovascular complication with optimal metabolic control.

Achieving excellent glycemic control is more difficult in children and adolescents because of the following factors:

- Insulin deficiency is often more complete
- Variable food intake
- Recurrent infections during childhood
- Variable exercise patterns
- Varying rates of growth and development
- Hormonal changes during puberty, necessitating high and changing insulin requirements
- Behavioral problems associated with psychosocial difficulties
- Difficulty with adherence to diabetes regime.

Indicators of poor Glycemic Control

- Polyuria, polydipsia
- Enuresis and nocturia
- Blurred vision
- Weight loss or failure to gain weight with growth
- Poor growth
- Pubertal delay
- Skin infections (Staphylococcal and Candida)
- Deteriorating school performance
- Signs of diabetic complications
- Elevated HbA1c and lipids.

Glycemic goals: The National Institute of Clinical Excellence guideline type 1 diabetes (childhood): Diagnosis and Management of type 1 diabetes in primary and secondary care makes the following recommendations:

- Children with type 1 diabetes and their parents should be inferred that the optimal target for long-term glycemic control is an HbA1c <7% without an increase in hypoglycemia.

- A preprandial blood glucose level is between 72–144 mg/dL
- A postprandial blood glucose level of less than 180 mg/dL

Glycemic targets need to take into account additional factors

- Hypoglycemia unawareness
- Unpredictability of hypoglycemia in some children
- Past history of recurrent severe hypoglycemia
- Ability to comply with blood glucose monitoring
- Presence of psychological or psychiatric disturbances
- Presence of any coexisting disease (Epilepsy).

Patients during the puberty may have particular difficulties in maintaining good control due to physiological and psychological changes and therefore, frequently require special counseling services and support.

Blood Glucose Monitoring

Blood glucose measurement is essential in management of children and adolescents with diabetes for the following reasons:

- To monitor daily control at different times of the day preprandially and postprandially in order to obtain a profile over the 24 hours, before, during and after sport, during intercurrent illness and during and after treatment of hypoglycemia.
- To detect hypoglycemic and hyperglycemic episodes
- To make possible the safe management of acute illness at home.

If the diabetes is very stable, then the frequency of testing may be reduced (e.g. to obtain a profile over the day several times a week).

Medical Nutrition Therapy

Today, there is no one "diabetic diet". The current nutrition recommendations can be defined simply as a "nutrition prescription based on assessment and treatment goals and outcomes", the distribution of calories from carbohydrates and fat be based on nutrition assessment and on blood glucose, weight and lipid goals, with continued emphasis on a diet with fewer than 10% of calories from saturated fats with 10–20% of calories from proteins.

Goals in Type 1 Diabetes

The primary goals of therapy for persons with type 1 diabetes are as follows:

- Provision of an individualized meal plan based on usual food intake and life style. This is used as basis for integrating insulin therapy into the usual eating and exercise pattern.
- Consistency of carbohydrate intake to allow the synchronization of mealtimes with times of insulin action for persons receiving fixed insulin regimes.
- Determination of premeal insulin dose and postprandial blood glucose response by monitoring of blood glucose levels and adjusting insulin doses for the amount of total carbohydrate consumed for persons receiving intensive insulin therapy.
- Prevention of weight gain is desirable. The attention is paid to total caloric intake from carbohydrate, protein and fat for persons with improved glycemia control.

- Adjustment of rapid- or short-acting insulin for deviations from usual eating and exercise habits is preferred choice for prevention of hypoglycemia. Additional carbohydrate may be needed for unexplained exercise.

Calories

Prescribing enough calories (kilocalories) to achieve and maintain a desirable weight should be carefully considered. Caloric needs vary with patient's weight, age, gender activity level and genetic background. Persons with type 1 diabetes are often thin when the diagnosis is first made, and the diet should include enough calories to ensure normal growth and development and to sustain the usual level of physical activity. For infants, children and adolescents, caloric intake should maintain consistent growth curves based on energy needs during periods of growth and sexual maturation.

A reasonable goal is to try to achieve and maintain a weight close to ideal body weight. When considering a dietary strategy that will help to achieve this it is useful to think in terms of over-all caloric intake, and composition of the diet in terms of carbohydrate, protein and fat content.

Carbohydrate

Diabetic diets or food plans should include unrefined carbohydrate rather than simple sugars such as sucrose. The carbohydrate is absorbed relatively slowly from fiber-rich foods, but when refined sugars are eaten, the blood glucose may rise rapidly. For example, the glucose peak seen in the blood after eating an apple is much flatter than that seen after drinking the same amount of carbohydrate as apple juice. No more than 40% of total daily caloric intake should come from carbohydrates, which should be mainly low-glycemic index foods such as vegetables, or processed grains and starchy food and white potatoes should be avoided or consumed in limited amounts.

All complex carbohydrates and all simple carbohydrates (or sugars) traditionally were thought to generate different blood glucose responses based on molecular structure. It is suggested that the blood glucose and insulin response to a food could be expressed as glycemic index, which quantifies the postprandial glucose response to a standard amount of glucose, or an attempt to classify foods by the extent to which they raise the blood glucose levels. Glucose alone produces the largest increase in blood glucose level and is assigned a glycemic index of 100. Fiber rich foods, acidic foods and high fat foods after have low-glycemic indexes. The glycemic index of sucrose, disaccharides made of glucose and fructose is lower than that of some starches, such as potatoes because sucrose contains less pure glucose. Low-glycemic index diets have been shown to improve glucose, lipids and insulin levels in people with diabetes.

Premeal boluses of insulin are calculated more accurately by carbohydrate (CHO) counting, insulin to carbohydrate ratio (ICR) and correction bolus. CHO counting is a meal planning where in the patients identifies the CHO in the meal, estimates the total CHO amount in the meal and calculates the insulin to balance the CHO using ICR thereby controlling postprandial glucose levels more accurately. It is done by two methods, CHO exchange (1 CHO serving = 15 g carb portions) and CHO gram counting (food is weighted and CHO is calculated). ICR is the amount of insulin required to cover a specified number of CHO grams. This is calculated by 500/300 rule [500/total daily dose of insulin (TDD) for children aged 5 years and above and 300/TDD for preschool children]. Correction bolus is the amount of extra, fast-acting insulin added to or subtracted from a bolus to correct a blood glucose that is above or below target (90–140 mg). This is calculated by [Current blood glucose—Target blood glucose/insulin sensitivity factor (ISF)]. ISF is how much unit of insulin will lower the blood glucose by. This is calculated by 1,500 or 1,800 rule (1500/TDD for short-acting and 1800/TDD for rapid-acting insulin.[22] Further adjustment of insulin or food intake may be made based on anticipation of special circumstances, such as increased exercise and intercurrent illness.

Sucrose

Consumption of modest amount of sucrose by persons with diabetes is acceptable as long as both metabolic control and weight are maintained. Available studies have allowing children and adults with diabetes to feel less constrained by allowing diet of their peers. Realistic guidelines for inducing sucrose-containing food in the diet also improve patient's adherence to overall dietary management. However, sucrose, doses encourage the development of dental carries, and sucrose-containing foods may contain a significant number of calories, especially when combined with fat in dessert foods such as baked goods, ice-cream and chocolate bars.

Fiber

Several studies have demonstrated that diet particularly high in fiber (20–30 g/daily) especially soluble fiber is associated with lower blood glucose and serum lipids levels. Water soluble fibers such as the pectin, gums, starch, polysaccharides and a few hemicelluloses found in fruits, legumes, roots, tubers, oats and oat bran, have little influence on fecal bulk, but may reduce serum levels of glucose and insulin.

Protein

The quantity of protein required by diabetic patients varies with age, weight and activity of the case as well as with the condition of the kidneys. It is a safe rule at the beginning of the treatment to increase the protein gradually up to the same quantity as that required by normal individual. This is approximately 1–1.5 g/kg body weight for adults but for children it may reach 3 g. For those with type 1 diabetes, possible increase in the protein content of the diet, which seems to have a minimal impact on glucose concentrations, while decreasing the carbohydrate content, may improve and stabilize blood glucose excursions.

Fat

People with type 1 diabetes who maintain good control of blood glucose with insulin have plasma lipids levels similar to those of the general population of the same age and gender. Monounsaturated fats are liquid at room temperature and derived from oleic acid. The nonessential fatty acids (NEFAs) help to lower low density lipoprotein-cholesterol (LDL-C) levels and possibly raise HDL-C levels. Major dietary sources are olive and peanut oils and nuts. Generally, about 10–15% of total calories may come from monounsaturated fatty acids.

Polyunsaturated fats are liquid at room temperature and derived from linoleic, linolenic and arachidonic acids. Major dietary sources are corn, sunflower, sesame and soybean oils.

These essential fatty acids are known to lower both LDL-C and plasma cholesterol levels. Omega-3 fatty acids, a type of polyunsaturated fats, lower plasma triglycerides and very low density lipopolysaccharide cholesterol (VLDL-C) levels. Major dietary sources are fatty fish, flaxseed and other vegetables oils and partially hydrogenated margarines.

Saturated fats are mostly solid at room temperature and synthesized in the body from acetate. Many dietary sources are animal products such as butter meat, whole milk, cheese, sour cream, cream cheese and tropical oils such as coconut, palm oil. These NEFAs increase total serum cholesterol and LDL-C levels.

Trans fats are semisolid at room temperature. The chemical process of hydrogenation causes unsaturated fatty acids to become more saturated and alters the position of hydrogen atoms around the double bond (on opposite sides; or trans). This process increases the shelf life of foods. Major dietary sources are polyunsaturated vegetables oils in solid margarines, salad dressings and many baked-foods. Trans fats increase LDL-C and decrease HDL-C and are associated with an increases risk of coronary heart disease.

A diet history should be taken, and review of a complete 3-day diet, diary, including all snacks, can lead many patients to recognize previously unappreciated sources of excess calories. A daily sodium intake of 2–3 g per day is recommended to limit the risk of hypertension. All patients of type 1 diabetes usually require snacks between meals and at bed-time, as injected insulin may linger in the blood. Foods that are labeled diabetic not recommended, as they usually contain nonglucose refined sugars such as sucrose or fructose. Artificial sweeteners are useful and could be used an alternative to sugars; concerns that they cause cancer have not been confirmed. Patients on insulin should be advised to eat the same amount at the same time each day.

Exercise

All levels of physical activity can be undertaken by people with type 1 diabetes who do not have complications and have good glycemic control. Therapeutic regimes can be adjusted to allow safe participation consistent with an individual goals and abilities. Along with dietary change, there must be an emphasis on overall lifestyle change, particularly in respect of exercise. It is useful to point out that small changes in everyday activities can be useful.

Regular scheduled exercise, even if only walking, should be encouraged, perhaps even prescribed, the aim being at least a half-hour each day on average. It is to be emphasized that perhaps the greatest value of regular exercise, even when there is disappointingly little weight loss, is that it reduces insulin resistance. When planning an exercise regimes it is important to:

- Assess contradictions and limitations
- The realistic people will only continue to do what they enjoy
- Build up the amount of exercise gradually
- Advise about the risk of hypoglycemia
- Remember, any exercise is better than none.

Exercise guidelines in type 1 diabetes

General advice

- Exercise regularly; even walking has metabolic benefits
- Tailor exercise regime to fit individual needs and physical fitness

- Avoid hypoglycemia during exercise by:
  - Taking 20–40 g extra carbohydrate before and hourly during exercise
  - Reduce pre-exercise insulin doses 30–50% if necessary
  - Use non-exercising sites for injections
  - Avoid heavy exercise during peak from insulin injection.

Contraindication

- In those with proliferative retinopathy, strenuous exercise (due to the risk of possible hemorrhage.
- For those taking insulin, sports where hypoglycemia could be dangerous.

Cautions

- Take care if cardiovascular comorbidities are present.
- Those with peripheral neuropathy need to be aware of the potential for damage to the feet.

Prevention of Diabetic Ketoacidosis: Sick-day Rules

The cornerstones of sick-day management are—(a) never omit insulin, (b) prevent dehydration and hypoglycemia, (c) monitor blood glucose frequently, (d) monitor for ketosis, (e) provide supplemental fast-acting or rapid-acting insulin doses according to guidelines, (f) treat underlying triggers and (g) have frequent contact with the diabetes healthcare team to review clinical status.

Never Omit Insulin

Illness presents specific dilemmas for children and adolescents with diabetes and their families. Insulin must always be administered during illness even if the child or adolescent is not eating. Infection induces insulin resistance, therapy often necessitating increased or supplemental doses of insulin. Generally, the usually prescribed insulin dosage is supplemented by rapid- or short-acting insulin in the form of lispro, aspart, glulisine, or regular. The additional or supplemental dose is needed to manage the hyperglycemia and ketosis. The optimal supplemental dosage of insulin is calculated from the blood glucose levels and the presence or absence of ketones. In general, supplemental insulin dosage, generally 10–20% of the total insulin dosages is based on the blood glucose levels and the urinary (or blood) ketone results (Table 3).

Prevent Dehydration and Hypoglycemia

Fluid intake to prevent dehydration must be encouraged. Oral hydration is preferred but may be impossible at times of nausea and vomiting. In fact the presence of vomiting and the inability to hold down orally administered fluids may be the limiting factor for the continued home management of a sick day.

Blood glucose level determines whether sugar-containing or sugar-free fluids are used. When the patients in anorexic and usual solid food intake is curtailed or absent, sugar-containing drinks such as regular soda, clear juices or other glucose-containing drinks are suggested to provide for usual carbohydrate intake, especially when blood glucose is under 180 200 mg/dL volumes 3m^2 per day should be encouraged.

Table 3: Supplemental insulin dosages

Based on blood glucose and urine ketone results		
Blood glucose level	***Ketone (> traces)***	***Suggested extra insulin***
80–250 mg/dL	No or Yes	None
250–400 mg/dL	No	10% of TDD
	Yes	20% of TDD
>400 mg/dL	No or Yes	20% of TDD

- Total daily dose (TDD) is calculated by adding up all of the insulin administered on a usual day including rapid or fast-acting insulin and intermediate/long-acting insulin.
- Blood glucose and urine ketones should be monitored every 2–4 hours.
- Supplemental insulin boosters are repeated every 2–3 hours with aspart or lispro, and every 3–4 hours with regular insulin.
- If hyperglycemia and/or urine ketone do not improve after 2 hours supplemental dose, contact the healthcare team. The team may recommend intramuscular injection of supplemental regular insulin.
- If hypoglycemia is present (glucose <80 mg/dL) with or without ketone, consider omitting aspart lispro or regular and decreasing intermediate/long-acting insulin by 20%; contact healthcare team.

Alternative algorithm incorporating more complexity			
Blood glucose level	***Urine ketone***		
	Negative	***Small***	***Moderate/Large***
<250 mg/dL	No change	0–5%	0–10%
250–400 mg/dL	5%	10%	15–20%
400 mg/dL	10%	15%	20%

Source: Adapted from In: C Ronald Kahn, Gordon Weir, George King, Alan Jacobson, Robert Smith, Alan Moses (Eds). Joslin's Diabetes Mellitus, 14th edition, Chapter 42. Philadelphia: Lippincott Williams & Wilkins. pp. 729.

Sugar-free drinks are recommended when the patients are able to follows a usual meal plan or take in solids that provided adequate carbohydrate and calories. Antipyretics are important at times of fever in order to reduce any additional insensible fluid losses. Reassessment of hydration status is important to avoid decompensation.

Monitor Blood Glucose Frequently

Self-(or family) monitoring of blood glucose should be performed at least every 2–4 hours for sick-day management. More frequent monitoring is recommended if the glucose level is low.

Monitor for Ketones

Recommendations for urine testing for ketones have included testing at 2–4 hours intervals during illness, with stress or whenever the blood glucose is consistently greater than 300 mg/dL. Administration of supplemental insulin and hydration are generally adequate interventions for successful treatment of ketosis. If the patient fails to clear ketones within 12 hours, the diabetes healthcare teams must be contacted for assessment.

Provide Supplemental Fast-acting or Rapid-acting Insulin

During any intercurrent illness, the frequency of monitoring blood glucose and ketone levels should be increased to every 2–4 hours. When the blood glucose level is greater than

300 mg/dL on two or more consecutive occasions, patients and families should always monitor for the presence of ketones. Ketones in general, are markers of insulin deficiency and the need for supplemental insulin. However, in the setting of gastrointestinal illness with vomiting, diarrhea, increased transit times, and malabsorption, hypoglycemia may prevail in the presence or absence of ketones. Under such circumstances, especially when the blood glucose level is 80 mg/dL in the setting of possible ketones, increasing fluid intake with the provision of 10–15 g of carbohydrates should be encouraged until the blood glucose level increases. Recommendations include the continued administration of fluid until the ketone clear.

Supplemental doses of rapid-acting insulin should be administered in addition to usual insulin dosage whenever hyperglycemia and ketosis are present. Doses of supplemental insulin are generally calculated according to weight (0.1–0.3 U/Kg) as percentage of total insulin dosage (usually between 10% and 20% of the total daily insulin requirement in the basal state), or according to team-derived algorithms (Table 3).

Treat Underlying Precipitating Factors

Identify underlying infection and treat it. Symptomatic treatment with antipyretics and analgesics is beneficial. Patients with history of recurrent DKA (Diabetic Ketoacidosis), with known eating disorders or psychosocial problems, and with poor glycemic control are at risk for decompensation.

Patients and family members should be advised to look out for signs that medical attention is needed. These include vomiting that continues for more than 2–4 hours, blood glucose levels that exceed 300 mg/dL or presence of ketones for more than 12 hours. Signs of dehydration such as dry mouth, cracked lips, sunken eyes, weight loss or dry skin; or symptoms that DKA may be developing, such as nausea, abdominal or chest pain, vomiting, ketotic breath, hyperventilation or altered consciousness.

Behavioral Issues

Physicians involved in care of type 1 diabetes need to address the overall issues of child and adolescent growth, development, temperament and behaviors, as well as the issues of the natural course of diabetes itself—diagnosis, adaptation, ongoing disease progression and potential complications. Children and adolescents with type 1 diabetes face unique demands in dealing with diabetes both because of the nature of their being children and adolescents and because of the chronicity of the disease. The psychological challenges include an increased risk for psychiatric disorders, including depression, adjustment and adaptation problems, and eating disorders. A variety of psychosocial interventions have been shown to be effective.

Care of Children and Adolescents with Type 1 Diabetes in the School and Day Care Setting

Pediatric behavioral studies and clinical programs have consistently documented the challenges of achieving optimal metabolic control. The goal is to provide direction for the care during school. The children and adolescents with diabetes are not unlike their peers without diabetes they spend the majority of their walking hours in school. Because of the need for optimal glycemic control for the youth with diabetes, the tasks of diabetes self-management become a necessary part of the school setting in built on a foundation of good communication between the parent(s), child, school and healthcare team. The goals are to provide the care of children and adolescents during school. An individual care team provides the framework for addressing the needs of the child with diabetes in a school or day-care environment and state needs, responsibilities, and expectations of the school, the patients, and the child and adolescents during the school day and during school related extracurricular activities.

REFERENCES

1. International Diabetes Federation: Diabetes Atlas 2nd edition. Brussels, Belgium: IDF; 2003.
2. International Diabetes Federation. IDF Diabetes Atlas, 6th edition. Brussels, Belgium: International Diabetes Federation; 2013.
3. Imperatore G, Boyle JP, Thompson TJ, et al. Projections of type 1 and type 2 diabetes burden in the US population aged <20 years through 2050: dynamic modeling of incidence, mortality, and population growth. Diabetes Care. 2012;35(12):2515-20.
4. Menon PSN, Virmani A, Shah P, et al. Childhood onset diabetes mellitus in India: an overview. Int J Diab Dev Countries. 1990;10:11-16.
5. Ramachandran A, Snehalatha C, Krishnaswamy CV. Incidence of IDDM in children in urban population in Southern India. Madras IDDM Registry Group Madras, South India. Diabetes Res Clin Pract. 1996;34:79-82.
6. Kalra S, Kalra B, Sharma A. Prevalence of type 1 diabetes mellitus in Karnal district, Haryana state, India. Diabetol Metab Syndr. 2010;2:14.
7. Onengut-Gumuscu S, Concannon P. The genetics of type 1 diabetes: lessons learned and future challenges. J Autoimmun. 2005;25(Suppl):34-9.
8. Concannon P, Rich SS, Nepom GT. Genetics of type 1A diabetes. N Engl J Med. 2009;360:1646-54.
9. Grant SF, Hakonarson H. Genome wide association studies in type 1 diabetes. Curr Diab Rep. 2009;9:157-63.
10. Pociot F, Akolkar B, Concannon P, et al. Genetics of type 1 diabetes: what's next? Diabetes. 2010;59:1561-71.
11. Polychronakos C, Li Q. Understanding type 1 diabetes through genetics: advances and prospects. Nat Rev Genet. 2011;12:781-92.
12. Radha V, Vimaleswaran KS, Deepa R, et al. The genetics of diabetes mellitus. Indian J Med Res. 2003;117:225-38.
13. Concannon P, Rich SS, Nepom GT. Genetics of type 1A diabetes. N Engl J Med. 2009;360:1646-54.
14. Barrett JC, Clayton DG, Concannon P, et al. Genome-wide association study and meta-analysis find that over 40 loci affect risk of type 1 diabetes. Nat Genet. 2009;41:703-7.
15. Cooper JD, Howson JM, Smyth D, et al. Confirmation of novel type 1 diabetes risk loci in families. Diabetologia. 2012;55:996-1000.
16. Concannon P, Erlich HA, Julier C, et al; Type 1 Diabetes Genetics Consortium. Type 1 diabetes: evidence for susceptibility loci from four genome-wide linkage scans in 1,435 multiplex families. Diabetes. 2005;54:2995-3001.
17. Concannon P, Chen WM, Julier C, et al. Type 1 Diabetes Genetics Consortium. Genome-wide scan for linkage to type 1 diabetes in 2,496 multiplex families from the Type 1 Diabetes Genetics Consortium. Diabetes. 2009;58:1018-22.
18. Katz LE, Jawad AF, Ganesh J, et al. Fasting C-peptide and insulin like growth factor-binding protein-1 levels help to distinguish childhood type 1 and type 2 diabetes at diagnosis. Pediatr Diabetes. 2007;8:53-9.

19. Wenzlau JM, Hutton JC. Novel diabetes autoantibodies and prediction of type 1 diabetes. Curr Diab Rep. 2013;13:608-15.
20. Eisenbarth GS. Type I diabetes mellitus. A chronic autoimmune disease. N Engl J Med. 1986; 314:1360-8.
21. Birkebaek NH, Johansen A, Solvig J. Cutis/subcutis thickness at insulin injection sites and localization of stimulated insulin boluses in children with type 1 diabetes mellitus: need for individualization of injection technique? Diabet Med. 1998;15(11):965-71.
22. The Leeds Insulin Pump Workbook for Children and Young People, 1st edition. Yorkshire; UK; 2012. p.16.

8
CHAPTER

Management of Type 1 Diabetes Mellitus in Children

Bhavana Sole, Prasanna Kumar KM

INTRODUCTION

The management of type 1 diabetes is different from management of type 2 diabetes as it needs specialized skills, infrastructure and knowledge. These challenges include factors like the age of the patient, unpredictable physical activity and dietary patterns, psychosocial issues, hypoglycemia and ketoacidosis.[1,2] Lack of infrastructure, affordability, family support, social stigma and lack of comprehensive care in the primary care setting are obstacles that need to be overcome.

The care of a patient with type 1 diabetes mandates the involvement of a healthcare team which includes an endocrinologist/diabetologist, a nurse, dietician, diabetes educator, mental health specialist (psychiatrist/psychologist) with active age appropriate involvement from the patient, family/caregiver and the school. This comprehensive care includes initial management and follow up that ensures a smooth transition from pediatric care through adolescence and into adulthood.[1-3]

INITIAL MANAGEMENT

First time a child with type 1 diabetes is recognized, it is advisable to admit the child in a hospital which has facilities for comprehensive care of type 1 diabetes. Children with ketoacidosis definitely need admission, but others not in ketoacidosis also need admission for proper evaluation and education of the child and parents.

The aims of management of diabetes in children are:

- Achieve euglycemia and maintain the same throughout life
- Physical and psychological growth of the child appropriate to the child's age
- Prevent complications of diabetes
- The child should have quality and quantity of life which should be as good as a nondiabetic child.

Successful management of children with type 1 diabetes involves the formulation and execution of an individualized care plan. This comprises of setting of age appropriate goals and understanding the specific needs of each child. The goals should be realistic keeping in mind the child's age, mental maturity, socioeconomic and educational background of the parents, and the degree of involvement of the parents and practical barriers that may stand in the way of ideal care.[1-3] This includes the following:[1-4]

- *Imparting a basic understanding of diabetes to the patient and family*: The essentials of the pathophysiology of type 1 diabetes, insulin secretion and function in the body, importance of glycemic control and follow up, complications of diabetes and differences from type 2 diabetes need to be taught to the patient and family.
- *Treatment plan*: The age appropriate management plan which includes the insulin regimen, nutrition, exercise schedule, Self-monitoring of Blood Glucose (SMBG) and Diabetes Self-Management Education (DSME) should be discussed with the family.
- *Insulin administration skills*: The patient and the family must learn about the type of insulin being prescribed, duration and mechanism of action, storage of insulin, injection technique and site rotation. They must be trained to measure and inject insulin themselves with assistance to overcome the fear of injections.
- *Blood glucose testing*: The patient and the caregivers should be taught the importance of blood glucose testing, sites of testing, importance of maintaining records, storage of strips and the frequency and timing of testing. The use of glucometers and testing by finger prick need to be demonstrated.
- *Hypoglycemia and hyperglycemia*: Recognition of signs and symptoms of hypoglycemia, prevention, and treatment needs to be emphasized upon. Hyperglycemia, risk of ketoacidosis and sick-day rules need to be addressed.
- *Nutrition and exercise plan*: This needs to be incorporated into the management along with SMBG to help adjust the insulin dosage to achieve glycemic targets.
- *Social and psychological support*: This should be provided to address issues such as depression, eating disorders and social stigma associated with diabetes.

All children require an age appropriate comprehensive evaluation including a detailed history and physical examination, assessment of cardiovascular risk factors, screening for microvascular and macrovascular complications to aid in prevention and facilitate early interventions.[1,2] Screening for coexisting autoimmune disorders, like thyroid disease, is essential. Screening for celiac disease, Addison's disease and pernicious anemia may be considered when clinical suspicion is present.[1,2,5-7]

ON GOING CARE

After the initial management, the healthcare team should ensure adequate follow up, ongoing education and specific interventions to achieve strict normoglycemia and targets based on the age of the patient. The patients need to be screened for microvascular and macrovascular complications and risk reduction needs to be initiated when indicated to prevent the long-term complications of diabetes. Treatment of complications should be initiated with further emphasis on glycemic control as often as required. Smooth transition into adolescence and adulthood with a slow increase in autonomy should be ensured.[1,2,8]

Age Appropriate Care

- Challenges faced
- Management plan
- Neonates (<1 year)

Hypoglycemia due to erratic feeding can be difficult to detect and neonates present with nonspecific symptoms such as poor feeding or lethargy. Recurrent episodes lead to seizures and may have long-term deleterious effects on cognition.[1-3,9,10]

Toddler (1–3 years)

Toddlers can also present with hypoglycemic or hyperglycemia due to erratic feeding and unpredictable changes in the day-to-day physical activity.[1-3] Parents must be taught to recognize hypoglycemia from tantrums and mood swings. They must start taking responsibility in the day-to-day care of the patient. Caregiver burden and stress of implementing the care plan also need to be looked into by the healthcare team.

Preschool (3–6 years)

In addition to the challenges seen in a toddler, the child may not cooperate with the regimen. Difficulties may be faced as they attend preschool if there are no designated trained teachers or nurses at the school.[1-3]

In addition to the above, the child must be encouraged to cooperate with the treatment plan. School or day-care authorities must be trained to identify and treat hypoglycemia and must be actively involved in the education process.

School (7–11 years)

Flexible treatment regimens may be needed based on the school timings and physical activity. Psychosocial problems, like depression, social stigma, bullying and isolation of children with type 1 diabetes, are common problems in school and society, and need to be addressed seriously.[1-3]

Autonomy should be encouraged and the child should be actively involved in SMBG and should learn to master the insulin injection technique. This needs to be done under adult supervision and complete autonomy at this stage can lead to hypoglycemia or hyperglycemia. Education on diabetes, hypoglycemia and hyperglycemia should be included at every visit. Referral to a mental health specialist may be warranted to deal with the pressure of living with the social burden of diabetes.[1-3,11-14]

Adolescence (12–18 years)

Psychological problems dominate this period with problems like body image, eating disorders, peer pressure, smoking, alcohol, sex and need for independence in decision making. Conflict with family members and increased autonomy to the patient can worsen glycemic control. Insulin requirements may also increase during puberty (Box 1).[1-3,11-14]

Problems need to be approached by formulating a care plan that entrusts adequate responsibility to the patient and the family. The services of a mental health specialist may

Box 1: Age appropriate care[1-3,11-14]

Toddlers (1-3 years):
- Erratic feeding leading to hypo/hyperglycemia.
- Recognize hypoglycemia from tantrums and mood swings.

Preschool (3–6 years):
- Child may not cooperate with the regimen difficulties in preschool children lack of training in day-care center authorities

School (7–11 years):
- Psychosocial problems like depression, social stigma, bullying and isolation of children with type 1 diabetes.
- Flexible treatment regimens and child should be actively involved in SMBG and should learn to master the insulin injection technique.

Adolescence (12–18 years):
- Psychological problems dominate this period with problems like body image, eating disorders, peer pressure, smoking, alcohol, sex and need for independence in decision making.
- Can worsen glycemic control. Insulin requirements may increase.

be sought to deal with psychosocial problems. A continuum of strict glycemic control needs to be ensured with emphasis of education and prevention of complications.[1-3,11-14] The Box 2 summarizes the initial assessment and follow up of a patient with type 1 diabetes.

GLYCEMIC CONTROL

Lowering of hyperglycemia should be achieved as safely as possible, balancing the HbA1c targets versus the risk of hypoglycemia. The Diabetes Control and Complications Trial demonstrated that strict glycemic control and lowering of HbA1c lower the risk of retinopathy, nephropathy and neuropathy and also retard the progression of preexisting microvascular complications.[15-17] However, as HbA1c is lowered, the risk of hypoglycemia also increases. This risk is higher in younger children and those with hypoglycemic unawareness.

The American Diabetes Association (ADA) guidelines traditionally recommended higher HbA1c targets based on the age of the patient. This approach focused primarily on reduction of hypoglycemic episodes based on literature suggesting that recurrent hypoglycemia would lead to cognitive impairment. However, the recent position statement by the ADA has dismissed these reports of neurocognitive decline. *The ADA recommends an HbA1c less than 7.5% in all children aged less than 18 years and an HbA1c less than 7% in all adults.* Taking into account the burden of microvascular and macrovascular complications secondary to poor glycemic control prior to puberty, and evidence of white matter changes in the central nervous system due to hyperglycemia the guidelines on target HbA1c have been altered. Newer modalities of treatment such as the use of rapid-acting insulin, basal insulin and insulin pumps with a suspend feature on detecting low glucose have further aided in reducing hypoglycemia and in achieving more stringent glycemic targets. However, individualization of targets bearing in mind age, comorbidities, life span and hypoglycemic unawareness is recommended.[1,2,18-20]

Box 2: Summary of assessment at diagnosis and follow up[1,2]

Medical history

1. Age of onset of diabetes
2. Characteristics of onset (diabetic ketoacidosis or symptoms of hyperglycemia or symptomatic routine blood test)
3. Medication regimen
4. Eating patterns, exercise, growth charts in children, past glycemic control and weight patterns
5. Education status, financial status and family support
6. Assessment of knowledge on diabetes, SMBG, injection technique, hypoglycemia, hyperglycemia and sick-day rules
7. Hypoglycemia—review the frequency, severity, causes and treatment
8. History of microvascular and macrovascular complications, psychosocial issues, contraception use, desire for pregnancy for those in the child-bearing age
9. Smoking, alcohol consumption and drug abuse
10. Other intercurrent illness.

Clinical examination and assessment

- Initial assessment
- Annual evaluation:

1. Comprehensive foot exam, based on age (begin in teenagers with diabetes since childhood)
2. Retinal examination

   A dilated comprehensive fundus examination once the child reaches puberty, or age >10 years, whichever is earlier or duration of diabetes 3–5 years

   If Yes.

   More frequently based on the severity of retinopathy. Treatment involves control of diabetes, hypertension, cholesterol, smoking cessation and photocoagulation or interventions by the retinal specialist as and when needed.
3. Diabetes self-management
4. C-peptide

   If Yes at the time of diagnosis of diabetes

   GADA, IA2A, ZNT8, IAA

   May be considered to establish the diagnosis of autoimmunity.
5. Lipids

   After glycemic control is achieved. If there is no family history of premature cardiovascular disease, screen once the child attains puberty or at the time of diagnosis if the child is >10 years of age.

   Yes, if abnormal

   If low-density lipoprotein (LDL) <100 mg/dL, screen every 5 years and annually once the patient reaches adulthood.

   It may be considered in those >2 years of age with a family history of premature cardiovascular disease.[1]

   Statins may be used in those with an LDL >160 mg/dL or an LDL >130 mg/dL with an additional cardiovascular risk factor after initiation of MNT and lifestyle changes.[1]
6. Thyroid-stimulating hormone

   Yes, at the diagnosis of diabetes

   Every 1–2 years if it is normal

   Supplementation with thyroxin

   Antithyroid antibodies, may be considered at the diagnosis of diabetes.

   Antibodies to diagnose celiac disease

   May be considered at diagnosis of diabetes. If patient develops symptoms

   Diet free from gluten.
7. Urine albumin—creatinine ratio

   At puberty, or age >10 years whichever is earlier, once the duration of diabetes exceeds 5 years

   Yes

   If patient is on treatment for albuminuria to assist in the titration of medication.

   Treat with an angiotensin-converting-enzyme inhibitor titrated to normalize the albumin-creatinine ratio.

Abbreviations: SMBG, self-monitoring of blood glucose; GADA, Glutamic acid decarboxylase antibodies; IA_2A, Insulinoma antigen-2 antibodies; ZNT_8, Zinc transporter-8; IAA, Insulin autoantibodies; MNT, Medical nutritional therapy.

BLOOD GLUCOSE MONITORING

Self-monitoring of Blood Glucose

Self-monitoring of blood glucose is central to the management plan. It allows patients to assess if their glycemic targets are being achieved. It helps to readjust insulin dosage to achieve targets. It helps in detecting and prevention of hypoglycemia and in readjusting insulin dosages based on the dietary patterns and degree of physical activity.

Patients with type 1 diabetes need to monitor their blood glucose prior to meal, post-prandially, at bed time, pre-exercise or postexercise and if hypoglycemia is suspected. The frequency of SMBG and timing needs to be individualized to each patient.[21,22]

Continuous Glucose Monitoring

Measurement of interstitial fluid glucose levels using a real time Continuous Glucose Monitoring (CGM) device is beneficial for patients with type 1 diabetes. Studies have demonstrated that patients with type 1 diabetes on intensive insulin therapy and CGM have recorded a lowering of HbA1c by 0.5% compared to those on intensive insulin and SMBG. This reduction in A1c was indirectly proportional to the frequency of sensor use. Newer CGM devices approved by the FDA in 2013 have the ability to suspend the delivery of insulin when the blood glucose falls below a set threshold value. The Automation to Simulate Pancreatic Response trial showed that the use of CMG devices with the "low glucose suspend" feature reduces episodes of lower nocturnal hypoglycemia without increasing HbA1c. The development of closed loop insulin devices which deliver insulin and glucagon based on real time CGM values appears to be promising technological advances.[23-27]

Insulin in Type 1 Diabetes

Administration of exogenous insulin is the treatment of choice for type 1 diabetes. This replacement can never fully mimic physiological endogenous insulin secretion and hence may lead to inadequate control. The type of insulin used and the regimen used may vary with each patient and over time. This selection is based on the affordability, lifestyle, glycemic goals and is individualized to each person with the intention of lowering blood glucose and minimizing the hypoglycemic episodes. Insulin may be delivered via a syringe, a pen or an insulin pump.

- Rapid-acting insulin analogs and short-acting insulin are administered as a premeal bolus. Rapid-acting insulin may also be administered by a continuous subcutaneous insulin infusion (CSII) via an insulin pump.
- Intermediate acting Neutral Protamine Hagedorn may be given twice a day.
- Long-acting basal insulin may be given once or twice a day.

The insulin regimen is selected based on the time to onset, peak activity, duration of action of the insulin and is individualized to match the needs of the patient. The insulin regimen may be a conventional or an intensive regimen depending on the patient, family, physician's preference and the practicality of the regimen (Box 3).[1,2,15-17,28-31]

Box 3: Insulin regimen

- Neutral Protamine Hagedorn twice a day with short/rapid-acting insulin given twice or thrice as a premeal bolus or the use of premixed insulin constitutes this regimen.
- Basal insulin is administered along with premeal and presnack boluses of short/rapid-acting insulin—multiple daily injections
- Continuous subcutaneous insulin infusion of a rapid-acting insulin via an insulin pump. Mimics physiologic insulin secretion as closely as possible.

Glycemic Control and HbA1c in Intensive Insulin Therapy

Studies have demonstrated that those on conventional therapy do not fare as well as those on intensive therapy; they also have improved glycemic control and HbA1c compared to the conventional regimen. As the intensive regimen can achieve HbA1c targets with lesser glucose variability, complications can be delayed if not prevented.

It requires more frequent SMBG, injections, titration of insulin based on exercise, premeal blood glucose levels and carbohydrate content in the food. The benefits are not attained if the patient and the family are not proactive or if they do not possess the required education/skills to understand the regimen.

Insulin Pump

Insulin delivery via a subcutaneously placed catheter is useful in the following conditions:

- Patients with recurrent hypoglycemia
- Suboptimal control of diabetes
- Micro/macrovascular complications
- Brittle diabetes
- Multiple injections compromising the lifestyle of the patient
- Pregnancy
- Rare cases of subcutaneous insulin resistance.

Insulin pumps deliver a continuous basal dose of insulin and smaller doses of boluses premeal or presnack. The catheter site needs to be changed every 3–4 days. Studies have shown that there is a further reduction in HbA1c and hypoglycemic episodes in those who are on CSII compared to the multiple daily injection intensive regimens. However, patients on CSII are not exempt from SMBG and the frequency of SMBG may even increase. Patients using insulin pumps with real time CGMS, which is called sensor augmented pump therapy, can achieve greater reductions in A1c based on the frequency of the sensor usage.

The added "low glucose suspend threshold" which features in the recently approved pumps can further reduce hypoglycemia without worsening of A1c. The "artificial pancreas", which is a bihormonal closed-loop device, has shown promising results; though further study indicated before such devices are commercially introduced.[1]

Disadvantages of an Insulin Pump[1,29-31]

- Expensive—the cost of the pump, insulin, lancets, blood sugar monitoring strips, consumables and frequent health visits needs to be considered.
- Patient and family need to be proactive, educated and need to adhere to the treatment plan.
- As patients are on a short- or preferably a rapid-acting insulin, pump failure can lead to sudden ketoacidosis as there is no subcutaneous depot of basal insulin available.
- Infection at the site of subcutaneous insertion.

DOSE OF INSULIN

A patient with type 1 diabetes may need 0.5–1 unit/kg. It may vary with the age, with the pubertal stage of the child and during periods of stress, infection or ketoacidosis.[1]

Honeymoon Phase

A few patients following the diagnosis of type 1 diabetes and initiation of treatment with insulin experience recurrent episodes of hypoglycemia and a reduction of their insulin dosage. This is due to the production of endogenous insulin in the remaining beta cells. The exact duration of this phase is unknown. Rise in blood sugar levels, HbA1c and increase in the insulin requirement indicate that the honeymoon phase is over.

Inhaled Insulin

An inhaled dry powder formulation of insulin was approved by the FDA in 2014. This inhaled insulin is an ultra-rapid-acting insulin, onset of action in about 10–15 minutes, peak at 60 minutes and duration of 2–3 hours. It is indicated in type 1 diabetes in addition to basal insulin in those who are more than 18 years of age, without asthma, chronic obstructive pulmonary disease, cough, DKA or pregnancy. The risk if hypoglycemia and weight gain were found to be lower when compared to injectable insulin. This is not yet available commercially. However, it broadens the options available in the management of type 1 diabetes.

Other Modalities of Treatment

Metformin

Metformin alone has not been proven to be effective in children with type 1 diabetes. There are studies that show that it may be beneficial in improving glycemic control in addition to insulin in those who are overweight or obese. However, stronger evidence from larger studies is required before this can be recommended.[1,32]

Incretin-based Treatment

GLP-1 analogs and DPP4 inhibitors are being studied in patients with type 1 diabetes. A few studies have shown improvement in prandial blood sugar and increase in satiety. However, GLP-1 analogs are not yet FDA approved modality of treatment for type 1 diabetes studies are underway.

SGLT-2 Inhibitors

Though studies are sparse and not yet approved for type 1 diabetes, SGLT-2 inhibitors are likely to be the first oral antidiabetic agents for treatment of type 1 diabetes as their mechanism of action is independent of insulin.[33] Remogliflozin etabonate, an inhibitor of the sodium-glucose transporter 2, was found to be safe when administered with insulin in type 1 diabetes and reduces plasma glucose concentrations compared with placebo.[33]

Transplantation

Solid organ pancreas transplantation simultaneously in those who require a kidney transplant is the current recommendation by the ADA. Simultaneous pancreas kidney (SPK) transplants have a greater durability and function in comparison to a pancreas after kidney (PAK) transplant. Patients need lifelong immunosuppression. Islet cell transplant is an option for those who are not candidates for solid organ procedures. Most procedures are done for research purposes as an experiment and there is always a risk of autoimmunity setting in, in the transplanted organ.[1]

Nutrition

Consultation with a dietician, carbohydrate counting, formulation of a comprehensive meal plan and follow up of the height, weight, growth charts and BMI are the important part of the management plan during childhood.

Exercise

All children must be encouraged to participate in sports for an hour daily. The risk of hypoglycemia with excess physical activity during or even hours after the exercise should be explained to the patient. The school authorities or the coach should be taught to recognize and treat hypoglycemia. Frequent SMBG before, during or after exercise is recommended. Patients with a blood sugar less than 100 mg/dL prior to exercise should eat a snack before engaging in the sport. Exercise in stressful situations can also trigger hyperglycemia.[1,2]

Psychosocial Issues

Adolescents may suffer from eating disorders, depression and conflicts with family members over the need for increased autonomy and must be referred to a mental health specialist.[1,34]

HYPOGLYCEMIA

Patient education, SMBG and adjustment of insulin dosage based on food and exercise, is essential. Hypoglycemia can be a limiting factor in achieving glycemic targets. Recurrent hypoglycemia can lead to hypoglycemic unawareness due to autonomic failure or reduced sympathetic and adrenergic feedback. This unawareness can be reversed by avoidance of hypoglycemia. 15 g of glucose orally is the treatment for all patients who are conscious. Repeat SMBG after 15 minutes and repetition of the treatment is advised if hypoglycemia persists. If glucose is not available, patient may consume any carbohydrate. Glucagon injections may be prescribed for severe hypoglycemia and the family must be instructed on its usage. Patients with severe hypoglycemia and loss of consciousness should be shifted to the nearest hospital. Severe hypoglycemia in the hospital should be treated with intravenous dextrose.[1,2,35]

SICK-DAY RULES[1,2]

- Increase the frequency of SMBG.
- Continue intake of food and fluids.
- Never skip insulin, unless the patient is vomiting or is unable to eat. In such situations, based on the blood sugar level, insulin may be reduced to prevent hypoglycemia after contacting the healthcare provider.
- Short-acting insulin may be omitted and the dose of the basal/intermediate-acting insulin may be decreased by 10–20% of the total daily dose.
- Rest and supervision by parents.
- Treatment of underlying infection.
- Constant contact with the patient's physician is a must and hospital-based care to be instituted when required.

CONCLUSION

Treatment of type 1 diabetes is challenging and requires a coordinated effort from the multidisciplinary healthcare team. Age-based care, continuous patient education, family support, frequent SMBG, titration of insulin based on dietary patterns and exercise, screening for complications and regular follow up are essential.

REFERENCES

1. Chiang JL, Kirkman MS, Laffel LM, et al; Type 1 Diabetes Sourcebook Authors. Type 1 diabetes through the life span: a position statement of the American Diabetes Association. Diabetes Care. 2014;37:2034-54.
2. American Diabetes Association. Standards of medical care in diabetes. Diabetes Care 2014;37: S14-80.
3. Silverstein J, Klingensmith G, Copeland K, et al. Care of children and adolescents with type 1 diabetes: a statement of the American Diabetes Association. Diabetes Care. 2005;28:186.
4. Haas L, Maryniuk M, Beck J, et al. National Standards for Diabetes Self-Management Education and Support. Diabetes Care. 2014;37 (Suppl.1):S144-53.
5. Holmes GK. Coeliac disease and type 1 diabetes mellitus—the case for screening. Diabet Med. 2001;18:169-77.
6. Rewers M, Liu E, Simmons J, et al. Celiac disease associated with type 1 diabetes mellitus. Endocrinol Metab Clin North Am. 2004;33:197-214.
7. Kordonouri O, Deiss D, Danne T, et al. Predictivity of thyroid autoantibodies for the development of thyroid disorders in children and adolescents with type 1 diabetes. Diabet Med. 2002;19:518-21.
8. Peters A, Laffel L; American Diabetes Association Transitions Working Group. Diabetes care for emerging adults: recommendations for transition from pediatric to adult diabetes care systems: a position statement of the American Diabetes Association, with representation by the American College of Osteopathic Family Physicians, the American Academy of Pediatrics, the American

Association of Clinical Endocrinologists, the American Osteopathic Association, the Centers for Disease Control and Prevention, Children with Diabetes, The Endocrine Society, the International Society for Pediatric and Adolescent Diabetes, Juvenile Diabetes Research Foundation International, the National Diabetes Education Program, and the Pediatric Endocrine Society (formerly Lawson Wilkins Pediatric Endocrine Society). Diabetes Care. 2011;34:2477-85.

9. Ryan CM, Becker DJ. Hypoglycemia in children with type 1 diabetes mellitus. Risk factors, cognitive function, and management. Endocrinol Metab Clin North Am. 1999;28:883.
10. Perantie DC, Lim A, Wu J, et al. Effects of prior hypoglycemia and hyperglycemia on cognition in children with type 1 diabetes mellitus. Pediatr Diabetes. 2008;9:87.
11. Pattison HM, Moledina S, Barrett TG. The relationship between parental perceptions of diabetes and glycaemic control. Arch Dis Child. 2006;91:487.
12. Grey M, Cameron ME, Lipman TH, et al. Psychosocial status of children with diabetes in the first 2 years after diagnosis. Diabetes Care. 1995;18:1330.
13. Cameron FJ, Northam EA, Ambler GR, et al. Routine psychological screening in youth with type 1 diabetes and their parents: a notion whose time has come? Diabetes Care. 2007;30:2716.
14. Wu YP, Hilliard ME, Rausch J, et al. Family involvement with the diabetes regimen in young people: the role of adolescent depressive symptoms. Diabet Med. 2013;30:596.
15. The Diabetes Control and Complications Trial Research Group. The effect of intensive treatment of diabetes on the development and progression of long-term complications in insulin-dependent diabetes mellitus. N Engl J Med. 1993;329:977-86.
16. The Diabetes Control and Complications Trial/Epidemiology of Diabetes Interventions and Complications Research Group. Retinopathy and nephropathy in patients with type 1 diabetes four years after a trial of intensive therapy. N Engl J Med. 2000;342:381-9.
17. Martin CL, Albers J, Herman WH, et al.; DCCT/EDIC Research Group. Neuropathy among the diabetes control and complications trial cohort 8 years after trial completion. Diabetes Care. 2006;29:340-4.
18. Cato MA, Mauras N, Ambrosino J, et al.; Diabetes Research in Children Network (DirecNet). Cognitive functioning in young children with type 1 diabetes. J Int Neuropsychol Soc. 2014;20: 238-47.
19. Marzelli MJ, Mazaika PK, Barnea-Goraly N, et al.; Diabetes Research in Children Network (DirecNet). Neuroanatomical correlates of dysglycemia in young children with type 1 diabetes. Diabetes. 2014;63:343-53.
20. Donaghue KC, Fairchild JM, Craig ME, et al. Do all prepubertal years of diabetes duration contribute equally to diabetes complications? Diabetes Care. 2003;26:1224-9.
21. Rewers M, Pihoker C, Donaghue K, et al. Assessment and monitoring of glycemic control in children and adolescents with diabetes. Pediatr Diabetes. 2009;10 Suppl 12:71.
22. Miller KM, Beck RW, Bergenstal RM, et al. Evidence of a strong association between frequency of self-monitoring of blood glucose and hemoglobin A1c levels in T1D exchange clinic registry participants. Diabetes Care. 2013;36:2009.
23. Yates K, Hasnat Milton A, Dear K, et al. Continuous glucose monitoring-guided insulin adjustment in children and adolescents on near-physiological insulin regimens: a randomized controlled trial. Diabetes Care. 2006;29:1512.
24. Bergenstal RM, Tamborlane WV, Ahmann A, et al. Effectiveness of sensor-augmented insulin-pump therapy in type 1 diabetes. N Engl J Med. 2010;363:311.
25. Ly TT, Nicholas JA, Retterath A, et al. Effect of sensor-augmented insulin pump therapy and automated insulin suspension vs standard insulin pump therapy on hypoglycemia in patients with type 1 diabetes: a randomized clinical trial. JAMA. 2013;310:1240.
26. Bergenstal RM, Klonoff DC, Garg SK, et al.; ASPIRE In-Home Study Group. Threshold-based insulin-pump interruption for reduction of hypoglycemia. N Engl J Med. 2013;369:224-32.

27. Ziegler R, Heidtmann B, Hilgard D, et al. Frequency of SMBG correlates with HbA1c & acute complications in children and adolescents with type 1 diabetes. Pediatr Diabetes. 2011;12:11.
28. Murphy NP, Keane SM, Ong KK, et al. Randomized cross-over trial of insulin glargine plus lispro or NPH insulin plus regular human insulin in adolescents with type 1 diabetes on intensive insulin regimens. Diabetes Care. 2003;26:799.
29. Phillip M, Battelino T, Rodriguez H, et al. Use of insulin pump therapy in the pediatric age-group: consensus statement from the European Society for Paediatric Endocrinology, the Lawson Wilkins Pediatric Endocrine Society, and the International Society for Pediatric and Adolescent Diabetes, endorsed by the American Diabetes Association and the European Association for the Study of Diabetes. Diabetes Care. 2007;30:1653.
30. Doyle EA, Weinzimer SA, Steffen AT, et al. A randomized, prospective trial comparing the efficacy of continuous subcutaneous insulin infusion with multiple daily injections using insulin glargine. Diabetes Care. 2004;27:1554.
31. Conwell LS, Pope E, Artiles AM, et al. Dermatological complications of continuous subcutaneous insulin infusion in children and adolescents. J Pediatr. 2008;152:622.
32. Vella S, Buetow L, Royle P, et al. The use of metformin in type 1 diabetes: a systematic review of efficacy. Diabetologia. 2010;53:809-20.
33. Mudaliar S, Armstrong DA, Mavian AA, et al. Remogliflozin etabonate, a selective inhibitor of the sodium-glucose transporter 2, improves serum glucose profiles in type 1 diabetes. Diabetes Care. 2012;35(11):2198-200.
34. de Wit M, Snoek FJ. Depressive symptoms and unmet psychological needs of Dutch youth with type 1 diabetes: results of a web-survey. Pediatr Diabetes. 2011;12:172.
35. Cryer PE, Davis SN, Shamoon H. Hypoglycemia in diabetes. Diabetes Care. 2003;26:1902-12.

9
CHAPTER

Management of Type 2 Diabetes Mellitus

Arpit Agrawal, Neeraj Agrawal

INTRODUCTION

Diabetes is a complex, chronic illness requiring continuous medical care with multifactorial risk-reduction strategies beyond glycemic control. Ongoing patient self-management education and support are critical to preventing acute complications and reducing the risk of long-term complications. Significant evidence exists that supports a range of interventions to improve diabetes outcomes.

General practitioners continue to provide most of the medical care to people with type 2 diabetes. The complexity of care for this common disease requires systematic care from the practice team and the timely referral to community and hospital-based specialists. Management of the person with diabetes requires the skills of several professionals (general practitioner, specialist physician, diabetes educator, podiatrist, dietitian, ophthalmologist or optometrist, exercise professional and dentist) and the active participation of the patient. The aim of this chapter is to provide guidelines for management of type 2 diabetes.

The underlying aim is improvement in the duration and quality of life of patients.

1. Encourage patients to participate and take an active role in the management of their diabetes.
2. Ensure that all other preventive healthcare activities are included, while maintaining good diabetes healthcare.
3. Any guideline should be flexible: Management takes into consideration the patient's age, educational level, cultural background, the current scientific knowledge, the availability of resources and the range of particular preferences of the patient and professionals involved.
4. The overall goals in degree of control and lifestyle modification must be realistic.
5. Education of a partner or other responsible carers is an important factor in maintaining positive lifestyle changes in a patient. Similarly the general practitioner can ensure that management is individualized to the person's cultural, educational and financial status.

This chapter is intended to provide clinicians and other interested individuals with the components of diabetes care and general treatment goals with adjustments for individual preferences, comorbidities, and other patient factors. Specific issues relating to the treatment of diabetes will be highlighted in boxes throughout the chapter. The role of the general practitioner ideally involves initial diagnosis, treatment, coordination of consultant and allied professional care and continuing management (including education and counseling of the patient and carers). The current chapter plays an important role in providing a readable summary of current guidelines and recommendations from various sources on the management of type 2 diabetes in adults in the general practice setting. We hope that these guidelines will be helpful to ensure a high standard of care for the patients.

The goals of therapy for type 1 and type 2 diabetes mellitus are to:

- Eliminate symptoms related to hyperglycemia
- Reduce or eliminate the long-term microvascular and macrovascular complications of diabetes mellitus
- Allow the patient to achieve as normal a lifestyle as possible.

Update: The ADA (2015 Guidelines) now recommends a premeal blood glucose target of 80–130 mg/dL rather than 70–130 mg/dL, to better reflect new data comparing average actual glucose levels with A1C targets.

ADA 2015 recommendations for pharmacological therapy in type 2 diabetes:

1. Metformin, if not contraindicated, and if tolerated is the preferred initial pharmacological agent for type 2 diabetes (Fig. 1). (Level A)
2. In patients with newly diagnosed type 2 diabetes and markedly symptomatic and/or elevated blood glucose/A1C consider initiating insulin therapy with/without additional agents. (Level E)
3. If noninsulin monotherapy at maximum tolerated dose does not achieve or maintain the A1C target over 3 months, add a second oral agent, a glucagon-like peptide-1 (GLP-1) agonist or basal insulin. (Level E)
4. A patient-centered approach should be used to guide choice of pharmacological agents. Considerations include efficacy, cost, potential comorbidities, hypoglycemia risk and patient preferences. (Level E)
5. Due to progressive nature of type 2 diabetes, insulin therapy is eventually indicated for many patients with type 2 diabetes. (Level B).

MEDICAL NUTRITION THERAPY IN DIABETES

Goals for Nutrition Therapy in Type 2 Diabetes

1. To promote and support healthful eating patterns, emphasizing a variety of nutrient-dense foods in appropriate portion sizes, in order to improve overall health and specifically to—(A) Attain individualized glycemic, blood pressure and lipid goals; (B) Achieve and maintain body weight goals; (C) Delay or prevent complications of diabetes.
2. To address individual nutrition needs based on personal and cultural preferences, health literacy and numeracy, access to healthful food choices, willingness and ability to make behavioral changes, and barriers to change.
3. To maintain the pleasure of eating by providing positive messages about food choices while limiting food choices only when indicated by scientific evidence.
4. To provide the individuals with diabetes with practical tools for day-to-day meal planning rather than focusing on individual macronutrients, micronutrients and single food.

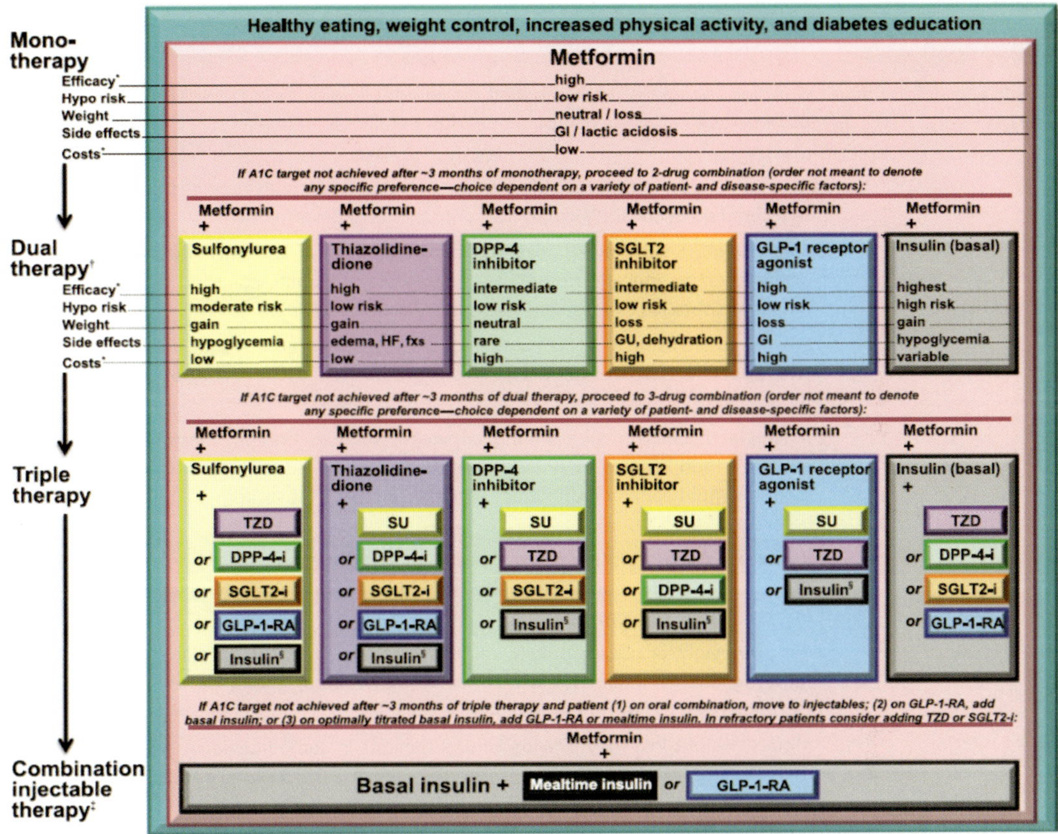

Fig. 1: Antihyperglycemic therapy in type 2 diabetes: general recommendedations (15). The order in the chart was determined by historical availability and the route of administration, with injectables to the right; it is not meant to denote any specific preference. Potential sequences of antihyperglycemic therapy for patients with type 2 diabetes are displayed, with the usual transition moving vertically from top to bottom (although horizontal movement within therapy stages is also possible, depending on the circumstances). DPP-4-i, DPP-4 inhibitor; fxs, fractures; GI, gastrointestinal; GLP-1-RA, GLP-1 receptor agonist; GU, genitourinary; HF, heart failure; Hypo, hypoglycemia; SGLT2-i, SGLT2 inhibitor; SU, sulfonylurea; TZD, thiazolidinedione. * See ref. 15 for description of efficacy categorization. † Consider starting at his stage when A1C is ≥ 9%. ‡ Consider starting at this stage when blood glucose is ≥300-350 mg/dL (16.7-19.4 mmol/L) and/or A1C is ≥ 10-12%, especially if symptomatic or catabolic features are present, in which case basal insulin + mealtime insulin is the preferred initial regimen. § Usually a basal insulin (NPH, glargine, detemir, degludec). Adapted with permission from Inzucchi et al. (15)

Nutrition therapy recommendations

Topic	*Recommendations*	*Evidence rating*
Effectiveness of nutrition therapy	Nutrition therapy is recommended for all people with type 1 and type 2 diabetes as an effective component of the overall treatment plan.	A
	Individuals who have diabetes should receive individualized medical nutrition therapy (MNT) to achieve treatment goals, preferably provided by a registered dietitian familiar with the components of diabetes MNT.	A
	For individuals with type 1 diabetes, participation in an intensive, flexible insulin therapy education program using the carbohydrate-counting meal planning approach can result in improved glycemic control.	A
	For individuals using fixed daily insulin doses, consistent carbohydrate intake with respect to time and amount can result in improved glycemic control and reduce hypoglycemia risk.	B
	A simple diabetes meal planning approach, such as portion control or healthful food choices, may be better suited to individuals with type 2 diabetes with health and numeracy literacy concerns. This strategy also may be effective for older adults.	C
	Because diabetes nutrition therapy can result in cost saving B and improved outcomes (e.g. A1C reduction) A, MNT should be adequately reimbursed by insurance and other payers. E	B, A, E
Energy balance	For overweight or obese adults with type 2 diabetes or at risk for diabetes, reducing energy intake while maintaining a healthful eating pattern is recommended to promote weight loss.	A
	Modest weight loss may provide clinical benefits in some individuals with diabetes, especially those early in the disease process. To Achieve modest weight loss, intensive lifestyle interventions with ongoing support are recommended.	A
Eating patterns and macronutrient distribution	Evidence suggests that there is not an ideal percentage of calories from carbohydrate, protein, and fat for all people with diabetes B; therefore, macronutrient distribution should be based on individualized assessment of current eating patterns, preferences, and metabolic goals. E	B,E
	Carbohydrate amount and available insulin may be the most important factors influencing glycemic response after eating and should be considered when developing the eating plan.	A
	Monitoring carbohydrate intake, whether by carbohydrate counting or experience-based estimation, remains critical in achieving glycemic control.	B
	Carbohydrate intake from vegetables, fruits, whole grains, legumes, and dairy products should be advised over intake from other carbohydrate sources, especially those that contain added fats, sugars, or sodium.	B
	Substituting low glycemic-load foods for higher glycemic-load foods may modestly improve glycemic control.	C
	Individuals at high risk for type 2 diabetes should be encouraged to achieve the U.S. Department of Agriculture recommendation for dietary fiber (14 g fiber/1,000 kcal) and to consume foods containing whole grains (one-half of grain intake).	C

Contd...

Contd...

	While substituting sucrose-containing foods for isocaloric amounts of other carbohydrates may have similar blood glucose effects, consumption should be minimized to avoid displacing nutrient-dense food choices.	A
	People with diabetes and those at risk should limit or avoid intake of sugar-sweetened beverages to reduce risk for weight gain and worsening of cardiometabolic risk profile.	B
Protein	In individuals with type 2 diabetes, ingested protein appears to increase insulin response without increasing plasma glucose concentrations. Therefore, carbohydrate sources high in protein should not be used to treat or prevent hypoglycemia.	B
	Evidence is inconclusive regarding an ideal amount of total fat for people with diabetes; therefore, goals should be individualized. C Fat quality appears to be far more important than quantity.B	C, B
	A Mediterranean-style eating pattern, rich in monounsaturated fatty acids, may benefit glycemic control and cardiovascular disease (CVD) risk factors and can therefore be recommended as an effective alternative to a lower-fat, higher-carbohydrate eating pattern.	B
Dietary fat	Increased consumption of foods containing long-chain omega-3 fatty acids (EPA and DHA), such as fatty fish, and omega-3 linolenic acid (ALA) is recommended.	B
	The consumption of fish (particularly fatty fish) at least two times (two servings) per week is recommended.	B
	The amount of dietary saturated fat, cholesterol, and trans fat recommended for people with diabetes is the same as that recommended for the general population.	C
	Evidence does not support recommending omega-3 supplements for people with diabetes for the prevention or treatment of cardiovascular events.	A
Micronutrients and herbal supplements	There is no clear evidence of benefit from vitamin or mineral supplementation in people with diabetes who do not have underlying deficiencies	
	Routine supplementation with antioxidants, such as vitamin E and C and carotene, is not advised due to insufficient evidence of efficacy and concerns related to long-term safety.	C
	There is sufficient evidence to support and routine use of micronutrients such as chromium, magnesium, and vitamin D to improve glycemic control in people with diabetes.	C
	There is insufficient evidence to support the use of cinnamon or other herbs/ supplements for the treatment of diabetes.	E
	It is recommended that individualized meal planning include optimization of food choices to meet recommended dietary allowance/dietary reference intake for all micronutrients.	E
Alcohol	If adults with diabetes choose to drink alcohol, they should be advised to do so in moderation (no more than one drink per day for adult women and no more than two drinks per day for adult men).	C

Contd...

Contd...

	Alcohol consumption may place people with diabetes at an increased risk for delayed hypoglycemia, especially if taking insulin or insulin secretagogues. Education and awareness regarding the recognition and management of delayed hypoglycemia are warranted.	B
Sodium	The recommendation for the general population to reduce sodium to less than 2,300 mg/day is also appropriate for people with diabetes.	B
	For individuals with both diabetes and hypertension, further reduction in sodium intake should be individualized.	B

ORAL ANTIDIABETIC AGENTS

History

The birth of oral antidiabetic agents dates back to the year 1926 when the guanidine derivative synthalin was given orally to treat diabetes mellitus for the first time. Subsequently, a sulfonylurea derivative (2254 RP) was found to have a significant hypoglycemic effect, a serendipitous observation. The sulfonylurea used in therapy since 1965, are all derived from this compound 2254 RP (glyprothiazole).

Drugs and their mode of action	
Mode of action	***Drugs***
1. Insulin secretagogues	a. Sulfonylurea b. Meglitinides c. Glucagon-like peptide-1 analogs
2. Insulin sensitizers	a. Biguanides b. Thiazolidinediones
3. Inhibitors of gastrointestinal (GI) glucose absorption	a. α-glucosidase inhibitors b. Amylin analogs
4. Insulin-mimetic agents	a. Insulin analogs

Biguanides (Metformin)

Mechanism of Action

- Reduction of excessive hepatic glucose output
- Stimulation of insulin mediated muscle glucose uptake (glycogen synthesis)
- Inhibition of lipolysis and of free fatty acid availability.

At Cellular Level

- Increased insulin binding
- Stimulation of insulin receptor tyrosine kinase activity
- Enhanced glucose transport (GLUT-4)
- Increased glycogen synthase (Fig. 2).

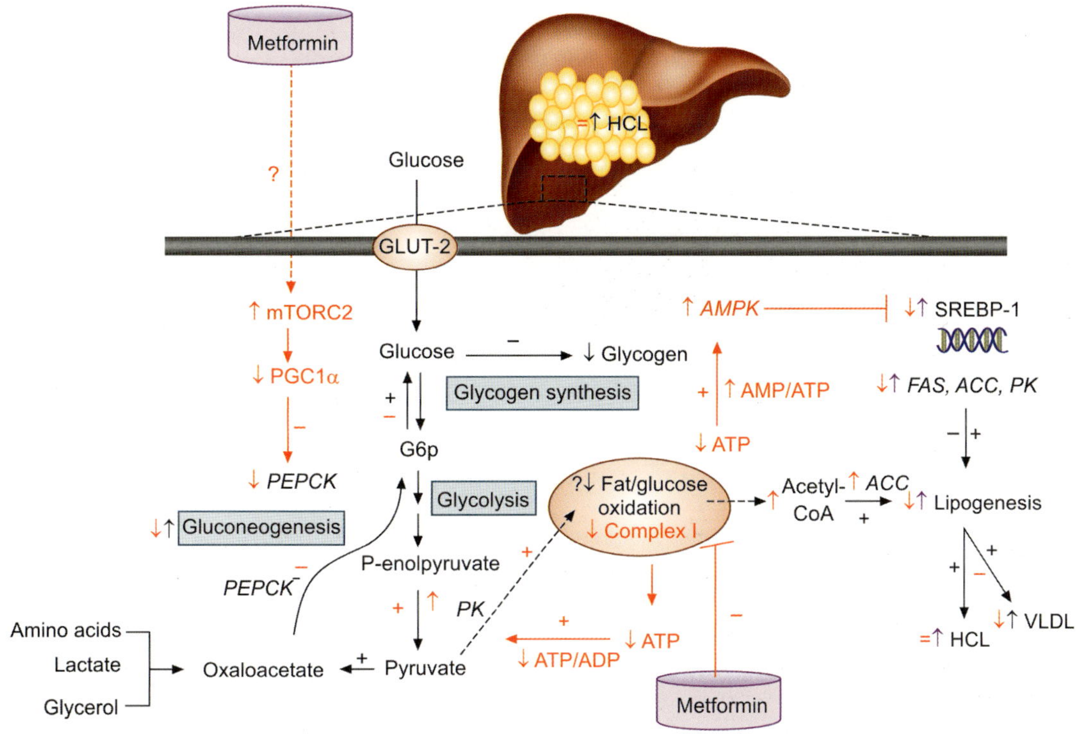

Fig. 2: Cellular effects of metformin. Black arrows/lines represent the metabolic situation in type 2 diabetes with increased endogenous glucose production (EGP) accompanied by greater hepatocellular gluconeogenesis, lipid content (HCL) and lower muscle glucose uptake. Red arrows/lines indicate metformin effects resulting from inhibition of mitochondrial complex I in liver and activation of AMPK in skeletal muscle and liver.

Abbreviations: ACC, acyl-CoA synthetase; G6P, glucose-6-phosphate; FAS, fatty acyl-CoA synthetase; mTORC2, mammalian target of rapamycin 2; PEPCK, phosphoenolpyruvate carboxykinase; PK, pyruvate kinase; PGC1α, PPARγ, Co-activator 1γα; SREBP, sterol regulatory element-binding protein; TG, triglyceride; VLDL, very-low density lipoprotein

Metformin decreases plasma glucose by an average of 25%. It reduces both fasting and postprandial blood glucose levels. Metformin in pharmacological doses does not reduce basal blood glucose concentration below the physiologic range in either diabetic or nondiabetic animals or humans, a distinct advantage over sulfonylureas. Hence, it is considered as an antihyperglycemic agent rather than a hypoglycemic agent. It lowers triglycerides by decreasing hepatic triglyceride synthesis.

Metformin activates AMP-dependent protein kinase and enters cells through organic cationic transporters (polymorphisms of these may influence response to metformin). Recent evidence indicates that metformin's mechanism for reducing hepatic glucose production is to antagonize glucagon's ability to generate cyclic adenosine monophosphate (cAMP) in hepatocytes. Metformin also has a favorable effect on fibrinolysis and platelet aggregation and causes weight loss.

Drugs

Metformin is available as 250 mg, 500 mg, 850 mg and 1 g tablets.

Indications

- Obese type 2 diabetes refractory to dietary treatment.
- Secondary failure to sulfonylureas.
- Type 2 diabetes patients with marked liability to blood glucose (brittle diabetes) can be stabilized by the addition of metformin.
- To reduce insulin requirements in case of true insulin resistance.
- Polycystic ovarian disease.
- Nonalcoholic steatohepatitis.

Contraindications

- Renal insufficiency (serum creatinine >1.5 mg/dL in men, >1.4 mg/dL in women; glomerular filtration rate <60 mL/min).
- Unstable congestive heart failure.
- Liver disease [serum transaminases >3 times upper limit of normal (ULN)].
- Severe hypoxemia.
- Type 1 diabetes.
- Patients with alcohol dependency or history of excessive alcohol intake.

Adverse Effects

- Common: Gastrointestinal—about 20% experience anorexia, nausea, vomiting and diarrhea, metallic taste and abdominal discomfort.
- Vitamin B12 malabsorption at doses 2000 mg or more.
- Lactic acidosis (rare).

Because of its relatively slow onset of action and gastrointestinal symptoms at higher doses, the initial dose should be low and then escalated every 2–3 weeks based on self-monitoring of blood glucose measurements.

Thiazolidinediones

Thiazolidinediones reduce insulin resistance by binding to PPAR-γ (peroxisome proliferator-activated receptor gamma) nuclear receptor (which forms a heterodimer with retinoid X receptor). The PPAR-γ receptor is found in highest level in adipocytes.*

Metabolic Effects of Thiazolidinediones

Adipose tissue

- Promote adipocyte differentiation
- Reduce hepatic fat accumulation

---

* The drugs under trial in this group are muraglitazar, tesaglitazar and ragaglitazar. They are supposed to have dual PPAR-γ and PPAR-γ agonist and simultaneously control glucose and lipid metabolism.

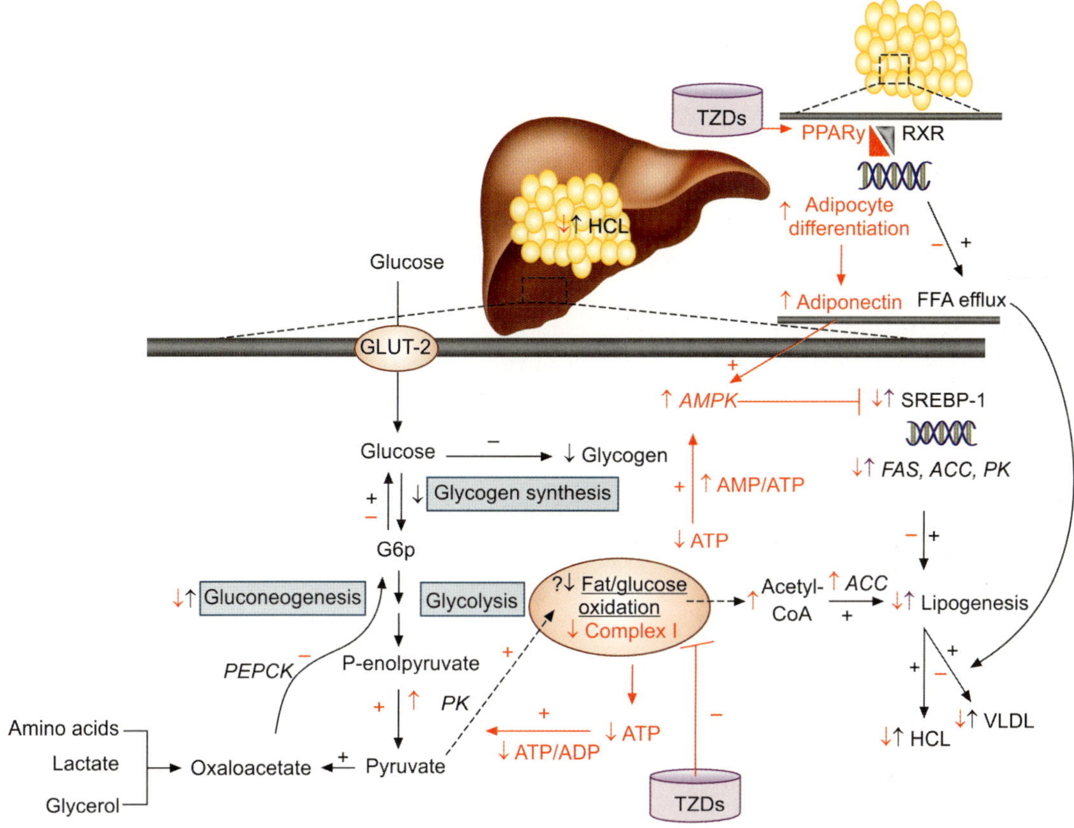

Fig. 3: Cellular effects of thiazolidinediones (TZD). Black arrows/lines represent the metabolic situation in type 2 diabetes with increased endogenous glucose production (EGP) accompanied by greater hepatocellular gluconeogenesis, lipid content (HCL) and free fatty acids (FFA) flux from adipose tissue. Red arrows/lines indicate TZD effects resulting from chronic PPARγ-mediated adipose tissue remodeling and increased adiponectin secretion. Direct TZDs inhibitory effect on Mitochondrial complex I activates 5′ AMP-activated protein kinase (AMPK).

Abbreviations: ACC, Acyl-CoA synthetase: aP2, adipocyte fatty acid binding protein; FAS, fatty acyl-CoA synthetase; FATP, fatty-acid transporter protein; PGC1α, PPARγ, co-activator 1γα; PK, pyruvate kinase; SREBP-1, sterol regulatory element-binding protein 1; TG, triglyceride; VLDL, very low density-lipoportein

- Promote fatty acid storage
- Redistribution of fat from central to peripheral location.

Circulating insulin levels decrease with the use of thiazolidinediones, indicating a decrease in insulin resistance. Pioglitazone has been shown to reduce inflammatory markers of atherosclerosis. Although, pioglitazone causes pedal edema and weight gain, studies have shown that low dose 7.5 mg/day is safe and efficacious compared to 15 mg/day dosing (Fig. 3).

Therapeutic Applications

- Important 2nd/3rd line Oral hypoglycemic agents (OHA).
- Potential single daily dose
- Decreases arterial blood pressure minimally

- Progressive increase in *high-density lipoprotein*
- Safer in moderate to severe renal failure
- Decreases microalbuminuria
- Decreases vascular intimal thickening.

Troglitazone

Withdrawn from the market due to reports of hepatotoxicity. FDA recommends measurement of liver function tests prior to initiating therapy.

Rosiglitazone

Rosiglitazone has been banned due to its adverse effects on cardiovascular system, i.e. increased incidence of myocardial infarction and heart failure.

Dosage

The starting dose of pioglitazone is 7.5 mg once daily and may be increased on follow up to 30 mg/day.

Adverse Effects

- Weight gain
- Peripheral edema and congestive heart failure
- FDA has launched an alert that rare patients with this agent may experience worsening of diabetic macular edema
- Increased risk of bony fractures
- Glitazones should not be used in patients with active hepatocellular disease and those with unexplained Alkaline transferase (ALT) levels >2.5 times of ULN
- US FDA recommends not to use pioglitazone in patients with active bladder cancer. Use pioglitazone with caution in patients with a prior history of bladder cancer.

Treatment goals for adults with diabetes[a]	
Index	***Goal***
Gycemic control[b]	
HbA_{1c}	<7.0%[c]
Preprandial capillary plasma glucose	4.4–7.2 mmol/L (80–130 mg/dL)
Peak postprandial capillary plasma glucose[d]	<10.0 mmol/L (<180 mg/dL)
Blood pressure	**<140/90 mm Hg**[e]
Lipids[f]	
Low-density lipoprotein	<2.6 mmol/L (100 mg/dL)[g]
High-density lipoprotein	>1 mmol/L (40 mg/dL) in men
	> 1.3 mmol/L (50 mg/dL) in women
Triglycerides	**<1.7 mmol/L (150 mg/dL)**

Contd...

Contd...

[a]As recommended by the American Diabetes Association; goals should be individualized for each patient (see text). Goas may be different for certain patient populations.[b] HbA_{1c} is primary goal.[c] Diabetes Control and Complications Trial-based assay.[d] 1–2 h after beginning of a meal.[e] Goal of <130/80 mmHg may be appropriate for younger individuals. [f]In decreasing order of priority. Recent guidelines from the American College of Cardiology and American Heart Association no longer advocate specific LDL and HDL goals.[g] Goal of <1.8 mmol/L (70 mg/dL) may be appropriate for individual with cardiovascular disease.

Abbreviation: HbA_{1c}, hemoglobin A1c
Source: Adapted from American Diabetes Association Diabetes Care 38(Suppl 1):S1. 2015.

INSULIN SECRETAGOGUES

Sulfonylureas

Insulin secretagogues stimulate insulin secretion by interacting with the adenosine triphosphate (ATP)-sensitive potassium channel on the beta cell (Fig. 4).

Sulfonylureas augment insulin response by binding to the receptor on the extracellular domain of ATP modulated potassium channels and causes its closure. This depolarizes the membrane leading to the entry of calcium through voltage dependent calcium channels and the resultant increase in intracellular calcium concentrations leading to fusion of insulin containing vesicles to the plasma membrane and subsequent rapid exocytosis of insulin from beta cells. In addition to this, some sulfonylureas are now known to directly activate the cAMP sensor Epac2 (exchange protein activated by cAMP 2) to induce Rap1 signaling which can induce the exocytosis of insulin containing vesicles.

First generation sulfonylureas, like glibenclamide, prevent cardioprotection induced by ischemia by interacting with mitochondrial KATP channels, whereas second generation sulfonylureas are thought not to interfere with ischemia preconditioning.

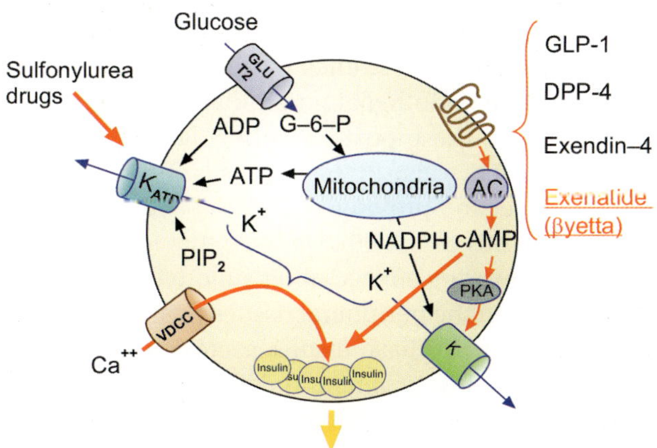

Source: ***Modified from:** PE Macdonald, MR Wheeler, Diabetologia. 2003; 48:1047-62 Holz, George, Diabetes. 2004; 53:5-13.

Fig. 4: Showing mechanisms of action of both insulin and exenatide

First Generation Sulfonylureas—(Not Available)

- Tolbutamide (short-acting)—dose 250–3000 mg/day in divided doses.
- Chlorpropamide (long-acting)—dose 50–5000 mg/day.

Second Generation Sulfonylureas

- Glibenclamide: 1.25–20 mg/day
- Glipizide: 2.5–40 mg/day
- Gliclazide: 80-240 mg/day.

Third Generation Sulfonylureas

Glimepiride: 1–8 mg/day short-term administration of sulfonylureas results in enhanced insulin release while paradoxically insulin biosynthesis is inhibited. The sulfonylureas during short-term treatment prime the beta cells and make them responsive to glucose stimulus (beta-cytotropic effect). On the other hand, chronic administration of sulfonylureas does not result in enhanced insulin release but the extra-pancreatic effect of increase in the number of receptors, an augmented post-receptor effect and increased insulin sensitivity manifests. The beneficial effect on the receptors also occurs during the short-term sulfonylurea therapy.

Therapeutic Applications

- *Glibenclamide*: Glibenclamide is also believed to result in release of duodenal insulin releasing agent (DIRA—a gut factor) which is probably responsible for the sustained effect of the drug. The incidence of secondary failure to glibenclamide is remarkably low.
- *Glipizide*: Its short duration of action necessitates multiple doses in a day. It results in better control of postprandial glucose. As this drug has a short duration of action and metabolized in liver, it can be used in diabetics with renal impairment.
- *Gliclazide*: It has a favorable influence over platelet aggregation and fibrinolysis. It might have a protective role in preventing the vascular complications of diabetes mellitus. Patients on gliclazide will not gain weight unlike with other sulfonylureas as the drug restores physiologic insulin secretion. Several studies have shown that gliclazide has antioxidant properties, reduces markers of endothelial inflammation, and prevents glucose mediated apoptosis of endothelial cells. These positive antioxidant effects are not confined to the vascular wall but they are effective also in the beta cells.
- *Glimepiride*: It has rapid onset and prolonged duration of action. It has more selectivity for beta cell KTP channels. It binds to the 65 kDa receptors leading to more rapid onset and longer duration of glucose lowering effects (other sulfonylureas target 140 kDa proteins). It has an insulin mimetic effect in the peripheral tissues possibly mediated by GLUT-4.
- Glimepiride does not restore first phase insulin secretion and it increases second phase insulin secretion, whole body glucose uptake and increases insulin sensitivity. Glimepiride treatment is associated with lower rates of hypoglycemia than other sulfonylureas.

Glimepiride versus Other Sulfonylureas

Glimepiride is therapeutically more advantageous because:

- It prevents postexercise insulin release and therefore has a reduced risk of hypoglycemia.

- It does not accumulate in the body with reducing renal function and its hydroxyl metabolite has negligible effects on blood glucose, hence can be safely used in mild renal failure and the elderly.
- It does not exhibit any drug interaction and due to poor binding to cardiac tissue, the interference with ischemic preconditioning as compared to other sulfonylureas.
- *Gliquidone,* which is predominantly metabolized in liver, can be used in renal impairment.
- *Glymidine,* a sulfapyrimidine derivative is useful when sensitivity to sulfonylureas should prove troublesome. Both the drugs are not available in our country. It is recommended that for better efficacy sulfonylureas be administered at least 30 minutes before food.

Sulfonylurea Failure

Primary Failure

Primary failure is when a diabetic who is strictly on a prescribed diet, with no occult or overt infection and put on maximum permissible doses of sulfonylureas, fails to achieve glycemic control within 1 month of initiation of therapy.

Secondary Failure

Secondary failure is defined as good glycemic response at least during the first month of therapy with eventual ineffectiveness. The annual reported incidence is 5–10%. Common causes of secondary failure to sulfonylureas are:

- Patient-related factors:
  - Overeating and weight gain
  - Poor patient compliance
  - Lack of physical activity
  - Stress
  - Intercurrent illness.
- Disease-related factors
  - Decreasing beta-cell function
  - Increasing insulin resistance.
- Therapy-related factors
  - Inadequate drug dosage
  - Desensitization to chronic sulfonylureas exposure
  - Impaired absorption of drugs because of hyperglycemia
  - Concomitant therapy with diabetogenic drugs (Modified from Groop et al.)

Adverse Effects and Contraindications

- Gastrointestinal—nausea, vomiting, heart burn, hepatitis and cholestasis.
- Insulin-dependent diabetes mellitus
- Pregnant women (glibenclamide was found to be safe)
- Patients with severe infections
- Allergy to sulfonylureas
- Patients with significant liver and kidney disease
- Worsening of ischemic preconditioning.

Nonsulfonylurea Secretagogues (Glinides)

- Meglitinide (Repaglinide)
- D-phenylalanine derivative (Nateglinide)

Repaglinide

Quick in onset and short-acting. It works by improving the insulin secretion in response to elevated glucose levels by regulating the ATP-sensitive potassium channels at a different binding site than sulfonylureas. Plasma half-life is less than 1 hour.

Dosage: 0.5–6 mg/day (maximum dose 16 mg/day).

The drug is given 15 minutes prior to meals. The drug should not be taken if the meal is skipped (no meal, no drug). The starting dose is 0.5 mg preprandial with each meal. The dose is doubled if control is not achieved. At least 1 week should elapse to assess the response and to increase the dose.

Nateglinide

It is faster acting than repaglinide and has a shorter duration of insulin secreting activity for postprandial glycemic control.

Dosage: 60 mg twice or thrice daily preprandial depending upon the meal pattern (maximum 360 mg/day). It is probably the only OHA that can be given in mild to moderate liver dysfunction.

Inhibitors of Gastrointestinal (GI) Tract Glucose Absorption α-glucosidase Inhibitors

- Acarbose (nitrogen containing pseudotetrasaccharide)
- Voglibose (valiolamine derivative)
- Miglitol (deoxynojirimycin derivative)
- Castanospermine (MDL 73945), an experimental compound α-glucosidase inhibitors reduce post-prandial hyperglycemia by delaying glucose absorption; they do not affect glucose utilization or insulin secretion. Therapy should be initiated at a low dose with evening meal and increased to a maximal dose over weeks to months.

Adverse Effects and Contraindications

- The major side effects (diarrhea, flatulence and abdominal distension) are related to increased delivery of oligosaccharides to the large bowel and can be reduced somewhat by gradual upward titration.
- Inflammatory bowel disease
- Gastroparesis
- Serum creatinine more than 177 μmol/L (2 mg/dL). This class of agents is not as potent as other oral agents in decreasing HbA1C levels but is unique because it reduces postprandial glucose rise even in patients with type 1 diabetes mellitus.

Dosage

- Acarbose: Started with 25 mg/day (maximum 200 mg/day)

- Miglitol: 25–200 mg/day
- Voglibose: 0.2–5 mg/day.

Bromocriptine

In vertebrates, body fat stores and insulin action are controlled by the temporal interactions of circadian neuroendocrine oscillations. Bromocriptine mesylate, an ergot derivative is a sympatholytic dopamine D2 receptor agonist that exerts inhibitory effects on serotonin turnover in the central nervous system (CNS). If administered systematically or into cerebral ventricle during early hours of the light cycle, prevents or reverses seasonal fattening insulin resistance and decreased endogenous (hepatic) glucose production in mammals.

Dosage: The recommended starting dose of bromocriptine is 0.8 mg daily and increased in 0.8 mg increments weekly until the target range (1.6 mg to 4.8 mg) or till maximal tolerance is reached. Doses should be administered once daily within 2 hours of waking in the morning and with food to reduce risk of GI adverse effects.

INSULIN THERAPY IN TYPE 2 DIABETES MELLITUS

History

Insulin since its discovery in 1921 (Banting and Best) has achieved many firsts in the field of medical research—the first protein known to have hormone action (Abel 1926); the first hormone to be sequenced (Frederick Sanger), chemically synthesized and produced by DNA recombinant technique.

Metabolic Effects of Insulin Therapy

- Reduces fasting and postprandial glucose levels
- Suppresses hepatic glucose production
- Stimulates peripheral glucose utilization
- Increases glucose oxidation/storage in skeletal muscles
- Improves abnormal lipoprotein composition
- Reduces glucotoxicity
- Improves endogenous secretory ability
- Reduces glycosylated end products.

Anticatabolic Effects of Insulin (Inhibits)

- Glycogenolysis
- Gluconeogenesis
- Fatty acid oxidation
- Ketogenesis
- Proteolysis in liver and skeletal muscle
- Amino acid output from skeletal muscle
- Lipolysis.

Rationality of Insulin in Type 2 Diabetes Mellitus

Insulin is secreted continuously by beta cells in a glucose-dependent manner throughout the day. It is also secreted in response to oral carbohydrate loads, including a large first-phase insulin release that suppresses hepatic glucose production followed by a slower second-phase insulin release that covers ingested carbohydrates.

Type 2 diabetes mellitus (T2DM) is associated with insulin resistance and slowly progressive beta-cell failure. By the time type 2 diabetes is diagnosed in patients, up to one-half of their beta cells are not functioning properly. Beta-cell failure continues at a rate of about 4% each year. Therefore, patients with type 2 diabetes often benefit from insulin therapy at some point after diagnosis.

Indications for Insulin Therapy

Insulin therapy is recommended for patients with T2DM and an initial A1C level greater than 9%, or if diabetes is uncontrolled despite optimal oral glycemic therapy. Insulin therapy may be initiated as augmentation, starting at 0.3 unit/kg, or as replacement, starting at 0.6–1.0 unit/kg. When using replacement therapy, 50% of the total daily insulin dose is given as basal, and 50% as bolus, divided up before breakfast, lunch and dinner. Augmentation therapy can include basal or bolus insulin. Replacement therapy includes basal-bolus insulin and correction or premixed insulin. Glucose control, adverse effects, cost, adherence and quality of life need to be considered when choosing therapy. Metformin should be continued if possible because it is proven to reduce all-cause mortality and cardiovascular events in overweight patients with diabetes. In a study comparing premixed, bolus and basal insulin, hypoglycemia was more common with premixed and bolus insulin, and weight gain was more common with bolus insulin. Titration of insulin over time is critical to improving glycemic control and preventing diabetes-related complications [Am Fam Physician. 2011;84(2):183-90].

Types of insulin				
	Insulin preparation	***Onset of action (Hr)***	***Peak of activity***	***Total duration of action (Hr)***
Short-acting	Regular	0.5–1	2–4	4–6
	Semilente	1–2	3–6	8–12
Intermediate-acting	Neutral Protamine Hagedorn (NPH)	3–4	10–16	20–24
	Lente	3–4	10–16	20–24
Long-acting	PZI	6–8	14–20	32
	Ultralente	6–8	14–20	32
Biphasic	Premixed (NPH + Regular	0.5	2–10	12–18
Analogs				
• Short-acting		Within a few minutes	1	4
– Lispro				
– Aspart		–	–	–

Contd...

Contd...

– Glulisine		–	–	–
• Long-acting	Peakless action for 24 hrs	–	–	–
– Glargine		–	–	–
– Detemir		–	–	–

Specific indications of insulin therapy
1. Type 1 diabetics
2. Pregnant women
3. Acute metabolic decompensation or major stress like surgery or sepsis
4. Liver and renal disease
5. Secondary diabetes (pancreatitis and corticosteroids)
6. Failure of oral antidiabetic drugs
7. Progressive complications threatening organ functions—proliferative retinopathy, maculopathy, severe neuropathy.
8. Weight loss of 10% body weight or BMI <19 kg/m^2.

Practical Aspects of Insulin Therapy

The initial dose required can roughly be taken as 0.5 U/kg for type 1 diabetes mellitus and 0.2 U/kg for T2DM. The other approximate method is to calculate the dose of intermediate-acting insulin required per day is given by the formula:

$$\frac{\textit{Fasting blood sugar—50}}{10}$$

Bolus insulin without basal insulin also commonly known as sliding scale therapy is used very commonly in hospital settings. This is associated with poor glycemic control. This does not mimic normal physiological insulin release and its use must be discouraged.

Special Situations

In certain situations, the fasting hyperglycemia may not be controlled despite increasing the dose of evening lente or neutral protamine hagedorn. This situation is referred to as "Dawn phenomenon". The fasting hyperglycemia is due secondary to early morning cortisol or growth hormone surge, or due to waning of insulin action in early hours. Here, shifting the same dose of lente insulin to bedtime is effective. Over insulinization may also result in posthypoglycemic—hyperglycemia called "Somogyi phenomenon". This can occur at any time of the day unlike Dawn phenomenon and it should be suspected if there are extreme fluctuations of blood sugar or urine sugar (+ to 4+) within the same day in the face of increasing insulin requirement. Somogyi phenomenon is due to the release of counter regulatory hormones like glucagon, catecholamines, etc. in response to hypoglycemia which the patient may not perceive.

Another situation in which extreme fluctuations in blood sugar can occur making the daily life of the patient unpleasant is "brittle diabetes". This may be true or idiopathic where no cause can be found or secondary to various causes that cause fluctuations in the blood sugar. The brittleness of diabetes itself apart from the mismatch between the usual insulin, food and exercise may be due to many other factors such as variable insulin absorption from injection sites, the residual endogenous insulin in the individual, various counter regulatory hormones imbalance or due to a neuropathic stomach in the elderly individuals (a delayed gastric emptying) and emotional disturbances.

Intensive Insulin Therapy

- *Multiple doses of insulin*: Recent reviews have shown that tight metabolic control can delay if not prevent the development of microvascular disease such as retinopathy and nephropathy as well as the neuropathic complications of diabetes. A tight control can be achieved by means of intensified conventional insulin therapy rather than by the injection regimen previously described.
- *Insulin pumps*: (A) Implantable and (B) portable implantable pumps deliver insulin into the peritoneal cavity or a central vein. They are still in experimental stages. Portable pumps provide a continuous subcutaneous insulin infusion via a thin needle that is periodically changed. There are two types of insulin infusion systems: (1) closed loop and (2) opened loop. Closed loop system requires a glucose sensor, a microprocessor and a pump (biostator). Such systems are not available at all places. In the open-loop system, there is a portable insulin infusion pump which delivers insulin at set rates as determined by the patient and physician, guided by periodic monitoring of blood glucose. These differ in size, shape, weight, insulin reservoir system and the degree of electromechanical complexity. The most common approach is to administer the regular insulin as a constant infusion throughout the day and night to mimic the basal pancreatic insulin secretion, and to give additional doses before meals (bolus doses). The dose can be changed either manually or by the program within the pump. For the pump therapy proper patient selection and education are required. Initial insulin doses calculated from the previous daily doses are usually in the range of 0.5–1 U/kg/day. The basal rate is about 40% of the total with a prebreakfast bolus of about approximately 20%, and prelunch and predinner injection of about 15% each, and 10% at bedtime.

Problems with Insulin Therapy

- Hypoglycemia
- Insulin edema
- Lipoatrophy
- Lipohypertrophy
- Insulin antibodies
- Insulin allergy
- Weight gain
- Immunologic insulin resistance

Newer Long-acting Insulin (Insulin Degludec)

Insulin degludec is new basal insulin that forms soluble multihexamer assemblies after subcutaneous injection. This results in an ultra-long action profile. It provides comparable glycemic control to insulin glaring. It might reduce dosing frequency due to its ultra-long action profile with thrice a week injections. It has a duration of action that lasts up to 40 hours.

Insulin Therapy in Future

Alternative routes of insulin therapy		
Routes	***Advantages***	***Disadvantages***
Intraperitoneal	• Portal absorption	• Pump required
	• Good bioavailability	• Catheter blockage
	• Physiological insulin profile	• Infection risk, cost
Intravenous	• Good bioavailability	• Pump required
	• Physiological insulin profile	• Catheter blockage, phlebitis
Intranasal	• Physiological insulin profile	• Interference with respiratory infection
	• Easy use	• Nasal irritation
Pulmonary	• Not available	
Transdermal	• Noninvasive	• Low bioavailability

Incretin-based Therapy

The Incretin Effect

The incretin effect seems to play a major role in the regulation of glucose metabolism in healthy subjects. "The incretin effect" implies that ingestion of carbohydrates (glucose) causes the release from the intestinal mucosa of substances that enhance insulin secretion beyond the release caused by the absorbed glucose itself.

The Incretin Hormones

Although there are probably many postprandially released hormones with an effect on insulin secretion, the available experimental evidence suggests that the two most important ones are:

- Glucose-dependent insulinotropic polypeptide
- Glucagon-like peptide-1.

Postprandially released hormones	
Glucagon-like peptide-1 (GLP-1)	***Glucose-dependent insulinotropic polypeptide (GIP)***
• GLP-1 is released from enteroendocrine L cells of intestine	• GIP is released from K cells in duodenum
• Stimulates insulin response from beta cells in a glucose-dependent manner	• Stimulates insulin response from beta cells in a glucose-dependent manner
• Inhibits gastric emptying	• GIP has a minimal effect on gastric emptying
• Inhibits glucagon secretion from alpha cells in a glucose-dependent manner	• Does not appear to inhibit glucagon secretion from alpha cells
• Reduces food intake and body weight	• GIP has no significant effect on satiety and body weight

Metformin and GLP-1 inhibit adenosine monophosphate (AMP) activated protein kinase (AMPK) in the hypothalamus and activate AMPK in peripheral tissues (Fig. 5). Hypothalamic AMPK activity is suppressed by leptin. Through metformin, low glucose-induced AMPK phosphorylation is inhibited, and the messenger ribonucleic acid expression of neuropeptide Y is suppressed in the hypothalamus. In peripheral tissues, activated AMPK inhibits 3-hydroxy-

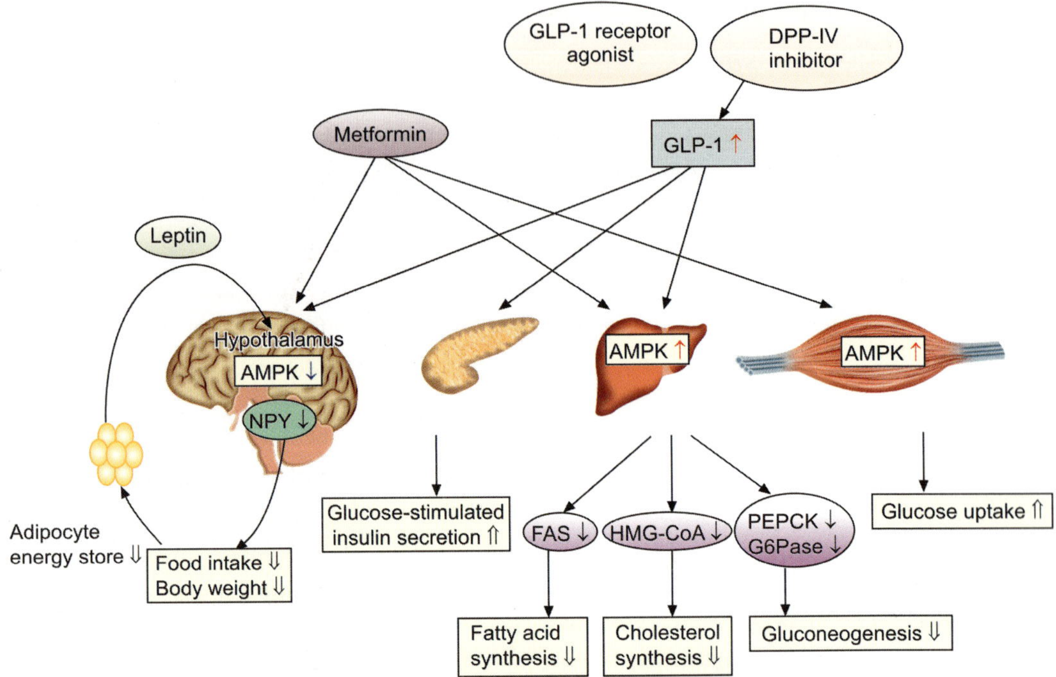

Fig. 5: Enzyme resistant glucagon-like peptide-1 (GLP-1) analog (incretin mimetic analog)

3-methylglutaryl-coenzyme A and suppresses fatty acid synthase expression, resulting in a decrease in fatty acid and cholesterol synthesis. AMPK also controls hepatic gluconeogenesis by inhibiting phosphoenolpyruvate carboxykinase and glucose-6-phosphatase. Additionally, metformin stimulates AMPK in muscle and induces glucose uptake (adapted from Indian Journal of Endocrinology and Metabolism).

Exenatide

Exenatide is a 39 amino acid peptide incretin mimetic agent that exhibits its glucoregulatory activities similar to the mammalian incretin hormone GLP-1. These actions include glucose-dependent enhancement of insulin secretion, restoration of first phase insulin response, suppression of inappropriately high glucagon secretion, slowing of gastric emptying and reduction of food intake.

Exenatide has acute effects on pancreatic beta-cell responsiveness to glucose and leads to insulin release only in the presence of elevated glucose concentrations. This insulin secretion subsides as blood glucose decreases and approach euglycemia. Exenatide's glucose-dependent enhancement of insulin secretion may be mediated by exenatide binding to the pancreatic GLP-1 receptor.

The collective glucoregulatory effects of exenatide complement the actions of existing therapies, making it an excellent treatment option for combination therapy. The effects of exenatide on the beta cell to enhance glucose-dependent insulin secretion and to restore first phase insulin secretion are unique. It is also apparently cleared in the kidneys only by glomerular filtration.

Dosage: Exenatide therapy should be initiated at 5 mcg per dose administered twice daily (bid) at any time within the 60 minute period before the morning and evening meals (or before the two main meals of the day, approximately 6 hours or more apart). Exenatide should not be administered after a meal. Based on clinical response the dose of exenatide can be increased to 10 mcg bid after 1 month of therapy.

Precautions

- Exenatide is not a substitute for insulin in insulin requiring patients.
- Exenatide should not be used in patients with type 1 diabetes or for treatment of diabetic ketoacidosis.
- The concurrent use of exenatide with insulin, thiazolidinediones, D-phenylalanine derivatives, meglitinides or alpha-glucosidase inhibitors has not been established.
- It has not been used in pediatric patients.
- It is not recommended for use with renal impairment, hepatic impairment or severe gastrointestinal disease.
- Acute pancreatitis has been reported in some patients.

Liraglutide

Liraglutide is a potent, long-acting GLP-1 analog. It has half-life of 11–13 hours making it suitable for once daily injections. The long half-life of liraglutide is believed to be based on albumin binding and an ability to form micellar-like aggregates in the subcutis, resulting in prolonged absorption and elimination as well as DPP-IV stability.

It has been proved that liraglutide provides 24-hour glycemic control. No effect of gender or age has been seen with the pharmacokinetics of liraglutide. In addition to the actions of exenatide, liraglutide has been shown to promote increased beta-cell mass in animal models of T2DM.

Liraglutide as an add-on therapy to metformin was evaluated by Nauck et al. following 5 weeks of treatment; HbA1C was significantly reduced relative to baseline in all the groups except the group receiving metformin as monotherapy.

Dosage: The starting dose is 0.6 mcg daily and the dose can be increased to 1.2 mcg. The maximum dose is 1.6 mcg/day.

Adverse Effects

- Mild nausea and vomiting which disappears after continuing the drug for 1–2 weeks.
- As a precautionary measure, liraglutide is contraindicated in any patient who has an underlying thyroid nodule or thyroid malignancy.
- The US FDA has issued a black box warning against pancreatitis for liraglutide.

Long-acting preparations of exenatide and liraglutide which can be given once a week is available in some countries.

Other drugs in this category under trial are Taspoglutide and Albiglutide.

DPP-IV Inhibitors (Incretin Enhancers)

Inhibitors of DPP-IV have also proved effective in protecting endogenous GLP-1 from degradation DPP-IV inhibitors improve beta-cell function and peripheral tissue sensitivity. This reduces both fasting and postprandial glucose concentration and thus HbA_{1C}. DPP-IV inhibitors are given orally. DPP-IV inhibitors do not cause nausea and are weight neutral. Sitagliptin can also be combined with insulin to reduce the dose requirement but this combination is not approved by FDA. (Vildagliptin has been approved to be combined with insulin).

Comparisons of DPP-IV inhibitors

Properties	***Sitagliptin***	***Saxagliptin***	***Alogliptin***	***Vildagliptin***	***Linagliptin***
Dosage	100 mg once daily	2.5, 5.0,10 mg once daily	12.5, 25 mg once daily	50 mg twice daily	5 mg daily
Half-life	12.4 hrs	2.2–3.8 hrs	12.5–21.1 hrs	2 hrs	>100 hrs
24-hr DPP-IV inhibition	80%	5 mg = 55%	25 mg = 78%	50%	80%
Elimination	Kidney (mostly unchanged)	Liver and kidney active metabolite	Kidney (mostly unchanged)	Liver and kidney	Bile (mostly unchanged)
Dose adjustments for renal impairment	Yes	Yes	Yes	None for mild impairment; for moderate to severe impairment drug not recommended	No
Selectivity for DPP-IV	>2,600-fold vs DPP-8, >10,000 fold vs DPP-9	>400-fold vs DPP-8, >100 fold vs DPP-9	>10,000 fold vs DPP-8/9	100 fold vs DPP-8, >1,000 fold vs DPP-2	>10,000 fold vs DPP-8/9
Drug interaction potential	Low	Strong CYP3A4/5 inhibitors	Low	Low	CYP3A4/5 inhibitors

Adverse effects: Upper respiratory tract infections, peripheral edema, osteoarthritis, anorexia, headache, drowsiness and dizziness

NOVEL ANTIDIABETIC DRUGS

Sodium-Glucose Cotransporter Inhibitors (SGLT-2 Inhibitors)

- All glucose excreted through glomerular filtration is subsequently reabsorbed via active transport mechanisms. Glucose transportation in the body is mainly mediated by two types of transporters—sodium-glucose linked transporters (SGLTs) and facilitative GLUTs. SGLT are members of sodium substrate co-transporters, the solute carrier family 5A (SLC5A).
- SGLT-1 and SGLT-2 have been identified that cause glucose to be reabsorbed. SGLT-2, which is found only in the proximal tubule of kidney, accounts for the most of the resorption of glucose. Almost all glucose is reabsorbed via SGLT-2 until blood glucose level reaches to its threshold value for glucose excretion. Increasing the glucose excretion by inhibiting the SGLT-2 is the novel approach for the treatment of diabetes (Fig. 6).

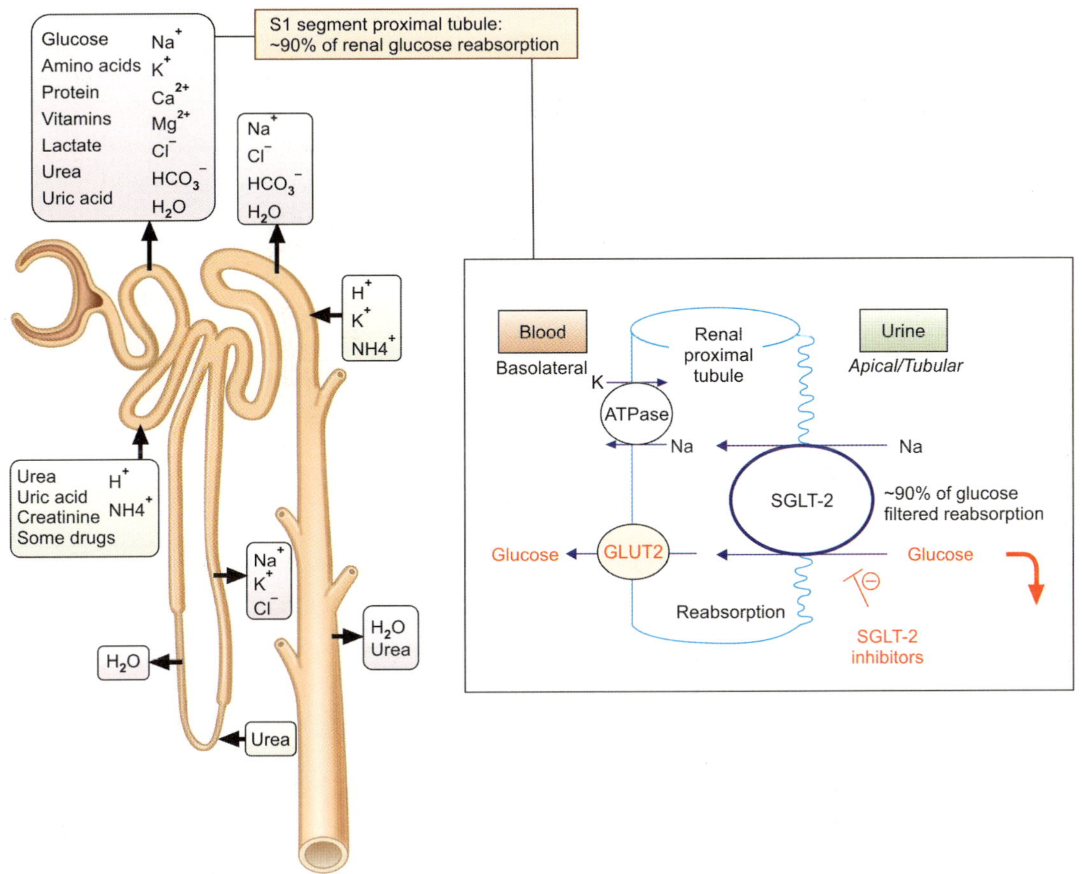

Fig. 6: Mechanism of action of SGLT-2 inhibitors

SGLT-2 inhibitors are:

- Dapagliflozin
- Canagliflozin
- Sergliflozin
- Remogliflozin etabonate
- AVE-2268
- KGT-1681
- TS-033
- YM-543

Amylin Analogs (Pramlintide)

Pramlintide, a soluble analog of amylin that does not aggregate and accumulate in islet tissue, has been shown to improve glycemic control in type 1 and type 2 diabetes when injected subcutaneously before meals (Fig. 7).

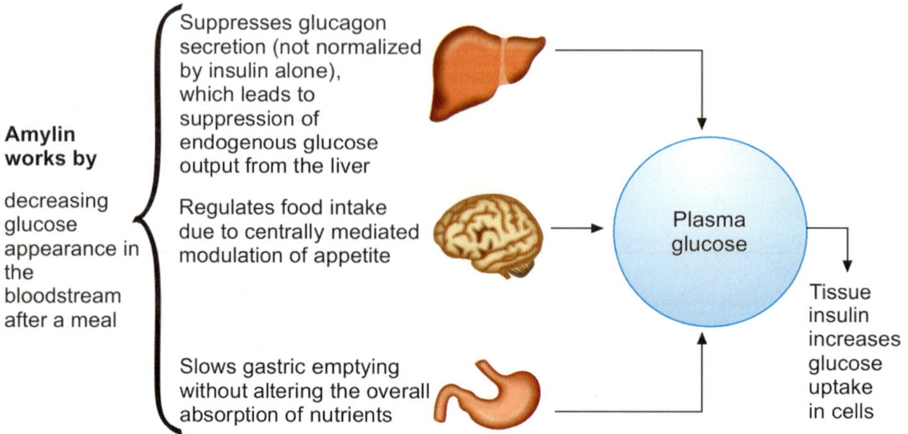

Fig. 7: Mechanism of action of amylin analogues

Physiological Actions of Amylin or Pramlintide

- Inhibition of food intake (by a central mechanism)
- Slowing of gastric motility and inhibition of gastric emptying
- Inhibition of postprandial glucagon secretion
- Suppression of postprandial hepatic glucose production
- Suppression of arginine-stimulated glucagon secretion
- Inhibition of gastric acid secretion and gastroprotection.

Administration

Diluent is injected into the vial, which the patient should agitate thoroughly to reconstitute the drug. Once in solution, the formulation can be withdrawn back into the syringe, and air bubbles should be removed. Once reconstituted and in the syringe, the once-weekly formulation must be administered immediately. It is best to inject at a different injection site each week but to use the same region of the body (e.g. arm, thigh and abdomen).

Patients receiving either the once-weekly exenatide formulation or liraglutide should be counseled to report any symptoms potentially associated with thyroid tumors (e.g. dyspnea, dysphagia, hoarseness, a lump in the neck). Patients receiving a DPP-IV inhibitor or GLP-1 agonist should be instructed to report any symptoms consistent with pancreatitis, including severe abdominal pain (especially if it radiates to the back), nausea, or vomiting. If any of these occur, the patient should discontinue the drug and contact a healthcare professional. Although the risk of bladder cancer with pioglitazone is a matter of debate and continued evaluation, patients should be educated to report blood in the urine, urinary urgency, abdominal pain, or pain on urination.

Both men and women, and particularly those with osteoporosis or osteopenia, should be warned of the possible increased risk of bone fractures with pioglitazone use. Patients should be told of the more common fracture sites associated with its use, which mainly involve the distal upper and lower limbs as previously described.

SUMMARY

- Many challenges face the general practitioner in their efforts to optimize pharmacotherapy for their patients with T2DM. New data continue to emerge regarding how to treat hyperglycemia associated with T2DM. As a result, guidelines/recommendations, new indications for existing medications, new therapeutic entities and safety issues continue to evolve.
- The ADA recently updated its therapeutic recommendations in the treatment of T2DM hyperglycemia. It recommends a patient-centered approach to care and a need to evaluate the advantages and disadvantages of the various agents used to treat hyperglycemia when making therapeutic changes to patients.
- The various guidelines differ in their recommendations in treating hyperglycemia, and the general practitioner should be aware of these differences.
- The DPP-IV inhibitors are a viable option to add to metformin when the latter no longer provides adequate glycemic control. They have a very low rate of adverse effects, are weight neutral, and provide a modest decrease in A1C.
- The GLP-1 agonists are also good options to add to metformin when metformin no longer controls hyperglycemia. They offer significant decreases in A1C and modest weight loss. Nausea, vomiting and the need for self-injection are potential drawbacks to their use.
- Bromocriptine and colesevelam have limited efficacy in treating T2DM hyperglycemia, but the clinical pharmacist should be aware of their use and adverse effect profile.
- Insulin offers a very effective addition to oral medications, and it may be used without oral medication. Pharmacists should be proficient in developing basal/bolus therapy recommendations or plans to optimize hyperglycemic control.
- General practitioner needs to be vigilant of the increased risk of bladder cancer and bone fracture with pioglitazone use and keep abreast of any new data regarding the risk of pancreatitis or thyroid carcinoma with GLP-1 agonists.
- New agents and new formulations of existing agents in the treatment of hyperglycemia continue to evolve.

SUGGESTED READING

1. American Diabetes Association. In: Wolfsdorf JI (Ed). Intensive Diabetes Management, 4th edition. Alexandria, VA: American Diabetes Association; 2009.
2. American Diabetes Association. Standards of Medical Care in Diabetes--2012. Diabetes Care. 2012;35 (Suppl 1):S11-63.
3. American Diabetes Association. Standards of Medical Care in Diabetes-2015: Abridged for Primary Care Providers. Clinical Diabetes. 2015.
4. Anderson SL, Marrs JC. Dapagliflozin for the treatment of type 2 diabetes. Ann Pharmacother. 2012;46:590-8.
5. Aubert RE, Herrera V, Chen W, et al. Rosiglitazone and pioglitazone increase fracture risk in women and men with type 2 diabetes. Diabetes Obes Metab. 2010;12:716-21.
6. Bennett WL, Maruthur NM, Singh S, et al. Comparative effectiveness and safety of medications for type 2 diabetes: an update including new drugs and 2-drug combinations. Ann Intern Med. 2011;154:602-13.

7. Buse JB, Rosenstock J, Sesti G, et al. Liraglutide once a day versus exenatide twice a day for type 2 diabetes: a 26-week randomised, parallel-group, multinational, open-label trial (LEAD-6). Lancet. 2009;374:39-47.
8. Defronzo RA. Bromocriptine: a sympatholytic, d2-dopamine agonist for the treatment of type 2 diabetes. Diabetes Care. 2011;34:789-94.
9. Desai NR, Shrank WH, Fischer MA, et al. Patterns of medication initiation in newly diagnosed diabetes mellitus: quality and cost implications. Am J Med. 2012;125:302e1-302e7.
10. Dormandy JA, Charbonnel B, Eckland DJ, et al. PRO active Investigators. Secondary prevention of macrovascular events in patients with type 2 diabetes in the PROactive Study (prospective pioglit Azone Clinical Trial in macrovascular Events): a randomised controlled trial. Lancet. 2005;366:1279-89.
11. Gastaldelli A, Ferrannini E, Miyazaki Y, et al. Beta-cell dysfunction and glucose intolerance: results from the San Antonio metabolism (SAM) study. Diabetologia. 2004;47(1):31-9.
12. Holman RR, Paul SK, Bethel MA, et al. 10-year follow-up of intensive glucose control in type 2 diabetes. N Engl J Med. 2008;359:1577-89.
13. Inzucchi SE, Bergenstal RM, Buse JB, et al .Management of hyperglycemia in type 2 diabetes, 2015: a patient-centered approach. Update to a position statement of the American Diabetes Association and the European Association for the Study of Diabetes. Diabetes Care. 2015;38:140-9.
14. Karagiannis T, Paschos P, Paletas K, et al. Dipeptidylpeptidase-4 inhibitors for treatment of type 2 diabetes mellitus in the clinical setting: systematic review and meta-analysis. BMJ. 2012;344:e1369.
15. Mooradian AD, Bernbaum M, Albert SG. Narrative review: a rational approach to starting insulin therapy. Ann Intern Med. 2006;145:125-34.
16. Ritzel RA, Bulter PC. Physiology of glucose homeostasis and insulin secretion. In: Leahy JL, Cefalu WT (Eds). Insulin Therapy. New York, NY: Marcel Dekker; 2002. pp. 61-72.
17. UK prospective diabetes study 16. Overview of 6 years' therapy of type II diabetes: a progressive disease. U.K. Prospective Diabetes Study Group. Diabetes. 1995;44(11):1249-58.
18. UK Prospective Diabetes Study (UKPDS) Group. Effect of intensive blood-glucose control with metformin on complications in overweight patients with type 2 diabetes (UKPDS 34). Lancet. 1998;352:854-65.
19. UK Prospective Diabetes Study (UKPDS) Group. Intensive blood-glucose control with sulphonylureas or insulin compared with conventional treatment and risk of complications in patients with type 2 diabetes (UKPDS 33). Lancet. 1998;352:837-53.
20. Yeh H-C, Brown TT, Maruthur N, et al. Comparative effectiveness and safety of methods of insulin delivery and glucose monitoring for diabetes mellitus: a systematic review and meta-analysis. Ann Intern Med. 2012;157:336-47.

10
CHAPTER

Acute Metabolic Complications in Diabetes

Dheeraj Kapoor

INTRODUCTION

Complications due to diabetes may be either acute or chronic. Acute complications are due to acute severe hyperglycemia while chronic complications are due to vascular damage. Diabetes is frequently associated with acute metabolic complications. Acute complications occurring in diabetes can broadly be divided into metabolic and nonmetabolic. The nonmetabolic complications include severe infections such as sepsis, malignant externa otitis, etc. While acute metabolic complications include: diabetic ketoacidosis (DKA), hyperglycemic hyperosmolar nonketotic state (HHNS), hypoglycemia and lactic acidosis. Among these, nowadays, lactic acidosis rarely occurs now because phenformin, a type of biguanide and the commonest causative drug agent, is no longer in use. However, lactic acidosis can still occur in some clinical situations like shock, cardiac, hepatic or renal decompensation, especially in the patients receiving metformin (biguanide) for treatment of diabetes.[1]

The incidence of diabetic complications is increasing worldwide. The outcomes are especially poor in the absence of immediate and optimal management. The mortality associated with these disorders is still very high, and with DKA can reach almost 10% even in the best of hands. HHNS has a mortality which approaches almost 50%.

DIABETIC KETOACIDOSIS

Diabetic ketoacidosis results from lack of insulin and it is considered a medical emergency as it has a mortality rate of approximately 5%, mostly because of late recognition and frequently suboptimal management. DKA can be the first manifestation of type 1 diabetes in a previously undiagnosed patient or can occur in a patient with type 1 diabetes when insulin requirements rise during medical stress.

Noncompliance with insulin administration is another common cause of DKA. Although DKA is much more common in type 1 diabetes, it can also occur in patients with type 2 diabetes who have a predominant insulin secretory defect under severe medical stress. DKA is clinically defined by absolute insulin deficiency with hyperglycemia (glucose levels usually >250 mg/dL) with increased lipolysis, increased ketone production, hyperketonemia (ketone levels positive at 1:4 dilution of serum or greater or beta hydroxybutyrate >0.5 mmol/L), and acidosis (pH ≤7.3 or bicarbonate ≤15 mEq/L). Normoglycemic ketoacidosis has been reported and milder forms of ketoacidosis have also been described with bicarbonate levels between 15 mEq/L and 18 mEq/L. It is important to precisely define DKA in epidemiologic studies to accurately assess and compare morbidity and mortality.

Pathophysiology

Diabetes is often referred to as "starvation in the midst of plenty" and the progression of events that results from acute insulin deficiency holds this concept to be valid (Flow chart 1).

Precipitating factors for diabetic ketoacidosis with established diabetes include infection and other acute illnesses

Lack of diabetes education and training, noncompliance, poor self-care, inadequate glucose monitoring, psychological problems and indeterminate causes. *Infection is a most common precipitating factor*. Very often, no known precipitating factor can be identified, but under these circumstances, it is most likely related to poor compliance, poor self-care habits and unrecognized subclinical illness.

Clinical Presentation

Diabetic ketoacidosis may itself be the initial manifestation of diabetes, particularly for insulin-dependent diabetes mellitus, in 20–30% of cases of DKA. Patients are often noted to have a recent history of polyuria, polydipsia, fatigue, nausea, vomiting and abdominal pain often accompanied by symptoms of an underlying infection, such as urinary tract infection, pneumonia or gastroenteritis. Although symptoms suggestive of uncontrolled diabetes can

Flow chart 1: Pathophysiology of ketoacidosis[2]

Acute insulin deficiency

↓

impaired peripheral glucose uptake

↓

energy stores in fat and muscle are rapidly broken down

↓

In the liver there is conversion to glucose and ketones (beta-hydroxybutyrate and acetoacetate)

↓

Counter-regulatory hormones such as glucagon, catecholamines, cortisol and growth hormone rise

↓

contributing to hyperglycemia and ketonemia

↓

Hyperglycemia causes osmotic diuresis with an ensuing reduction of intravascular volume

↓

Hyperosmolality develops which, when severe (over 320 mosm/kg)

↓

Cardiac output and vascular tone can be greatly diminished by acidemia, thereby leading to shock be present for days, the metabolic changes typical of DKA evolve rapidly (usually within a day). On physical examination, patients with DKA can have signs of dehydration, tachycardia, hypotension, fruity breath (due to exhaled acetone) and abdominal tenderness, as well as symptoms and signs like fever specific to the precipitating factor (e.g. infection). They may breathe rapidly and deeply to compensate for acidemia (Kussmaul respirations). Mental status changes may be seen in severe DKA (due to an elevated osmolality). In the absence of timely treatment, DKA progresses to coma and death.

Acute cerebral edema, a complication in about 1% of DKA patients, occurs primarily in children. Headache and fluctuating level of consciousness herald this complication in some patients, but respiratory arrest is the initial manifestation in others. The cause is not well understood but may be related to too rapid reductions in serum osmolality or to brain ischemia. It is most likely to occur in children less than 5 year when DKA is the initial manifestation of diabetes mellitus. Children with the highest blood urea nitrogen (BUN) and lowest $PaCO_2$ at presentation appear to be at greatest risk. Delays in correction of hyponatremia and the use of HCO_3 during DKA treatment are additional risk factors.

Laboratory Evaluation and Diagnosis

In patients suspected of having DKA, serum electrolytes, BUN and creatinine, glucose, ketones and osmolarity should be measured. Urine should be tested for ketones. Patients who appear significantly ill and those with positive ketones should have arterial blood gas measurement. DKA is diagnosed by an arterial pH <7.30 with an anion gap >12 and serum ketones in the presence of hyperglycemia (usually over 250 mg/dL). A presumptive diagnosis can be made when urine glucose and ketones are strongly positive. Urine test strips and some assays for serum ketones may underestimate the degree of ketosis because they detect acetoacetic and not β-hydroxybutyric acid, which is usually the predominant ketoacid. Symptoms and signs of a triggering illness should be pursued with appropriate studies (e.g. cultures, imaging studies). Adults should have an ECG to screen for acute myocardial infarction (MI) and to help determine the significance of abnormalities in serum K. Other laboratory abnormalities include hyponatremia, elevated serum creatinine, and elevated plasma osmolality. Hyperglycemia may cause dilutional hyponatremia, so measured serum Na is corrected by adding 1.6 mEq/L for each 100 mg/dL elevation of serum glucose over 100 mg/dL.

Prevention and Management

Prevention remains the most important aspect of managing DKA in known diabetic persons. This can be accomplished through appropriate education, improved self-care and compliance, and self-monitoring of blood glucose. In ambulatory programs having improved patient access to medical care and providing outpatient education, there has been a 40–50% reduction in diabetes hospitalizations among patients who attended classes. More attention in the ambulatory care setting to diabetes education, self-care and self-blood glucose monitoring should result in decreased frequency of DKA and decreased hospitalizations for the condition. Ways to prevent DKA include frequent blood glucose monitoring, continuous insulin administration even when unable to eat, knowledge about "sick day" management and monitoring for the presence of ketones. Traditionally, patients are advised to check for urine ketones when their blood glucose is over 250 mg/dL or feeling ill. Reducing hospitalizations by taking preventive actions for DKA will decrease the cost burden of healthcare delivery in diabetes and which is most required for developing country like India.

Appropriate treatment of DKA requires (1) restoration of volume and solute homeostasis, (2) correction of insulin deficiency and (3) search for precipitating factors.

Management of DKA is summarized in Table 1.

Table 1: Management of diabetic ketoacidosis

Fluid administration	• Start with 0.9% saline at 15 (10–20) cc/kg/hr (total 2–3 L) for the first 2 (1–3) hours, then 0.45% saline at 7.5 cc/kg/hr (total 250–500 mL/hr). • Decrease the rate as the intravascular volume is repleted. • Add D5W (150–250 mL/hr) when the blood glucose level is 250 mg/dL.
Insulin replacement	• Administer an intravenous (IV) bolus of 10–20 units of regular insulin initially (0.1–0.3 units/kg). • Start a continuous IV infusion of regular insulin at 0.1 units/kg/hr. • Monitor serum blood glucose levels hourly and double infusion rate after 2 hours if there is no improvement in serum glucose. • Glucose levels should not decrease by more than 100 mg/dL per hour to prevent cerebral edema. • IV infusion of regular insulin should be continued until ketoacidosis resolves, then regular insulin should be given subcutaneously. Dose and frequency of subcutaneous insulin should be calculated based on insulin drip requirements and oral/IV intake.
Potassium replacement	• Serum potassium can be normal or elevated with diabetic ketoacidosis because of extracellular shifts of potassium with the metabolic acidosis, but total body potassium stores are depleted. • As the metabolic acidosis is corrected, there is an intracellular shift of potassium and a drop in serum potassium levels. • If the patient is normokalemic initially, then potassium supplementation should be started at 20 mEq/L. • If the patient is hypokalemic initially, if initial k+-<3.3 mmol/L, do not administer insulin, then potassium supplementation should be started at 40 mEq/L. • Potassium replacement should be held in patients with renal failure or persistent hyperkalemia.
Bicarbonate	• If pH <7.0 or pH <7.1 with associated hypotension or arrhythmia, then ADA recommends 50 mmol/L 200 mL of sterile water in first 2 hours • Do not mix sodium bicarbonate with normal saline.
Work-up for precipitating factors	• Complete blood count, blood cultures, urine analysis and urine cultures • Chest X-ray • ECG • Further diagnostic testing as needed.

Elements of Therapy

- Intravenous (IV) 0.9% saline
- Intravenous insulin (as long as serum K is ≥3.3 mEq/L)
- Correction of any hypokalemia
- Rarely IV $NaHCO_3$ (if pH <7 after 1 hour of treatment).

Treatment should occur in intensive care settings because clinical and laboratory assessments are initially needed every hour or every other hour with appropriate adjustments in treatment. Intravascular volume should be restored rapidly to raise BP and ensure glomerular perfusion; once intravascular volume is restored, remaining total body water deficits are corrected more slowly, typically over about 24 hours. Initial volume repletion in adults is typically achieved with rapid IV infusion of 1–3 L of 0.9% saline solution, followed by saline infusions at 1 L/hr or faster as needed to raise BP, correct hyperglycemia and keep urine flow adequate. Adults with DKA typically need a minimum of 3 L of saline over the first 5 hours. When BP is stable and urine flow is adequate, normal saline is replaced by 0.45% saline. When plasma glucose falls to <200 mg/dL (11.1 mmol/L), IV fluid should be changed to 5% dextrose in 0.45% saline. For children, fluid deficits are estimated at 60–100 mL/kg body weight. Maintenance fluids (for ongoing losses) must also be provided.[3] Initial fluid therapy should be 0.9% saline (10–20 mL/kg) over 1–2 hours, followed by 0.45% saline once BP is stable and urine output (0.5 mL/kg/hr) is adequate. The remaining fluid deficit should be replaced over 36 hours, typically requiring a rate (including maintenance fluids) of about 2–4 mL/kg/hr, depending on the degree of dehydration. Hyperglycemia is corrected by giving regular 0.1 unit/kg IV bolus initially, followed by continuous IV infusion of 0.1 unit/kg/hr in 0.9% saline solution.

Insulin should be withheld until serum K is ≥3.3 mEq/L. Insulin adsorption onto IV tubing can lead to inconsistent effects, which can be minimized by preflushing the IV tubing with insulin solution. If plasma glucose does not fall by 50–75 mg/dL (2.8–4.2 mmol/L) in the first hour, insulin doses should be doubled. Children should be given a continuous IV insulin infusion of 0.1 unit/kg/hr or higher with or without a bolus. Ketones should begin to clear within hours if insulin is given in sufficient doses. However, clearance of ketones may appear to lag because of conversion of β-hydroxybutyrate to acetoacetate (which is the "ketone" measured in most hospital laboratories) as acidosis resolves. Serum pH and HCO_3 levels should also quickly improve, but restoration of a normal serum HCO_3 level may take 24 hours. Rapid correction of pH by HCO_3 administration may be considered if pH remains <7 after about an hour of initial fluid resuscitation, *but HCO_3 is associated with development of acute cerebral edema* (primarily in children) and should not be used routinely. If used, only modest pH elevation should be attempted (target pH of about 7.1), with doses of 50–100 mEq over 30–60 minutes, followed by repeat measurement of arterial pH and serum K. When plasma glucose becomes <200 mg/dL (<11.1 mmol/L) in adults, 5% dextrose should be added to IV fluids to reduce the risk of hypoglycemia. Insulin dosage can then be reduced to 0.02–0.05 unit/kg/hr, but the continuous IV infusion of regular insulin should be maintained until the anion gap has narrowed and blood and urine are consistently negative for ketones. Insulin replacement may then be switched to regular 5–10 units SC q 4–6 hours. When the patient is stable and able to eat, a typical split mixed or basal bolus insulin regimen is begun. IV insulin should be continued for 1–4 hours after the initial dose of SC insulin is given. Children should continue to receive 0.05 unit/kg/hr insulin infusion until SC insulin is initiated and pH is >7.3.

Hypokalemia prevention requires replacement of 20–30 mEq K in each liter of IV fluid to keep serum K between 4 mEq/L and 5 mEq/L. If serum K is <3.3 mEq/L, insulin should be withheld and K given at 40 mEq/hr until serum K is ≥3.3 mEq/L; if serum K is >5 mEq/L, K supplementation can be withheld. Initially normal or elevated serum K measurements may reflect shifts from intracellular stores in response to acidemia and belief the true K deficits that almost all DKA patients have. Insulin replacement rapidly shifts K into cells, so *levels should be checked hourly or every other hour in the initial stages of treatment.* Hypophosphatemia often develops during treatment of DKA, but phosphate repletion is of unclear benefit in most cases. If indicated (e.g. if rhabdomyolysis, hemolysis or neurologic deterioration occurs), K phosphate, 1–2 mmol/kg of phosphate, can be infused over 6–12 hours. If K phosphate is given, the serum Ca level usually decreases and should be monitored.

Treatment of suspected cerebral edema is hyperventilation, corticosteroids and mannitol, but these measures are often ineffective after the onset of respiratory arrest.

Essential to the management of DKA is the search for a precipitating cause and an evaluation that includes a chest X-ray, blood cultures, urine cultures and ECG. If mental status changes are present in the absence of a significant elevation in serum osmolality (over 320 mosm/kg), then other causes for the mental status changes should be entertained.

HYPERGLYCEMIC HYPEROSMOLAR NONKETOTIC STATE (HHNS)

Hyperglycemic hyperosmolar nonketotic state (HHNS) is an acute complication sharing many symptoms with DKA, but an entirely different origin and different treatment. *Hyperglycemia, hyperosmolality and dehydration without ketosis are the hallmarks of the HHNS.* As with DKA, urgent medical treatment is necessary. It occurs rarely and is clinically associated with noninsulin-dependent diabetes mellitus (NIDDM). Typically, in clinical practice, HHNS is seen in patients with NIDDM and residual insulin secretion and is most commonly seen in individuals age above 65 years. Mortality for HHNS is much higher than DKA (approximately 50%) mainly because of the advanced age of the patients and the presence of comorbid conditions. HHNS associated with congestive heart failure or renal failure carries a worse prognosis. Mental status changes, such as lethargy and confusion, develop when the serum osmolality raises over 300 mosm/kg.

Pathophysiology

The basic pathophysiology of HHNS is similar to that of DKA (Flow chart 2). Deficient insulin action due to:

Flow chart 2: Pathophysiology of HHNS[2]

Insulin deficiency relative to increased insulin resistance

↓

Reduces glucose uptake by muscle and adipose

↓

Increases hepatic gluconeogenesis

↓

Increases production of glucagon and other counter regulatory hormones

↓

The resultant hyperglycemia causes glucosuria and osmotic diuresis

↓

High blood glucose levels, water is osmotically drawn out of cells into the blood

↓

Kidneys eventually dump glucose into the urine.
This results in loss of water and an increase in blood osmolarity

↓

Eventually lead to dehydration

However, lipolysis and subsequent ketone production are prevented by the presence of small amounts of insulin in type 2 diabetics. Mental status changes that occur with a rise in serum osmolality over 320 mosm/kg, severe mental changes characterized by coma can occur because of fluid shifts within the brain.

It can be precipitated in patients with type 2 diabetes by acute stress (infection, stroke, MI and surgery), hyperglycemic-inducing drugs (glucocorticoids and thiazide diuretics), or worsening of concomitant chronic disease (kidney failure).

Clinical Presentation

Polyuria, polydipsia, generalized weakness and reduced fluid intake all may herald the onset of HHNS by days. The primary symptom is altered consciousness varying from confusion or disorientation to coma, usually as a result of extreme dehydration with or without prerenal azotemia, hyperglycemia, and hyperosmolality. In contrast to DKA, focal or generalized seizures and transient hemiplegia may occur. On physical examination, signs of dehydration (decreased skin turgor, dry mucous membranes and orthostatic hypotension) can be present along with mental status changes.

Laboratory Evaluation and Diagnosis

Measurement of serum electrolytes, BUN and creatinine, glucose, ketones, and plasma osmolality should be done. Urine should be tested for ketones. Exceptionally elevated serum glucose levels can be found ranging from 800 mg/dL to 2400 mg/dL. Serum K levels are usually normal, but Na may be low or high depending on volume deficits. BUN and serum creatinine levels are markedly increased. Arterial pH is usually >7.3, but occasionally mild metabolic acidosis develops due to lactate accumulation. Acidemia is generally not present with HHNS.

The average fluid deficit is 10 L, and acute circulatory collapse is a common cause of death. Widespread thrombosis is a frequent finding on autopsy, and in some cases bleeding may occur as a consequence of disseminated intravascular coagulation. Other complications include aspiration pneumonia, acute renal failure, and acute respiratory distress syndrome.

Prevention and Management

Prevention of HHNS in known diabetic persons is accomplished through education, self-monitoring of blood glucose, self-care, avoidance of dehydration, and awareness and avoidance, if possible, of medications that may precipitate the disorder such as steroids and thiazides.

Patients with HHNS respond well to hydration and small doses of insulin to correct hyperglycemia. Hospitalization is usually short unless there is some underlying or comorbid condition that prolongs the stay. Some patients with HHNS may be treated in the ambulatory care setting before they lapse into more severe mental status disorientation.

Elements of Therapy

- Intravenous 0.9% saline
- Correction of any hypokalemia
- Intravenous insulin (as long as serum K is ≥3.3 mEq/L).

Fluid replacement is critical in treating HHNS. Fluid replacement should be done cautiously in patients with cardiac disease to avoid fluid overload. Fluid replacement alone can dramatically lower glucose levels. Treatment is 0.9% saline solution 1 L IV over 30 minutes, then at 1 L/hr to raise BP and improve circulation and urine output. It can be replaced by 0.45% saline when BP becomes normal and plasma glucose reaches 300 mg/dL. The rate of infusion of IV fluids should be adjusted depending on BP, cardiac status, and the balance between fluid input and output.

Insulin should be administered judiciously as only small amounts may be required to correct hyperglycemia compared with DKA. Insulin is given at 0.1 unit/kg IV bolus followed by a 0.1 unit/kg/hr infusion after the first liter of saline has been infused. Hydration alone can sometimes precipitously decrease plasma glucose, so insulin dose may need to be reduced. A too quick reduction in osmolality can lead to cerebral edema. Occasional patients with insulin resistant type 2 DM with HHNS require larger insulin doses. Once plasma glucose reaches 300 mg/dL, insulin infusion should be reduced to basal levels (1–2 units/hr) until rehydration is complete and the patient is able to eat. Target plasma glucose is between 250 mg/dL and 300 mg/dL. Addition of 5% dextrose infusion may occasionally be needed to avoid hypoglycemia.

After recovery from the acute episode, patients are usually switched to adjusted doses of subcutaneous insulin. Most patients can resume using oral antihyperglycemic drugs once their condition is stable. Electrolytes should be monitored and repleted. K replacement is similar to DKA: 40 mEq/hr for serum K <3.3 mEq/L; 20–30 mEq/hr for serum K between 3.3 mEq/L and 4.9 mEq/L, and none for serum K ≥5 mEq/L.

As in DKA, essential to the management of HHNS is the search for a precipitating cause and an evaluation that includes a chest X-ray, blood cultures, urine cultures and ECG. If mental status changes are present in the absence of a significant elevation in serum osmolality (over 320 mosm/kg), then other causes for the mental status changes should be entertained.

HYPOGLYCEMIA

Hypoglycemia, or abnormally low blood glucose, is an acute complication of several diabetes treatments. It is rare otherwise, either in diabetic or nondiabetic patients, characterized by low plasma glucose level, symptomatic sympathetic nervous system stimulation and central nervous system (CNS) dysfunction.

Clinical Presentation

The surge in autonomic activity in response to low plasma glucose causes sweating, nausea, warmth, anxiety, tremulousness, palpitations, and possibly hunger and paresthesias. Insufficient glucose supply to the brain causes headache, blurred or double vision, confusion, difficulty in speaking, seizures and coma.

In controlled settings, autonomic symptoms begin at or beneath a plasma glucose level of about 60 mg/dL, whereas CNS symptoms occur at or below a glucose level of about 50 mg/dL. However, symptoms suggestive of hypoglycemia are far more common than the condition itself. Most people with glucose levels at these thresholds have no symptoms, and most people with symptoms suggestive of hypoglycemia have normal glucose concentrations.

Furthermore, reduced sympathoadrenal responses can cause hypoglycemia unawareness. The concept of hypoglycemia-associated autonomic failure (HAAF) in diabetes that recent incidents of hypoglycemia cause both defective glucose counter regulation and hypoglycemia unawareness.[4] By shifting glycemic thresholds for the sympathoadrenal (including epinephrine) and the resulting neurogenic responses to lower plasma glucose concentrations, antecedent hypoglycemia leads to a vicious cycle of recurrent hypoglycemia and further impairment of glucose counter regulation. In many cases (but not all), short-term avoidance of hypoglycemia reverses hypoglycemia unawareness in affected patients, although this is easier in theory than in clinical experience.

Laboratory Evaluation and Diagnosis

Patients with NIDDM who develop hypoglycemia while on sulfonylurea therapy are usually age above 60 years and may have some mild renal insufficiency. It is, therefore, important to treat individuals age above 60 years cautiously with sulfonylureas and modify the dosage upward, as needed, for glycemic control. It is rarely necessary to aggressively treat elderly patients to precipitously correct hyperglycemia to normal glycemia. Patients do not usually require hospitalization for hypoglycemia unless it is extremely severe and/or the patient becomes unresponsive.

- Blood glucose level correlated with clinical findings.
- Response to dextrose (or other sugar) administration.

In principle, diagnosis requires verification that a low plasma glucose level (<50 mg/dL) exists at the time hypoglycemic symptoms occur and that the symptoms are responsive to dextrose administration. If a practitioner is present when symptoms occur, blood should be sent for glucose testing. If glucose is normal, hypoglycemia is ruled out and no further testing is needed. If glucose is abnormally low, serum insulin, C-peptide and proinsulin measured from the same tube can distinguish insulin mediated from noninsulin mediated and factitious from physiologic hypoglycemia and can obviate the need for further testing.

Prevention and Management

Frequent self-monitoring of blood glucose should reduce the frequency of hypoglycemic reactions, but not necessarily, as noted in the DCCT study. It is important for the patient with diabetes to avoid missing meals after taking insulin. Also, adjustments for exercise, either by additional food intake or adjustment of insulin dosage, will need to be made to avoid hypoglycemia. Multiple daily doses of insulin make it possible to adjust the insulin program for possible delays in meals or unplanned exercise. Prevention of hypoglycemia depends on appropriate education regarding diabetes management and self-care, self-monitoring of blood glucose, and awareness of factors that may precipitate hypoglycemia.

Elements of Therapy

- Oral sugar or IV dextrose
- Sometimes parenteral glucagon.

Immediate treatment of hypoglycemia involves provision of glucose. Patients able to eat or drink can drink juices, sucrose water, or glucose solutions; eat candy or other foods; or chew on glucose tablets when symptoms occur. Infants and younger children may be given 10% dextrose solution 2–5 mL/kg IV bolus. Adults and older children unable to eat or drink can be given glucagon 0.5 (<20 kg) or 1 mg (≥20 kg) SC or IM or 50% dextrose 50–100 mL IV bolus, with or without a continuous infusion of 5–10% dextrose solution sufficient to resolve symptoms. The efficacy of glucagon depends on the size of hepatic glycogen stores; Glucagon has little effect on plasma glucose in patients who have been fasting or who are hypoglycemic for long periods.

Underlying disorders causing hypoglycemia must also be treated. Islet cell and nonislet cell tumors must first be localized, and then removed by enucleation or partial pancreatectomy. Diazoxide and octreotide can be used to control symptoms while the patient is awaiting surgery or when a patient refuses or is not a candidate for a procedure. Drugs that cause hypoglycemia, including alcohol, must be stopped. Treatment of hereditary and endocrine disorders; hepatic, renal and heart failure; and sepsis and shock should be initiated.

Metabolism of Glucose during Shock Septicemia and Trauma in Diabetes

Significant alterations to glucose metabolism occur under conditions of stress such as trauma, burn, major surgery and sepsis. Stress-induced hyperglycemia is the result of increased sympathomimetic activity and increased release of counter regulatory hormones and proinflammatory cytokines. Counter regulatory hormones enhance glycogenolysis and gluconeogenesis to increase glucose production. For instance, epinephrine enhances glycogenolysis in the liver and skeletal muscles and increases gluconeogenesis in the kidneys. Growth hormone inhibits peripheral glucose uptake and stimulates gluconeogenesis. Proinflammatory cytokines are inflammatory mediators that also contribute to increasing glucose production by stimulating gluconeogenesis and glycogenolysis and by indirectly increasing the release of counter-regulatory hormones such as glucagon and cortisol. Furthermore, proinflammatory cytokines contribute to insulin resistance by inhibiting insulin release. The end result of these physiologic changes is increased endogenous glucose production coupled with insulin resistance that leads to stress-induced hyperglycemia.

Long-term Impact of Acute Complications of Diabetes

Acute complications of diabetes and especially hypoglycemia have huge long-term impact on the health and well-being of patients, healthcare cost to the community. DKA, HHNS and hypoglycemia results in the use of significant healthcare resources. It is estimated that 50% of these hospitalizations could have been prevented by better adherence to self-care and compliance with diabetes management programs.

Hypoglycemia can cause severe morbidity and even death on long-term basis. A possible link between hypoglycemia and acute vascular events like angina, MI and acute cerebrovascular disease has been proposed by several studies. In addition, some studies have highlighted an increased risk of death and microvascular complications when glucose levels are intensively controlled.

Sympathoadrenal stimulation and release of counter regulatory hormones during acute hypoglycemia causes hemodynamic changes including white blood cell activation and inflammatory mediators and cytokines release. Changes in regional blood flow, localized vasoconstriction, an increased risk of intravascular and endothelial damage, could provoke tissue ischemia. Recurrent exposure to hypoglycemia may contribute to this process by aggravating established micro- and macrovascular complications. In addition, hypoglycemia could potentially increase the sudden death through inducing either ischemic or other electrocardiographic changes (increased QTc), which in turn may predispose the diabetic subjects to ventricular arrhythmias.

A new research suggests a possible association between severe acute complication of diabetes and cognitive dysfunction. It is suggested that early exposure to severe hypoglycemia could have clinically relevant effects on cognition many years later.

In type 2 diabetes, study in elderly patients revealed that severe hypoglycemia episodes are associated with an increased risk of dementia in this population, although the impact of mild episodes on dementia risk remains unknown.

Hypoglycemia and quality of life studies reported that severe hypoglycemia can have a significant impact on patients' health-related quality of life, treatment satisfaction and cost of diabetic management.[5] The well-being of patients may be affected both directly from the effects of hypoglycemia and indirectly from fear of recurrence.

REFERENCES

1. Tripathi BK, Srivastava AK. Diabetes mellitus: Complications and therapeutics. Med Sci Monit. 2006;12(7):RA130-47.
2. Fishbein HA, Palumbo PJ. Acute metabolic complications in diabetes. In Diabetes in America. National Diabetes Data Group, National Institutes of Health; 1995. pp. 283-91.
3. Kishore P. Merck Manual for Professional. New Jersey: Merck & Co., Inc; 2014 June.
4. Shafiee G, Tehrani MM, Pajouhi M, et al. The importance of hypoglycemia in diabetic patients. J Diabetes Metabol Disord. 2012;11:17.
5. Liu S, Zhao Y, Hempe JM, et al. Economic burden of hypoglycemia in patients with Type 2 diabetes. Expert Rev Pharmacoeconomics Outcomes Res. 2012;12(1):47-51.

11
CHAPTER

Diabetes and Its Complications—An Overview

Rajeev Chawla

INTRODUCTION

The prevalence of diabetes is rapidly rising globally at an alarming rate and the disease is now amongst the most common noncommunicable diseases globally. According to the World Health Statistics 2012 report 1 in 6 adults is obese, 1 in 10 diabetic and 1 in 3 has raised blood pressure. Although, diabetes has been known since the ancient times, it is the last 30 years where a changing status has been observed; from being considered as a relatively mild disorder, seen predominantly in the elderly population, diabetes has become a major cause of morbidity and mortality, worldwide. It has been found to affect not only the elderly population but also the youth and middle aged subjects.

GLOBAL BURDEN: FACT SHEET[2]

- In 2012, 371 million people had diabetes; the numbers is likely to increase to 552 million by 2030.
- There is a rising incidence of type 2 diabetes globally.
- 80% of diabetic subjects live in low- and middle-income countries.
- The greatest number of people with diabetes is between 40 years and 59 years of age.
- Almost 50% (183 million) diabetics are undiagnosed.
- Diabetes caused 4.6 million deaths in 2011.

Although, both type 1 and 2 diabetes contribute to this burden, and prevalence of type 1 diabetes has also increased over the years; type 2 diabetes is the major contributor to the epidemic, contributing more than 90% of all cases of diabetes. 78,000 children develop type 1 diabetes every year.

New figures for diabetes prevalence in India indicate that the epidemic is progressing rapidly across the nation, reaching a total of 62.4 million persons with diabetes in 2011 and 77.2 million people are on the threshold, with prediabetes as per India Diabetes (ICMR-INDIAB) study.

DIABETES-RELATED COMPLICATIONS IN INDIA[1,4]

It has been found in various studies that over 50% of diabetic subjects in India have a poor glycemic control and a substantial proportion amongst these also have diabetes related complications (Table 1).[3]

Table 1: Prevalence of diabetes-related complications in various trials

Author (Year)	*City*	*Prevalence*
• Retinopathy		
– Rema et al., 1996	Chennai	34.10%
– Dandona et al., 1999	Hyderabad	22.60%
– Ramachandran et al., 1999	Chennai	23.70%
– Rema et al., 2000	Chennai	7.30%
– Narendran et al., 2002	Palakkad	26.8%
– Rema et al., 2005	Chennai	17.60%
• Nephropathy		
– John et al., 1991	Vellore	Microalbuminuria: 19.7% Diabetic nephropathy: 8.9%
– Gupta et al., 1991	New Delhi	Microalbuminuria: 26.6%
– Yajnik et al., 1992	Pune	Microalbuminuria: 23.0%
– Vijay et al., 1994	Chennai	Proteinuria: 18.7%
– Mohan et al., 2000	Chennai	Macroproteinuria with retinopathy: 6.9%
– Varghese et al., 2001	Chennai	Microalbuminuria: 36.3%
• Coronary artery disease		
– Mohan et al., 1995	Chennai	17.80%
– Ramachandran et al., 1999	Chennai	11.40%
– Mohan et al., 2001	Chennai	21.40%
• Peripheral vascular disease		
– Premalatha et al., 2000	Chennai	6.30%
• Peripheral neuropathy		
– Ramachandran et al., 1999	Chennai	27.50%
– Ashok et al., 2002	Chennai	19.10%
– Pradeepa et al.	Chennai	26.10%

This is apart from the presence of other life style disorders such as uncontrolled hypertension and dyslipidemia. These complications (both macrovascular and microvascular) cause significant morbidity and mortality among diabetic subjects.

Data from The Chennai Urban Population Study (CUPS) and The Chennai Urban Rural Epidemiology Study (CURES) provide valuable insight into the prevalence of various diabetes-related complications. The prevalence of coronary artery disease (CAD) was 21.4% among diabetic subjects and 14.9% in those with impaired glucose tolerance (IGT). The CURES

Eye study demonstrated an overall prevalence of 17.6% for diabetic retinopathy. Another population-based study reported 2.2% prevalence of overt nephropathy in Indians while microalbuminuria was seen in 26.9% of the cohort.

In our own study from North Delhi Diabetes Center comprising 720 type 2 diabetics, retinopathy was seen in 21.2%, microalbuminuria in 41%, peripheral neuropathy in 15.3%, CAD in 7% and peripheral vascular disease (PVD) in 7.4% of patients.

The high rate of complications could be due to a variety of factors. It has been found that Asian Indians have higher genetic predisposition to developing type 2 diabetes and the related complications. A unique combination of clinical and biochemical parameters has been identified and labeled as the "Asian Indian phenotype". Delayed diagnosis of diabetes in India, lack of adequate healthcare facilities and lack of information on part of the patients are the other factors contributing to high complication rates of diabetes in the Indian population.

Acute Complications of Diabetes Mellitus[5,6]

Acute complications of diabetes mellitus comprise diabetic ketoacidosis (DKA), hyperglycemic hyperosmolar syndrome (HHS) and iatrogenic hypoglycemia. DKA and HHS result from absolute or relative insulin deficiency coupled with concomitant increase in counter-regulatory hormones. Iatrogenic hypoglycemia is often a result of overzealous glycemic control treatments.

Pathogenesis

The basic underlying mechanism for the pathogenesis of DKA and HHS involves a net reduction in circulating insulin levels coupled with a concomitant increase in counter-regulatory hormones like catecholamines, cortisol, glucagon and growth hormone. Metabolic derangements, which ensue in these settings, lead to hyperglycemia, hyperosmolarity of the extracellular space, ketonemia and metabolic acidosis. Hyperglycemia results in reduced glucose utilization coupled with increased gluconeogenesis and glycogenolysis. Ketoacidosis results from increase in ketogenesis due to increased lipolysis and increased supply of free fatty acids for hepatic fatty acid oxidation (Fig. 1).

Factors known to precipitate DKA and HHS include:
- Poor treatment compliance, vascular disease
- Injury or infection
- Medications such as corticosteroids, thiazides, sympathomimetic agents and second generation antipsychotics.

Chronic Complications of Diabetes

Microvascular and macrovascular complications[8] manifesting as chronic complications of diabetes, largely account for diabetes-related mortality and morbidity. Diabetes, especially type 2 (due to its increased prevalence) has become the principal cause for blindness and end-stage renal disease in western countries. About 30–45% of all diabetic subjects suffer from microvascular complications. Patients with diabetes are at 2–4 times increased risk of coronary heart disease, cardiovascular disease and related deaths than those in the general population. Patients with diabetes are at four times higher risk of developing PVD and are at 15–40% higher risk of amputations as compared to general population (Table 2).

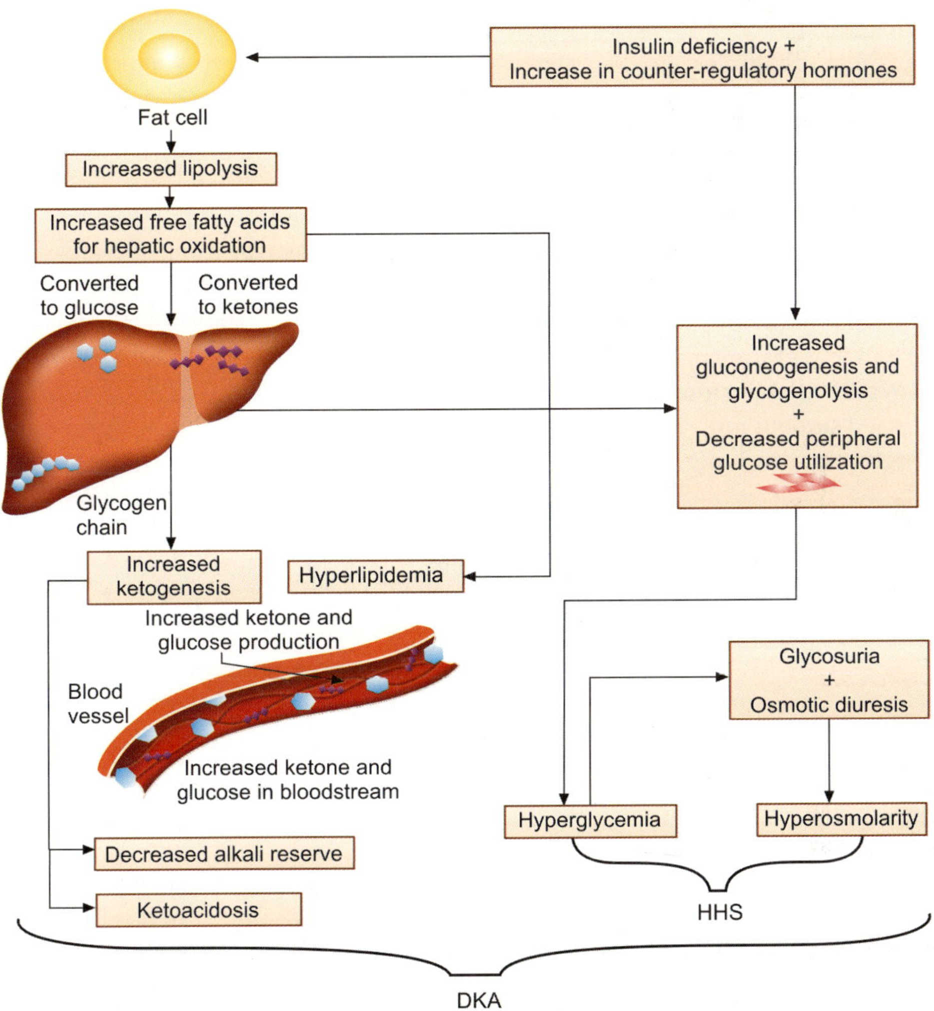

Fig. 1: Schematic representation of pathogenesis of diabetic ketoacidosis (DKA) and hyperglycemic hyperosmolar syndrome (HHS)[7]
***Source*:** In: Rajeev Chawla (Ed). Complications of Diabetes, 1st edition. New Delhi: Jaypee Brothers Medical Publishers; 2012.

Table 2: Chronic complications of diabetes

Macrovascular complications	*Microvascular complications*
Cerebrovascular disease	Diabetic neuropathy
Coronary artery disease	Diabetic retinopathy
Peripheral artery disease	Diabetic nephropathy
Erectile dysfunction	—

Pathogenesis[10,11]

Numerous clinical studies have implicated endothelial dysfunction as the principal cause of macrovascular and microvascular complications seen in both type 1 and type 2 diabetes. Endothelial cells regulate vascular tone by releasing endothelium-derived relaxing factors (EDRF), which include nitric oxide, prostacyclin and endothelium derived hyperpolarizing factor.

Mechanisms underlying impaired endothelium-derived vasodilatation

- Decreased production of EDRF
- Increased inactivation of EDRF
- Impaired EDRF diffusion to underlying smooth muscles
- Decreased smooth muscle responsiveness to EDRF.

Hyperglycemia induces a variety of metabolic changes, which include activation of polyol pathway, activation of diacylglycerol-protein kinase C and increased oxidative stress. Hyperglycemia inflicts cumulative long-term structural and functional changes in important macromolecules through advanced glycation end-products (AGEs). Endothelial dysfunction in diabetes is more often described in the context of oxidative stress (Fig. 2) (Flow chart 1).

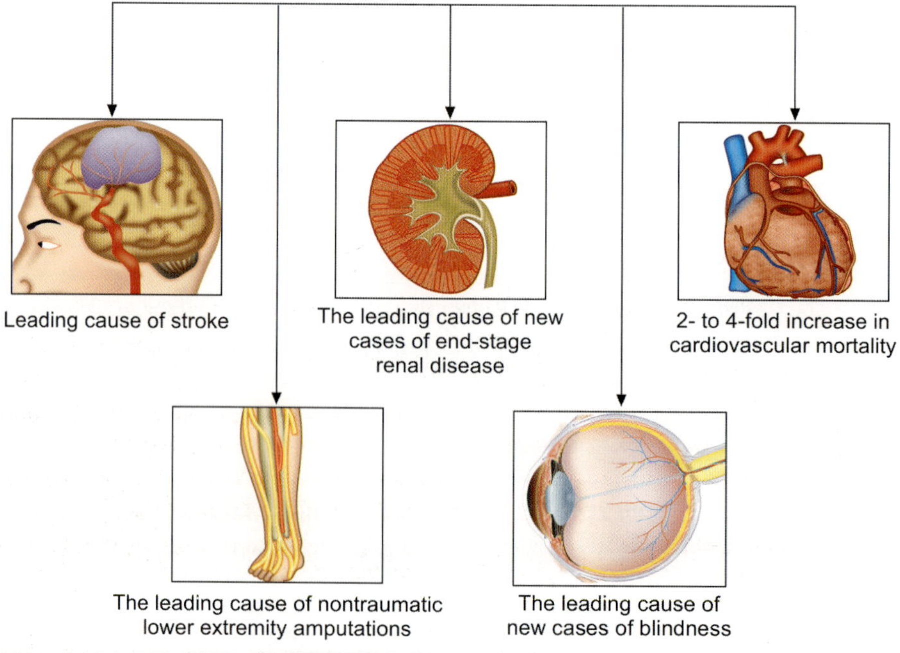

Fig. 2: Mechanisms of diabetes induced endothelial dysfunction[10]

Flow chart 1: Endothelial dysfunction in diabetes[8]

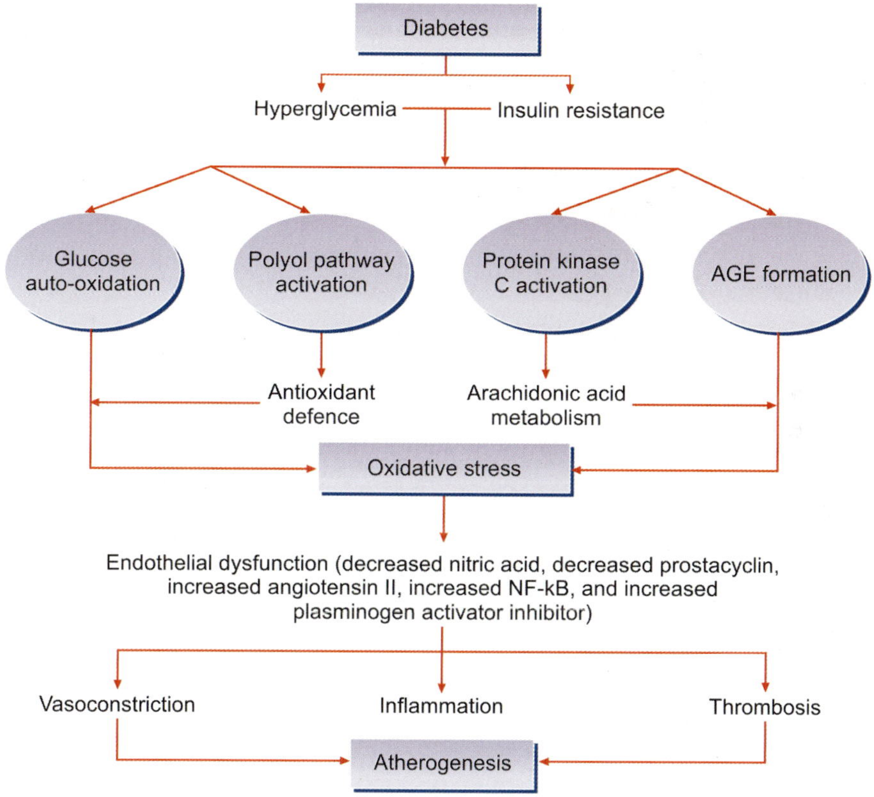

Diabetes

Hyperglycemia — Insulin resistance

Glucose auto-oxidation

Polyol pathway activation

Protein kinase C activation

AGE formation

Antioxidant defence

Arachidonic acid metabolism

Oxidative stress

Endothelial dysfunction (decreased nitric acid, decreased prostacyclin, increased angiotensin II, increased NF-kB, and increased plasminogen activator inhibitor)

Vasoconstriction

Inflammation

Thrombosis

Atherogenesis

Abbreviations: AGE, advanced glycation end-product; NF-κB, nuclear factor-κB.
Source: In: Rajeev Chawla (Ed). Complications of Diabetes, 1st edition. New Delhi: Jaypee Brothers Medical Publishers; 2012.

Pathogenesis of Diabetic Neuropathy[9,13-15]

Pathogenesis of diabetic neuropathy involves an interaction of metabolic and ischemic factors. Hyperglycemia-mediated activation of polyol pathway, glucose auto-oxidation and activation of protein kinase C are all known to contribute to development of diabetic neuropathy. These metabolic changes, which are associated with endothelial dysfunction in vascular beds, are associated with abnormal Schwann cell and axonal metabolism. Hyperglycemia causes endoneurial hypoxia by increasing endoneurial vascular resistance. Endoneurial hypoxia impairs axonal transport and reduces nerve sodium-potassium-ATPase activity. These impairments result in axonal atrophy and impaired nerve conduction (Flow chart 2).

Pathogenesis of Diabetic Nephropathy[17]

Hyperglycemia, hypertension and dyslipidemia are strong risk factors for diabetic nephropathy. The association of intense glycemic control to reduced microvascular complication, as reported by the Diabetes Control and Complications Trial, has emerged as a strong proof of concept for

Flow chart 2: Pathogenesis of diabetic neuropathy

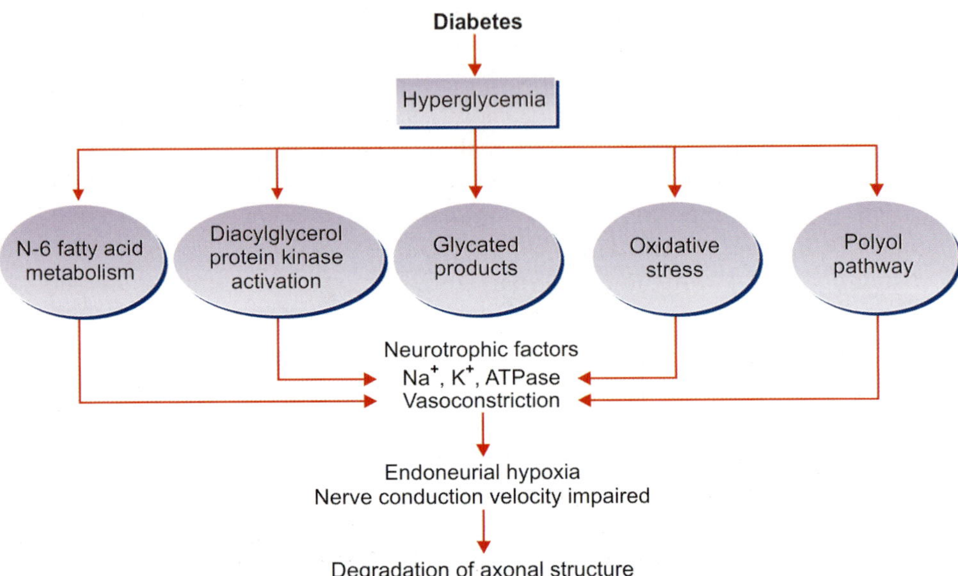

Source: In: Rajeev Chawla (Ed). Complications of Diabetes, 1st edition. New Delhi: Jaypee Brothers Medical Publishers; 2012.

Flow chart 3: Pathogenesis of diabetic nephropathy

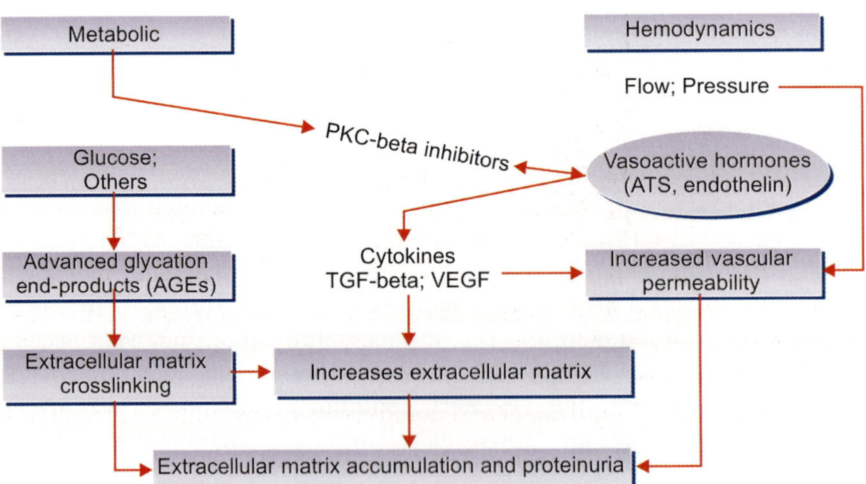

Abbreviations: PKC, protein kinase C; TGF-beta, transforming growth factor-beta; VEGF, Vascular endothelial growth factor; ATS, Angio tengin

Source: In: Rajeev Chawla (Ed). Complications of Diabetes, 1st edition. New Delhi: Jaypee Brothers Medical Publishers; 2012.

hyperglycemia as an important modifiable risk factor for diabetic nephropathy. Reduction in 10 mm Hg of systolic blood pressure[16] is associated with the 13% decrease in the microvascular complications with minimal risk in patient with systolic pressure <120 mm Hg (Flow chart 3).

This strand of data suggests that hypertension is another modifiable risk factor for diabetic nephropathy. Dyslipidemia with increased low-density lipoprotein (LDL) cholesterol and triglycerides is independently associated with diabetic kidney disease. The pathogenic mechanisms underlying diabetic nephropathy involve generation of mitochondrial reactive *protein kinase C* in a manner similar to pathogenesis oxygen species (ROS), accumulation of AGEs, and activation of intracellular signaling molecules such as *protein kinase C* in a manner similar to pathogenesis of other microvascular complications.

Diabetic Retinopathy[18,19]

Diabetic retinopathy, an ocular complication of diabetes, is the leading cause of severe visual impairments in adults. Studies indicate a correlation between diabetic retinopathy and duration of diabetes. Retinopathy seems to affect 60% of patients with history of diabetes mellitus for more than 15 years and to 90% by 25 years of diabetes. Many visually compromised diabetic patients also have other comorbidities such as, renal failure, hypertension and cardiovascular disease, which lead to significant mortality and morbidity. Prolonged hyperglycemia causes microvascular damage in the eyes, especially in the small blood vessels of the retina, leading to diabetic retinopathy and consequent sight loss. Microvascular changes also lead to weakening of capillary walls and formation of aneurysms, which may rupture resulting hemorrhage. Ischemia and microinfarction of retinal tissue may lead to neovascularization, scar tissue formation and possible retinal detachment. Treatment of diabetic retinopathy includes tight glycemic control and management of blood pressure to reduce the risk of progression. Elevated serum cholesterol levels are associated with decrease in visual acuity and provide the rationale for management of dyslipidemia. Laser photocoagulation is an important treatment option, especially for focal and diffuse maculopathy and proliferative retinopathy.

Coronary Artery Disease and Diabetes[20]

Diabetes and CAD are comorbid diseases and frequently coexist. Patients with diabetes have two- to threefold increased risk of CAD as compared to nondiabetic controls. CAD is the leading cause of death in diabetes population (Fig. 3).

Prevalence of CAD has a positive correlation with age and duration of diabetes, and over 40% of diabetic patients over 20 years of age have CAD. High risk for CAD in diabetes happens irrespective of ethnicity, even after adjustments for age, sex and income. Diabetes is known to worsen both early and late outcomes in patients with acute coronary syndrome. Guidelines suggest diabetes as a CAD risk equivalent and mandate aggressive anti-atherosclerotic therapy for risk reduction.

Pathogenesis of CAD[21]

A causal relationship among hyperglycemia, coronary thrombosis and vascular degeneration is well known. Several metabolic alterations are known to contribute to diabetes associated atherosclerosis.

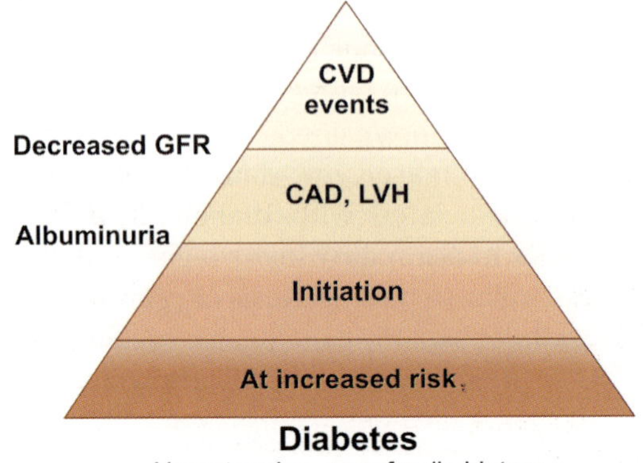

Fig. 3: The diabetes continuum

Abbreviations: GFR, glomerular filtration rate; CVD, cardiovascular disease, CAD, coronary artery disease; LVH, left-ventricular hypertrophy.

***Source*:** In: Rajeev Chawla (Ed). Complications of Diabetes, 1st edition. New Delhi: Jaypee Brothers Medical Publishers; 2012.

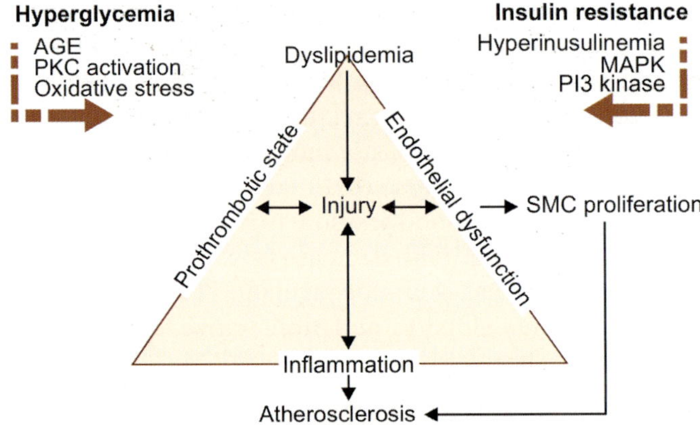

Fig. 4: Insulin resistance and hyperglycemia drive the atherosclerotic process

***Abbreviations*:** AGE, advanced glycation end-product; PKC, protein kinase C; MAPK, mitogen-activated protein kinases; SMC, smooth muscle cell

***Source*:** In: Rajeev Chawla (Ed). Complications of Diabetes, 1st edition. New Delhi: Jaypee Brothers Medical Publishers; 2012.

Though hyperinsulinemia does not necessarily cause CAD; it is an associated core defect in the metabolic syndrome. Metabolic syndrome is almost a well-established clinical concept, and its cluster risk components include insulin resistance leading to reduction in insulin-stimulated glucose uptake, glucose intolerance, hyperinsulinemia, hypertriglyceridemia, dyslipidemia (high levels of LDL cholesterol and low levels of high-density lipoprotein concentrations), hypertension, and high levels of plasminogen activator inhibitor-1. The exact mechanisms underlying the link between insulin resistance in diabetes and hypertension are still not clearly defined, but studies have shown hypertension as a comorbid risk factor (Fig. 4). Studies have revealed that inflammatory markers are high in patients with insulin resistance; diabetes and endothelial inflammation contribute to metabolic syndrome and may partly explain the high risk for CAD among diabetic subjects.

Peripheral Arterial Disease and Diabetes[24]

Peripheral arterial disease (PAD) is characterized by atherosclerotic occlusive disease of the lower extremities and is a relatively common complication associated with diabetes. Numerous studies have confirmed an association between diabetes and prevalence of PAD, and its presence not only adversely affects their quality of life but also is associated with substantial impairment due to intermittent claudication and results in progressive functional loss and long-term disability. Patients with diabetes and PAD are at higher risk of lower extremity amputation than those without diabetes. Furthermore, cardiovascular and cerebrovascular complications like myocardial infarction and stroke are higher in diabetic individuals with PAD than in nondiabetic population having PAD. However, PAD is still an under diagnosed and under treated condition despite its recognized complications.

Pathogenesis

Pathophysiological mechanisms of PAD seem similar in patients with or without diabetes. However, diabetes may have a higher propensity to affect peripheral vascular beds. Deranged metabolic states in diabetes may trigger proatherogenic changes, which include endothelial inflammation and alterations in blood cells and hemostatic factors. Development of PAD and elevated C-reactive protein (CRP) levels are correlated. CRP levels are very high in patients with IGT and diabetes, suggesting underlying endothelial inflammation (Fig. 5).

Diabetes impairs nitric oxide-mediated vasodilatation, increases production of vasoconstrictors such as endothelin-1, and enhances vascular smooth muscle cell migration, which is an important step in progression of advanced plaque. Hyperglycemia activates protein kinase C and nuclear factor kappa-B, leading to increased oxidative stress and development of atherosclerotic lesions.

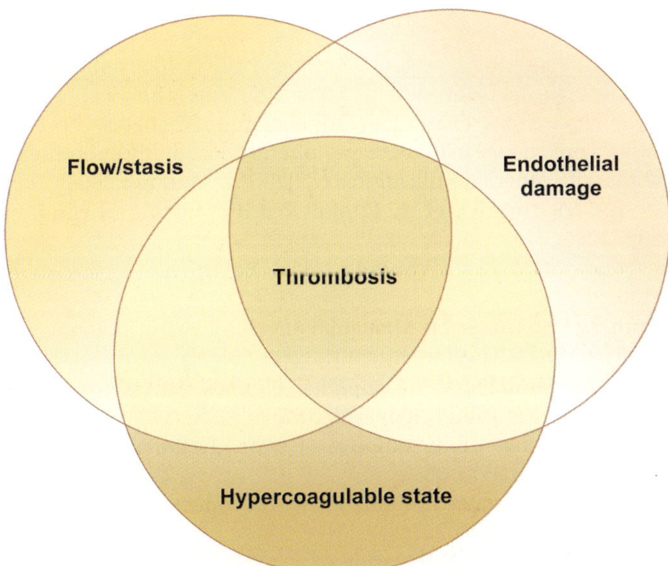

Fig. 5: Pathophysiology of peripheral arterial disease

Source: In: Rajeev Chawla (Ed). Complications of Diabetes, 1st edition. New Delhi: Jaypee Brothers Medical Publishers; 2012.

Cerebrovascular Disease and Diabetes

Cerebrovascular disease, most often manifesting as "stroke or cerebral infarction", is one of the most frequent causes of death worldwide, and frequent cause of disability. Though diabetic patients experience an unduly high rate of various types of vascular complications, stroke features as one of the prominent complications.

Pathogenesis

High risk of stroke in diabetes is due to complex interplay of various hemodynamic and metabolic factors. Cardiometabolic risk factors like hypertension and dyslipidemia often coexist with diabetes (e.g. in metabolic syndrome). Factors include insulin resistance, truncal obesity, IGT and hyperinsulinemia. Poor glycemic control leads to increased atherogenesis, and increasing levels of glycemia seem to be a continuous risk factor for fatality in stroke.

REFERENCES

1. Mohan V, Sandeep S, Deepa R, et al. Epidemiology of type 2 diabetes: Indian scenario. Indian J Med Res. 2007;125:217-30.
2. International Diabetes Federation. IDF Diabetes Atlas, 6th edition. Brussels, Belgium: International Diabetes Federation; 2013.
3. Anjana RM, Pradeepa R, Deepa M, et al. The Indian Council of Medical Research-India Diabetes (ICMR-INDIAB) study: methodological details. J Diabetes Sci Technol. 2011;5(4):906-14.
4. A Ramachandran, AK Das, SR Joshi, et al. Current status of diabetes in India and need for novel therapeutic agents. JAPI. 2010 (Suppl);58:7-9.
5. In: Rajeev Chawla (Ed). Complications of Diabetes, 1st edition. New Delhi: Jaypee Brothers Medical Publishers; 2012.
6. Acute Metabolic Complications in Diabetes. [online] NIH website. Available from http://diabetes.niddk.nih.gov/dm/pubs/america/pdf/chapter13.pdf. [Accessed August 2015].
7. Kitabchi A, Umpierrez GE, Murphy MB. Diabetic ketoacidosis and hyperglycemic hyperosmolar state. In: De Fronzo RA, Ferrannini E, Keen H, Zimmet P (Eds). International Textbook of Diabetes Mellitus, 3rd edition. Chichester: John Wiley & Sons; 2004. pp. 1101-19.
8. Fowler M. Microvascular and macrovascular complications of diabetes. Clin Diab. 2003;21:186-7.
9. Rajeev Chawla. Study of prevalence of diabetic peripheral neuropathy by biothesiometric evaluation and its coassociations with other complications. NNDU Proceedings; 2004.
10. Esper RJ, Nordaby RA, Vilarino JO, et al. Endothelial dysfunction: a comprehensive appraisal. Cardiovasc Diabetol. 2006;5:4.
11. De Vriese AS, Verbeuren TJ, Van de Voorde J, et al. Endothelial dysfunction in diabetes. Br J Pharmacol. 2000;130:963-74.
12. Yamagishi S, Fukami K, Ueda S, et al. Molecular mechanisms of diabetic nephropathy and its therapeutic intervention. Curr Drug Targets. 2007;8:952-9.
13. Thornalley PJ. Glycation in diabetic neuropathy: characteristics, consequences, causes, and therapeutic options. Int Rev Neurobiol. 2002;50:37-57.
14. Sheetz MJ, King GL. Molecular understanding of hyperglycemia's adverse effects for diabetic complications. JAMA. 2002;288:2579-88.
15. Eichberg J. Protein kinase C changes in diabetes: is the concept relevant to neuropathy? Int Rev Neurobiol. 2002;50:61-82.
16. Adler AI, Stratton IM, Neil HA, et al. Association of systolic blood pressure with macrovascular and microvascular complications of type 2 diabetes (UKPDS 36): prospective observational study. BMJ. 2000;321:412-9.

17. Raile K, Galler A, Hofer S, et al. Diabetic nephropathy in 27,805 children, adolescents, and adults with type 1 diabetes: effect of diabetes duration, A1C, hypertension, dyslipidemia, diabetes onset, and sex. Diabetes Care. 2007;30:2523-8.
18. Kowluru RA, Chan PS. Oxidative stress and diabetic retinopathy. Exp Diabetes Res. 2007;2007:43603
19. Matthews DR, Stratton IM, Aldington SJ, et al. Risks of progression of retinopathy and vision loss related to tight blood pressure control in type 2 diabetes mellitus: UKPDS 69. Arch Ophthalmol. 2004;122:1631-40.
20. Calkin AC, Allen TJ. Diabetes mellitus-associated atherosclerosis: mechanisms involved and potential for pharmacological invention. Am J Cardiovasc Drugs. 2006;6:15-40.
21. Deepa R, Arvind K, Mohan V. Diabetes and risk factors for coronary artery disease. Current Science. 2002;83:1497-505.
22. Reaven GM. Multiple CHD risk factors in type 2 diabetes: beyond hyperglycemia. Diabetes Obes Metab. 2002;4:S13.
23. Suzuki LA, Poot M, Gerrity RG, et al. Diabetes accelerates smooth muscle accumulation in lesions of atherosclerosis: lack of direct growth-promoting effects of high glucose levels. Diabetes. 2001;50:851-60.
24. Carr ME. Diabetes mellitus: a hypercoagulable state. J Diabetes Complications. 2001;15:44-54.

12

CHAPTER

Pharmacology of Insulins

Sanjay Kalra

INTRODUCTION

The name "insulin" was coined much before its discovery in Belgium by JD Meyer and by Sharpey Schafer in 1916 in Britain. Insulin was discovered in 1921 by an orthopedic surgeon turned researcher, Dr Frederick Banting and an intern in the University of Toronto, Charles Best, along with support of Professor JJR Macleod and JB Collip, a biochemist. In January 1922, Leonardo Thompson, a 14-year-old diabetic patient was the first to receive pancreatic extract made by Banting and Best. This, however, turned out to be a clinical failure. The first injections were administered by Dr Ed Jeffery. After few days, a new series of injections were given to Leonardo, his glycosuria and ketonuria disappeared, and his blood sugar level returned to normal. Various landmarks in the history of pharmacology are listed in Table 1.[1]

Table 1: Landmarks in the history of insulin pharmacology

Year	*Achievements*
1889	Oscar Minkowski and Joseph von Mering: Note development of severe diabetes mellitus after total pancreatectomy in experimental animals, thinking a mysterious substance is responsible for metabolic control
1906–1914	Zuelzer: Administer active insulin, but with no clear evidence to reduce glycosuria and acidosis because of contaminants and life-threatening actions
1921–1922	Frederick Banting, Charles Best supported by JJR Macleod and JB Collip: Isolate insulin in a form which could be used for therapeutic purposes
1922–1924	Walden (supported by Clowes): Develop large scale processes using isoelectric precipitation
1936	DA Scott and AM Fisher: Develop protamine insulinate
1948	HC Hagedorn: Neutral protamine Hagedorn (NPH)
1951	Hallas-Møller: Develop zinc complexed insulins (lente series of insulin)
1953	Novo: Formulate lente porcine and bovine insulins by adding zinc for longer lasting insulin
1964	Novo: Porcine insulin mixtard launched

Contd...

Contd...

Year	Achievements
1978	Genentech produce human insulin in Escherichia coli using recombinant DNA
1981	Novo Nordisk: Chemically and enzymatically convert bovine to human insulin
1983	Lilly: Produce recombinant human insulin
1988	Novo Nordisk: Produce recombinant human insulin
1989	Novo Nordisk: Biphasic human Insulin "Mixtard" launched
1996	Eli Lilly: Insulin lispro approved
2000	Novo Nordisk: Insulin aspart approved by USFDA
2003	Aventis: Insulin glargine approved in USA
2003	Novo Nordisk: Biphasic insulin aspart launched in India
2006	Novo Nordisk: Insulin detemir approved in USA
2006	Aventis: Insulin glulisine approved in USA
2012	Novo Nordisk: Insulin degludec approved in Japan and European countries
2014	MannKind: Afrezza (inhalable human insulin) approved USA
2014	Novo Nordisk: Insulin Ryzodeg approved in India

STRUCTURE OF INSULIN

Insulin is a 51 amino acid protein produced by beta cells of the pancreatic islet. It is composed of two peptide chains, A and B linked by two disulfide bridges. A chain has 21 amino acids while the B chain has 30 amino acids. A chain also has an intrachain disulfide bridge linking residues 6 and 11 (Fig. 1). The composition of the insulin molecule differs from species to species but the differences are generally not sufficient to affect the biologic activity of particular insulin. These differences can make the insulin antigenic if injected for a prolonged period into another species and the anti-insulin antibodies formed may inhibit the action of injected insulin. Earlier pork and beef insulins were available but this is of historical importance now. Pork insulin is more homologous to human insulin than beef insulin. The difference in the amino acid sequence of insulin of other animal species is mentioned in Table 2.

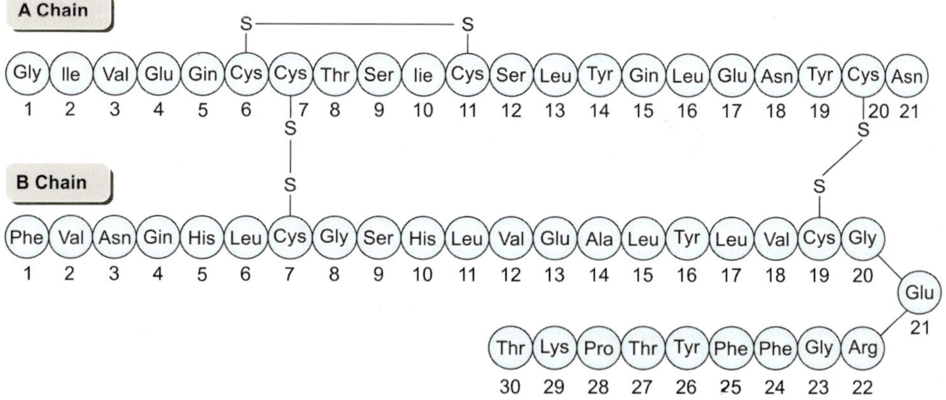

Fig. 1: Structure of human insulin

Table 2: Difference in amino acid sequence of insulin of different species

Species	*A Chain*		*B chain*
Different amino acid	8th amino acid	10th amino acid	30th amino acid
• Human	• Thr	• Ileu	• Thr
• Pork, Dog	• Thr	• Ileu	• Ala
• Beef	• Ala	• Val	• Ala

BIOSYNTHESIS OF INSULIN

Insulin is derived from pre-proinsulin (110 AA), from which 24 AAs are first removed to produce proinsulin. This is structurally similar to insulin-like growth factors I and II, which bind weakly to the insulin receptor. A connecting "C" peptide (35 AA) is split off from proinsulin by proteolysis in Golgi apparatus, to form insulin. Both insulin and C-peptide are stored in granules within the cell. The C-peptide is secreted in the blood along with insulin. C-peptide is generally found in amounts equal to insulin. It does not affect blood glucose levels in the body but serves as an indicator of how much insulin is being secreted by the pancreas.

Granules in the B cells store insulin in the form of crystals which consists of six molecules of insulin and two atoms of zinc. Insulin monomers aggregate to form dimers and hexamers with the help of zinc.

INSULIN SECRETION

Insulin is secreted from the beta cells in response to various stimuli as mentioned in Table 3. Glucose is the most important messenger for the secretion of insulin. Insulin release occurs when glucose is taken up by beta cells through glucose transport (GLUT)-2 receptors, and glucose concentration exceeds 90 mg/dL. With the increase in glucose concentrations, adenosine triphosphate (ATP) levels increase inside the beta cells causing closure of K+ATP channels on beta cell membrane which further causes membrane depolarization, opening of voltage gated Ca^{2+} channels, leading to Ca^{2+} influx, an increase in calcium concentration and hence exocytosis of insulin granules and insulin release. The amount of insulin secreted in the basal state is about 1 U/h with a fivefold to tenfold increase following ingestion of food. Therefore, the average amount secreted per day in a normal human is about 40 U (287 nmol).

Table 3: Various agents affecting insulin secretion

Insulin stimulants		*Insulin suppressants*
Physiological	*Pharmacological*	
Glucose	*Sulfonylureas*: Glimepiride, glibenclamide and gliclazide	Norepinephrine
Amino acids: Arginine and Leucine	*GLP-1 analogs*: Exenatide and liraglutide	Somatostatin
Cholecystokinin		
Incretins: Glucagon-like peptide (GLP-1) and glucose-dependent insulinotropic peptide (GIP)		

MECHANISM OF ACTION OF INSULIN

Insulin circulates in the blood stream until it binds to the GLUT4 receptors, and stimulates the uptake of glucose into the skeletal muscle, liver and adipose tissue. Insulin receptor is a transmembrane receptor that is activated by insulin. Insulin receptor consists of two subunits, alpha and beta. Insulin binds to the extracellular portion of alpha subunits of insulin receptor causing conformational change in the insulin receptor. This further activates the kinase domain residing on the intracellular portion of the beta subunits which autophosphorylates tyrosine residues on the C-terminus of receptor as well as tyrosine residues on the insulin receptor substrate 1 (IRS-1) protein. The phosphorylated IRS-1 then serves as a type of docking center for recruitment and activation of other enzymes that further mediate insulin's effects.

The main action of insulin is to decrease the blood glucose levels. There are three ways in which this action is accomplished. Firstly, insulin signals the cells of insulin-sensitive peripheral tissues, primarily skeletal muscle, to increase their uptake of glucose. Secondly, insulin acts on the liver to promote glycogenesis. Finally, insulin simultaneously inhibits glucagon secretion from pancreatic α-cells, thus signaling the liver to stop producing glucose via glycogenolysis and gluconeogenesis. Other important actions include stimulation of fat synthesis, promotion of triglyceride storage in fat cells, promotion of protein synthesis in the liver and muscle, and proliferation of cell growth (Fig. 2).

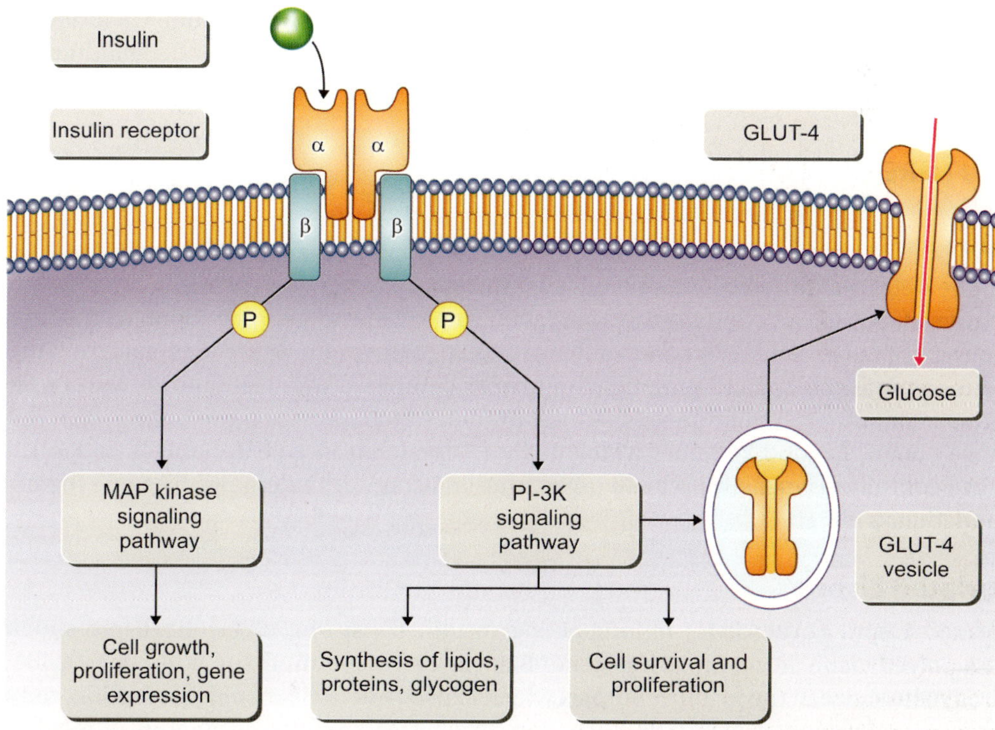

Fig. 2: Action of insulin

METHODS OF INSULIN PRODUCTION

Animal insulin refers to the insulin taken from the pancreas of animals, usually pigs (porcine or pork insulin) and cows (bovine or beef insulin). This is then purified further to reduce the chance of insulin users developing an allergic reaction. Animal insulins are no longer in commercial production.

Human insulins refer to the synthetic insulin which is laboratory grown to mimic the insulin in humans. Recombinant human insulin is laboratory created by growing insulin proteins either in yeast (usually *Saccharomyces cerevisiae*) or *Escherichia coli*. It is, currently available in two forms, a short acting (regular) form and an intermediate acting (NPH) form. Other pharmaceutical preparations, like lente, ultralente and semilente, have been discontinued.

Insulin analog refers to the genetically modified human insulins in which some changes have been made in the structure of the human insulin. Many insulin analogs are now available broadly classified as rapid acting (prandial insulins) and long acting (basal insulins). They can be manufactured as premixed preparations and coformulations as well. Insulins can be classified according to the type of preparations (Table 4) as well as type of regimen.

PHARMACOKINETICS OF INSULIN

The pharmacokinetics of various insulin preparations are listed in Table 5, while their mechanism of action and compatibility with intravenous solutions is detailed in Tables 4 and 6. The onset of action, time of peak action and duration of action allow insulins to be classified as rapid-acting, long-acting, ultra-long-acting and premixed insulins. Understanding of the pharmacology allows appropriate use of these insulin in clinical practice.

FUTURE DEVELOPMENTS

U300

Glargine U300 is a new formulation with glargine at a concentration of 300 U/mL rather than the usual 100 U/mL. It contains the same active ingredient as glargine. Upon subcutaneous injection, U300 forms a compact subcutaneous depot with a smaller surface area to produce a more gradual and prolonged release as compared with glargine. So, it has a flatter pharmacokinetic and pharmacodynamics profile which provides prolonged tight blood glucose control beyond 24 hours which is dose dependent in type 1 diabetes patients, and glucose control was evident up to 36 hours after injection. It undergoes the same metabolic degradation as glargine.

Pegylated Lispro

Pegylated Lispro (LY2605541) is long-acting insulin consisting of insulin lispro modified with a polyethylene glycol moiety at lysine B28 via a covalent urethane bond, increasing the hydrodynamic size of the insulin complex which causes a delay in insulin absorption, reduces clearance, and prolongs its duration of action. LY2605541 has a lower binding affinity for the insulin receptor and insulin-like growth factor-1 receptor than lispro, and a lower mitogenic potency than human insulin. The half-life is 24–45 hours and duration of action exceeds 36 hours, and are unaffected by renal impairment. A hepatoselective action on glucose metabolism has been suggested by animal studies.

Table 4: Various insulin preparations

Name of insulin	*Modification from human insulin*	*Mechanism of action*
Short-acting conventional (human) insulin		
Regular insulin	Buffered solution of unmodified human insulin stabilized by a small amount of zinc	At the concentration of injectable solution, insulin molecules self-aggregate to form hexamers around zinc ions. After subcutaneous injection, insulin monomers are released gradually by dilution, so that absorption occurs slowly
Rapid-acting insulin analogs		
Insulin aspart	A single proline amino acid at B28 has been replaced with an aspartic acid residue	Modification removes interaction at monomer-monomer surface. Repulsion between the charged aspartic acid and nearby glutamic acid B21 may also contribute to rapid dissociation into monomers
Insulin lispro	Position of two amino acids inverted. In lispro, lysine is at B28 and proline at B29 position	Inversion of lysine and proline from their respective position blocks formation of insulin dimer and hexamer, so more monomeric insulin is available for postprandial hyperglycemia
Insulin glulisine	Asparagine at position B3 is replaced by lysine and lysine in position B29 is replaced by glutamic acid	Rapid absorption and shorter duration of action is achieved
Intermediate-acting conventional (human) insulin		
NPH	Protamine is added to the unmodified human insulin sufficient to complex all insulin molecules	On subcutaneous injection, the complex dissociates slowly to yield an intermediate duration of action.[3]
Long-acting insulin analogs		
Insulin detemir	Threonine at position B30 deleted and an aliphatic fatty acid added to lysine at B29	This enables detemir to bind with albumin reversibly and facilitate formation of multimers within subcutaneous tissue which prolongs the duration of action
Insulin glargine	Acidic long-acting analog with substitution of asparagine with glycine at A21, and at B30, there is addition of two arginine residues	When injected into skin at neutral pH, there it forms precipitates which delays its absorption hence longer duration of action.[5]
Ultra-long-acting insulin analogs		
Insulin degludec	Deletion of threonine at B30, and addition of 16 chain carbon fatty di-acid to lysine at B29 with glutamic acid as a spacer	Allows degludec to form multiple hexamers which dissociate slowly after subcutaneous injection and are responsible for its ultra-long duration of action

Abbreviation: NPH, neutral protamine Hagedorn.

Table 5: Pharmacokinetic properties of various insulins

Preparation of insulin	*Appearance*	*Onset of action (hrs)*	*Peak (hrs)*	*Duration of action (hrs)*	*Time of administration*
Conventional human insulin					
Short-acting • Regular insulin	Clear	0.5–1.0	2–3	6–8	30 minute before meal
Intermediate-acting • NPH	Cloudy	2–3	7–12	Up to 18	Need not be given with meal
Premixed human insulins*					
70/30: 70% NPH, 30% regular insulin	Cloudy	0.5–1.0	Dual	10–16	30 minute before meal
50/50: 50% NPH, 50% regular insulin	Cloudy	0.5–1.0	Dual	10–16	30 minute before meal
Rapid-acting insulin analogs					
Insulin aspart	Clear	<0.25	0.5–1.5	3–5	At the time of meal
Insulin lispro	Clear	<0.25	0.5–1.5	3–4	At the time of meal
Insulin glulisine	Clear	<0.25	0.5–1.5	<3	At the time of meal
Long-acting insulin analogs					
Insulin detemir	Clear	1–4	Minimal peak activity	16–24	Need not be given with meal
Insulin glargine	Clear	1–4	Minimal peak activity	Up to 24	Need not be given with meal
Ultra-long-acting insulin analogs					
Insulin degludec	Clear		Peakless profile	Up to 42	Need not be given with meal
Premixed insulin analogs*					
70/30: 70% protamine aspart, 30% aspart	Cloudy	<0.25	1.5	Up to 10–16	At the time of meal
50/50: 50% protamine aspart, 50% aspart	Cloudy	<0.25	1.5	Up to 10–16	At the time of meal
75/25: 75% protamine lispro, 25% lispro	Cloudy	<0.25	1.5	Up to 10–16	At the time of meal
50/50: 50% protamine lispro, 50% lispro	Cloudy	<0.25	1.5	Up to 10–16	At the time of meal
Coformulations					
I Deg Asp: 70% insulin degludec, 30% insulin aspart	Clear	<0.25	1.5	24 hrs	At the time of meal
I Deg Lira: insulin degludec + liraglutide	Clear	<0.25	–	24 hrs	At any time
I Glar Lixi: insulin glargine + lixisenatide	Clear	1-4	–	24 hrs	At time of meal

*Premixed insulins: A single vial or cartridge contains a fixed ratio of insulin (% of short-acting vs % of intermediate-acting insulin)

Abbreviation: NPH, neutral protamine Hagedorn.

Table 6: Compatibility of different insulin preparations with various intravenous fluids/in infusion pumps

Type of insulin	*5% Dextrose*	*Ringer solution*	*Normal saline*	*Infusion pumps*
Regular	√	√	√	√
Aspart	√	√	√	√
Lispro	√	√	√	√
Glulisine	X	X	√	√
Premixed	X	X	X	X
Basal	X	X	X	X

REFERENCES

1. Shah SN, Joshi SR, Parmar DV. History of Insulin. J Asso of Physicians Ind. 1997;45(Suppl 1):4-9.
2. Boehm BO, Home PD, Behrend C, et al. Premixed insulin aspart 30 vs. premixed human insulin 30/70 twice daily: a randomized trial in Type 1 and Type 2 diabetic patients. Diabet Med. 2002;19(5):393-9.
3. McNally PG, Dean JD, Morris AD, et al. Using continuous glucose monitoring to measure the frequency of low glucose values when using biphasic insulin aspart 30 compared with biphasic human insulin 30: a double-blind crossover study in individuals with type 2 diabetes. Diabetes Care. 2007;30:1044-8.
4. Raskin PR, Hollander PA, Lewin A, et al. Basal insulin or premix analogue therapy in type 2 diabetes patients. Eur J Intern Med. 2007;18(1):56-62.
5. Strojek K, Bebakar WM, Khutsoane DT, et al. Once-daily initiation with biphasic insulin aspart 30 versus insulin glargine in patients with type 2 diabetes inadequately controlled with oral drugs: an open-label, multinational RCT. Curr Med Res Opin. 2009;25(12):2887-94.
6. Luzio S, Dunseath G, Peter R, et al. Comparison of the pharmacokinetics and pharmacodynamics of biphasic insulin aspart and insulin glargine in people with type 2 diabetes. Diabetologia. 2006;49:1163-8.
7. Heise T, Heinmann L, Hovelmann U, et al. Biphasic Insulin Aspart 30/70: Pharmacokinetics and pharmacodynamics. Compared With Once-Daily Biphasic Human Insulin and Basal-Bolus Therapy. Diabetes Care. 2009;32(8):1431-3.
8. Garber AJ, Wahlen J, Wahl T, et al. Attainment of glycaemic goals in type 2 diabetes with once-, twice-, or thrice-daily dosing with biphasic insulin aspart 70/30 (The 1-2-3 study). Diabetes Obes Metab. 2006;8(1):58-66.
9. Heinemann L, Heise T, Jorgensen LN, et al. Action profile of the rapid acting insulin analogue: human insulin B28Asp. Diabet Med. 1993;10:535-9.
10. Wang F, Surh J, Kaur M. Insulin degludec as an ultralong-acting basal insulin once a day: a systematic review. Diabetes Metab Syndr Obes. 2012;5:191-204.
11. Kalra S, Baruah MP, Niazi AK. Degludec: a novel basal insulin. Recent Pat Endocr Metab Immune Drug Discov. 2012;6:18-23.
12. Keating GM. Insulin degludec and insulin degludec/insulin aspart: a review of their use in the management of diabetes mellitus. Drugs. 2013;73:575-93.

13

CHAPTER

Diabetic Eye Disease and Its Complications

Prashant Bhushan, Arpit Agrawal, MK Singh, VP Singh, RP Maurya

INTRODUCTION

In recent years, diabetes mellitus has come up as a major cause of blindness; it can be avoided by the combined efforts of the endocrinologist and ophthalmologist. Major technological advances are now available to aid in making an accurate diagnosis of various stages of diabetic retinopathy. Anti-vascular endothelial growth factor inhibitors are now major adjuncts to treatment, besides panretinal photocoagulation (PRP) and surgical interventions.

Epidemiology and Trends of Diabetic Retinopathy in India and Worldwide

The prevalence of insulin dependent diabetes mellitus (IDDM) is only 10–15% of the diabetic population hence the majority is non-insulin dependent diabetes mellitus (NIDDM).[1] The global prevalence of diabetes among adults aged more than or equal 20 years was estimated in 2000 to be around 171 million (2.8% of the world's population), and is expected to rise to 366 million (4.4% of the estimated world population) by the year 2030. Asia is expected to be home to 61% of the total global projected number of people with diabetes by 2010, not only because it is the most populous continent on earth, but also because of increased urbanization and improved life expectancy. India, China and the USA are expected to have the highest numbers of people with diabetes in 2030.[2]

Various population based studies in the Western World have suggested the prevalence of diabetic retinopathy (DR) to be 28.7% whereas proliferative DR and macular edema account for 9% and 17%, respectively.[3]

The Wisconsin epidemiological study of diabetic retinopathy (WESDR) has proposed a prevalence of DR of 50.1% in IDDM patients while the diabetes control and complications trial (DCCT) suggests a prevalence of 54.2% in IDDM.[4,5] The United Kingdom prospective diabetes study (UKPDS) has in NIDDM proposed a prevalence rate of DR of 35–39% and marked severe retinopathy in 4–8%.[6]

Indian studies have suggested that European values are comparable to Indian populations.[7]

PATHOGENESIS OF PROLIFERATIVE AND NONPROLIFERATIVE DIABETIC RETINOPATHY

The metabolic pathway causing DR is still unknown, several theories have been proposed, some substantiated with evidences. It is believed that prolonged exposure to hyperglycemia leads to hypoxia through a number of biochemical and physiologic changes; this results in damage to the endothelium.[8] It is thought that, decreased levels of 2–3 diphosphoglycerate in the erythrocytes influences the oxygen dissociation curve of blood cells, leading to a hypoxia of the tissues; this effect is reinforced by greater oxygen holding capacity by glycosylated hemoglobin, which are naturally increased in uncontrolled diabetics.[9]

The polyol pathway of glucose metabolism, results in accumulation in cells of large amount of fructose and sorbitol. This has a profound osmotic effect, resulting in edema of retinal cells more so in the cells of macula.[10] This is one of the reasons of occurrence of diabetic macular edema (DME).[11]

High levels of aldose reductase, is supposed to cause an electrolyte imbalance, which causes changes in the pericytes, which in turn is responsible for leakages from microvessels and cell death leads to microaneurysm formation.[12]

In the normal eye, there is a balance between the vasoproliferative and vasoinhibitory factors in the retina and the vitreous; this leads to a stable vascular bed. A disbalance by a host of factors including mechanisms denoted above results in excess vascular endothelial growth factors (VEGFs) leading to proliferation of vessels.[13,14]

There are a host of risk factors which activate the above pathogenetic mechanisms; a few prominent ones being duration of diabetes, glycemic control, age and sex, hypertensive status, renal involvement, dyslipidemia, anemia, etc. Few general factors such as socioeconomic factor, puberty and pregnancy also play a major role.

The interplay of the above factors leads to:

- Increased platelet and erythrocyte aggregation
- Abnormal serum lipids
- Defective coagulation profile and blood viscosity
- Abnormal levels of growth hormone
- Raised levels of VEGF.

Terminologies, Definition of Diabetic Retinopathy and Types

- A *microaneurysm* is a red spot less than 125 microns (approximate width of vein at disk margin) with sharp margins.
- A *hemorrhage* is a red spot with irregular margins.
- *Flame shaped hemorrhages* are superficial hemorrhages just under the nerve fiber layer.
- *Blot hemorrhages* are deeper hemorrhages, which is a sign of retinal ischemia.
- *Hard exudates* are small, white or yellowish-white deposits with sharp margins, extravasations of lipoproteins located typically in the outer layers of the retina (Fig. 1).
- *Soft exudates* are fluffy white opaque areas caused by an accumulation of axoplasm in the nerve fiber layer of the retina.
- *Venous loop* is an abrupt curving deviation of a vein from its normal path.

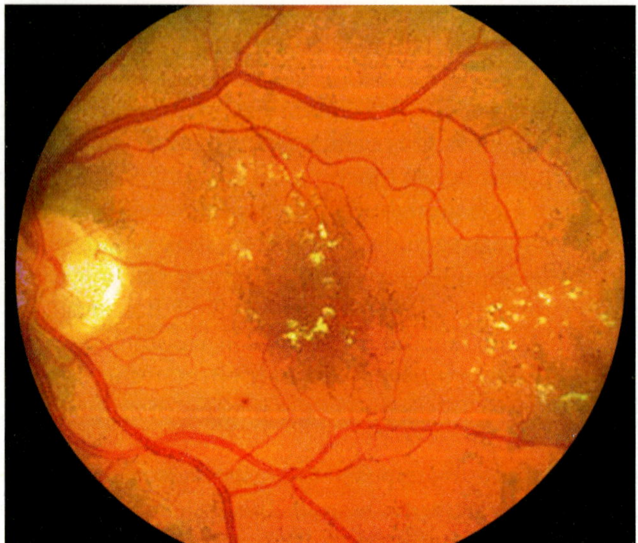

Fig. 1: Nonproliferative diabetic retinopathy with hard exudates

Reduplication is dilation of a preexisting channel or proliferation of a new channel adjacent to and approximately of the same caliber as the original vein.

Superior and inferior to the disk are multiple fine, new abnormal vessel formations, the hallmark of proliferative diabetic retinopathy (PDR) (Figs 2A and B). Along the disk toward the macula, there is extensive fibrosis extending superiorly and inferiorly. This fibrosis is in response to recurrent hemorrhages and repair from proliferation around the optic disk. This fibrotic band is anterior to the surface of the retina. Inferiorly, there is retinal hemorrhage that also involves the inferior macula. This hemorrhage is on the retinal surface. However, inferior to the hemorrhage between 4 o'clock and 5:30, there is a darker brownish area that would be consistent with hemorrhage more anteriorly extending into the vitreous (Fig. 3) (American College of Physicians, 2010).

The *early treatment diabetic retinopathy study (ETDRS)* has classified DR into the following categories (Fig. 3):[15]

1. None
2. Minimal nonproliferative diabetic retinopathy (NPDR)
3. Mild NPDR
4. Moderate NPDR
5. Severe NPDR
6. PDR
7. High-risk PDR.

The *International Clinical Diabetic Retinopathy and Diabetic Macula Edema Disease Severity Scale* proposes five levels for grading of DR; it is based on risk of progression:

1. None
2. Mild

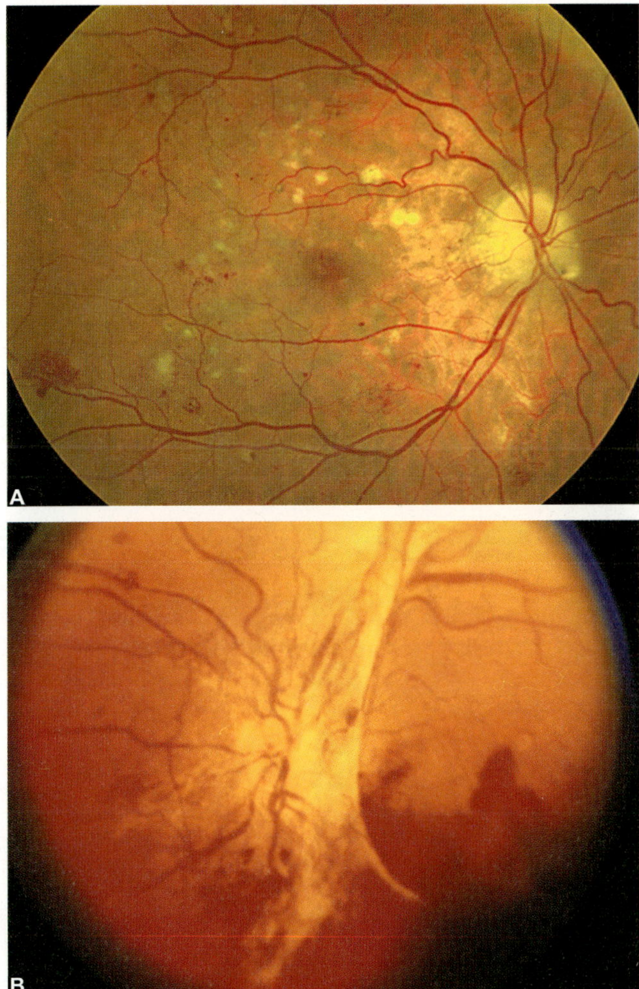

Figs 2A and B: Proliferative diabetic retinopathy. Notice the frond-like vessels coming from optic disk which represent neovascular vessels
Source: Adapted from Digital Journal of Ophthalmology, 2015.

3. NPDR
4. Moderate NPDR
5. Severe NPDR or PDR.

Presence and severity of DME is classified separately.

CLINICAL FEATURES OF DIABETIC RETINOPATHY

The clinical features of DR are broadly divided into NPDR and PDR. NPDR, also known as background DR indicates that the disease is limited to the confines of the retina, i.e. it is not beyond the internal limiting membrane. NPDR affects the vision by increased intraretinal

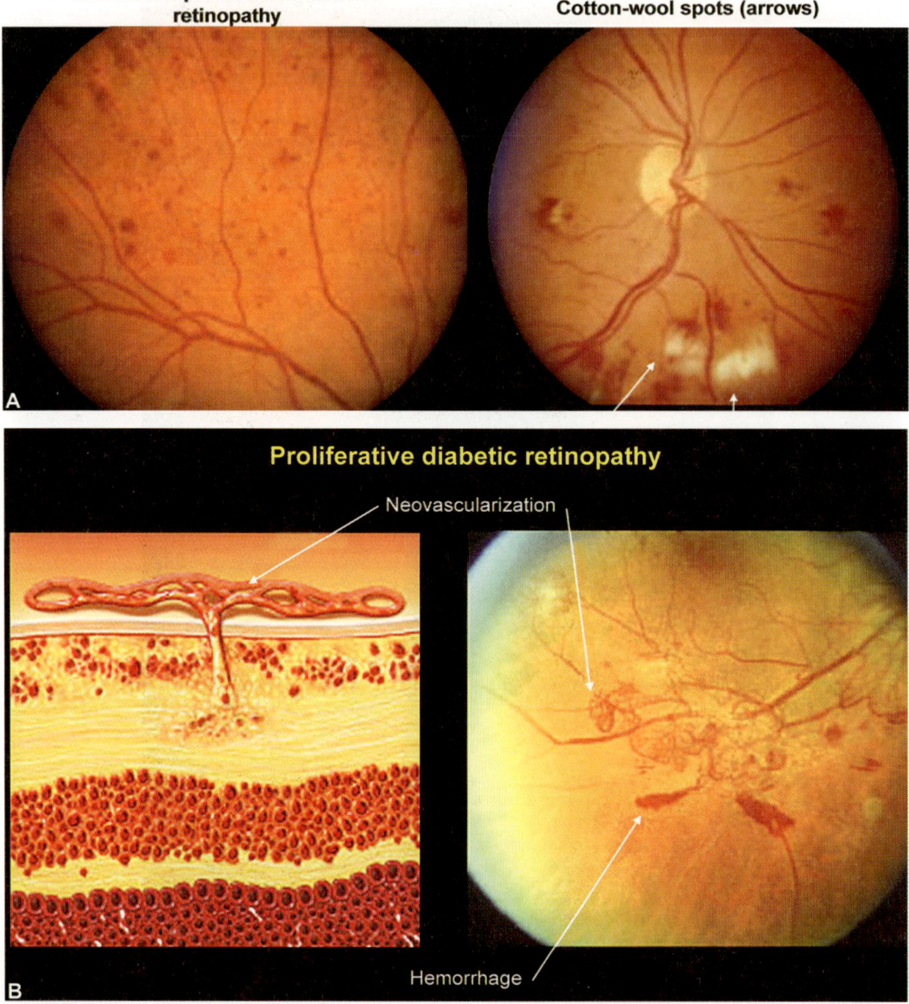

Figs 3A and B: Showing features of severe nonproliferative diabetic retinopathy and proliferative diabetic retinopathy (neovascular and hemorrhage)

vascular permeability, resulting in macular edema and variable degrees of intraretinal capillary closure resulting in macular ischemia. It includes:

- *Microaneurysms* (which are the first clinically detectable lesions of DR located in the inner nuclear layer of the retina), areas of capillary nonperfusion.
- *Nerve fiber layer infarcts* also known as soft exudates or cotton wool spots (these result from capillary occlusion of the retinal nerve fiber layer).
- *Intraretinal microvascular abnormalities (IRMAs)*: These arise close to areas of capillary closure and function as collateral channels.
- *Dot and blot hemorrhages* (which are located in the middle layers of retina).
- *Retinal edema* (characterized by accumulation of fluid between the outer plexiform layer and inner nuclear layer).

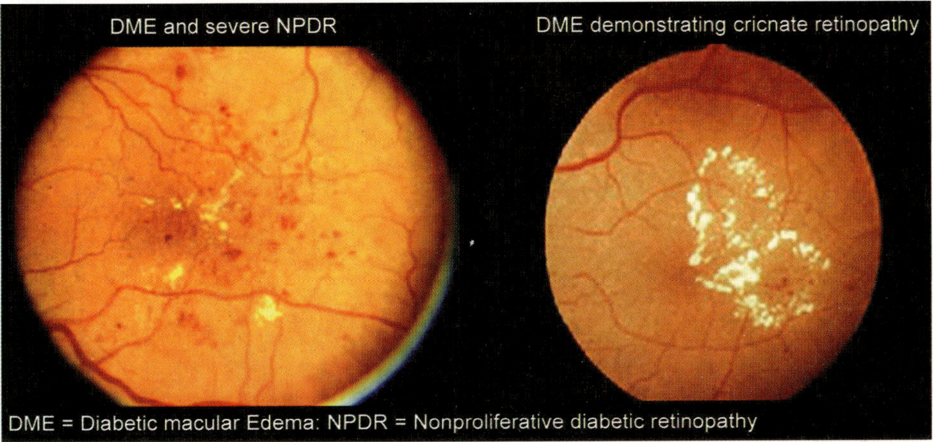

Fig. 4: Diabetic macular edema

- *Hard exudates* (which are located between the inner plexiform and inner nuclear layer of the retina), arteriolar abnormalities, and dilation and beading of retinal veins.

The proliferative diabetic retinopathy characterizes the process of revascularization. The new vessels are made up of tunica intima alone; they are leaky and fragile, and they may lead to sudden or slow vitreous hemorrhage and significant visual loss. They may be present at the optic disk [neovascularization of the disk (NVD)], or may be present elsewhere in the retina [neovascularization elsewhere (NVE)].

DIABETIC MACULAR EDEMA (FIG. 4)

This is the most frequent cause of moderate to severe vision loss in the stage of NPDR; it is due to fluid accumulation in the interstitial spaces of macula. It may be associated with cystoid spaces or lipid deposits, depending upon the duration of the disease. Clinically macular edema is defined as retinal edema within two disk diameters of the center of macula. The ETDRS has defined the clinically significant macular edema (CSME) as having any one of the following:

- Retinal thickening at or within 500 microns from the center of macula.
- Hard exudates at or within 500 microns from the center of macula associated with thickening of the adjacent retina.
- An area or areas of retinal thickening at least one disk area in size, at least a part of which is within one disk diameter of the center of macula.

Lenticular Changes in Diabetes

The clarity of the lens, its refractive index and accommodation ability are all affected by diabetes. Here, we are reminded of the hypothesis of polyol pathway, taught conventionally in pathology classes which states that there is an increase in the level of glucose in the vitreous and aqueous. Glucose enters the lens as it is independent of presence of insulin; it is converted to fructose and subsequently sorbitol by aldose reductase. Sorbitol is metabolized slowly by

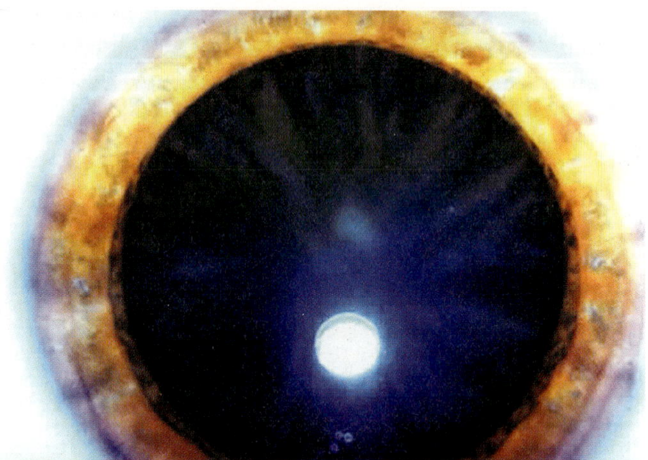

Fig. 5: Early snowflake and spoke cortical opacities
***Source*:** Manual B Datiles, Benjamin V Magno.

the lens and accumulates for a long time. This gives rise to tremendous osmolarity of the lens and subsequent water accumulation; this rate of hydration leads to changes and fluctuations of refractive power of the lens (hence frequent change of glasses). Acute myopic shifts may indicate poorly controlled diabetes.

The typical cataract of diabetes is a *"snowflake cataract";* it is bilateral subcapsular change of abrupt onset, so much so, that the patient may complain of appearance of symptoms over one week only. The initial cortical involvement sometimes gives a diurnal variation to the visual status. A cataract surgery under controlled circumstances is indicated.

DIABETES RELATED COMPLICATION IN ANTERIOR CHAMBER

In patients with advanced DR, small tufts of vessels are of common occurrence over the iris, referred to as rubeosis iridis; it may only be present with a subtle appearance at the angle of the anterior chamber detected only by careful gonioscopy. PRP is indicated in all progressive or nonprogressive cases, to stop further proliferation. Intracameral injection of anti-VEGFs helps in reducing proliferation temporarily, which is to be followed up by PRP. Secondary glaucoma due to proliferation may become intractable at times and may require advanced glaucoma surgeries which include trabeculectomy with adjuncts or valve placements.

DIABETES RELATED COMPLICATION IN POSTERIOR SEGMENT

Vitreous Hemorrhage

The NVD and the NVE may develop into frond of vessels and become elevated structures that they will bleed or not depends on their location, supported by the vitreous and their own structure. NVD is more prone to subhyaloid and vitreous hemorrhage. If the vitreous has detached, chances of hemorrhage are low but partially attached vitreous leads to dynamicity with the ocular movement; the fragile nature of the new vessels gives way to bleeds, sudden appearance of even small hemorrhages extending upon the macula lead to sudden episode of diminution of vision in a diabetic patient. Larger hemorrhages are more vision-threatening. The diabetic retinopathy study (DRS) elaborates the role of vitrectomy as a treatment option for these cases.

Tractional Retinal Detachment

Other concurrent systemic complications of diabetes many a times become a hindrance to surgical treatment options. In such cases, resolving vitreous hemorrhage takes the shape of single or multiple bands in the vitreous which are attached either surface to surface over the retina or anteroposterior connecting the retinal surface to the back of the lens. With the movement of the eye such attachments lead to traction at the macula. The contraction of such an extensive fibrovascular sheath leads to distortion or dragging, fractional detachment of the retina or a hole formation giving rise to rhegmatogenous retinal detachment. In the end, PDR enters an involutional or burned-out stage with a regression of all signs of disease and limited visual potential.

TREATMENT OPTIONS

For the people with diabetes, an HbA1c level of less than 7% is considered good control, although some people may prefer their numbers to be closer to that of nondiabetics. For the people with risk of hypoglycemia, this may be taken to be less than 8%.[16]

The DCCT suggests that intensive control of blood sugar levels reduces the risk of progression and also slows down the progress of retinopathy. It also reported a higher level of lipids in patients of DR.[5] The ACCORD (action to control cardiovascular risk in diabetes) eye study also suggests that fenofibrate along with simvastatin show significant reduction in retinopathy than simvastatin alone.

MEDICAL MANAGEMENT

The goal of medical management is to control risk factors like hypertension and carotid occlusive disease, as both lead to an enhancement of retinal ischemia which is already present in the diabetics. Women with diabetes who become pregnant are at a greater risk of developing and progression of DR, so they require frequent observations. If PDR is imminent, photocoagulation may be instituted.

LASER TREATMENT

In 1945 there was a solar eclipse, and many people developed retinopathy; this gave Meyer-Schwickerath an idea of photocoagulation. The DRS conclusively demonstrated that PRP significantly reduced the risk of severe visual loss in 50% cases of PDR. It showed that treatment benefit outweighs risk for eye with high-risk PDR (50% 5-year rate of severe visual loss in such eyes without treatment was reduced to 20% by treatment). The ETDRS also concluded that focal photocoagulation (direct laser for focal leaks and grid laser for diffuse leaks on fundus fluorescein angiography) reduced the risk of moderate visual loss by 50% or more and

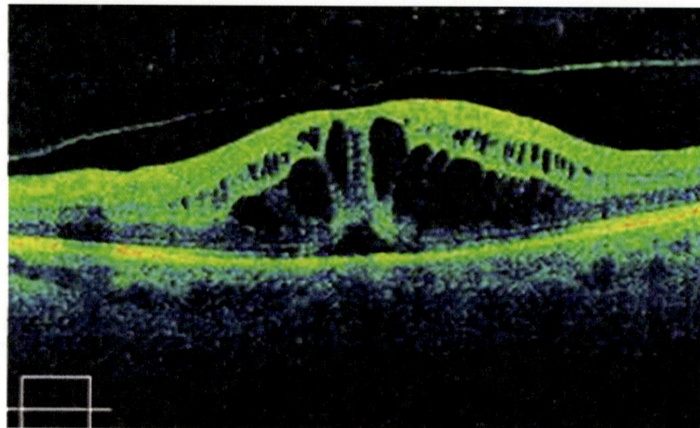

Fig. 6: OCT showing macular edema

increased the chance of small improvement of visual acuity. It also indicated the beneficial effects of early treatment in the form of low rates of severe visual loss.[17]

SURGICAL TREATMENT

The role of surgical pars plana vitrectomy is in cases of marked visual loss due to new or old vitreous hemorrhage especially where it appears that the hemorrhage is not likely to resolve soon.[18] Non-clearing vitreous hemorrhage which may be further complicated by tractional retinal detachment (TRD), combined TRD with rhegmatogenous retinal detachment, severe fibrovascular proliferation, anterior segment neovascularization, dense premacular hemorrhage, ghost cell glaucoma or cataract preventing the treatment of severe PDR warrants a vitrectomy surgery. Vitrectomy helps in decreasing the load of VEGFs, and inflammatory cytokines and thus retards the process of DME.

Vitrectomy is helpful in preventing retinal detachments, opaque membrane formations and rubeosis. It is helpful in delaying the final burned-out stage.[19]

Macular edema may be noted on fundus examination, but is much more easily appreciated using optical coherence tomography (OCT) (Fig. 6). OCT is a laser imaging technique which produces an image showing the individual layers of the retina and the shape of the retinal surface. Fluid accumulation between layers can be appreciated as black patches on the scan and irregular retinal surfaces may reflect the etiology behind a patient's visual abnormalities. It should be noted, however, that in the ETDRS (the study which is used to support the treatment for CSME), OCT was not used. CSME was diagnosed only by clinical appearance.[20]

MODERN TREATMENT OPTIONS

It is well known now that retinal ischemia, leads to changes in the microanatomy of the vasculature, this in turn causes release of growth factors. The VEGF thus released from the retinal pigment epithelium, pericytes and endothelial cells of the retina causes leukocyte adhesion and provokes the intracellular adhesion molecule-1 (ICAM-1) which is a precursor of inflammation. Intravitreal corticosteroids have been potent in reducing the effect of VEGF with the help of platelet derived growth factors, so these have been used in the form of triamcinolone acetonide and fluocinolone acetonide intravitreally.

More recently anti-VEGF agents like ranibizumab (Lucentis) and bevacizumab (Avastin) have shown favorable results and are now widely being used. They have been helpful in reducing the DME and the neovascularization; their dose dependent effect has led to their being used in the form of multiple injections.

Human trails are on with favorable results with oral protein kinase C, aldose reductase inhibitors and long-acting octreotide.

SCREENING

Sudden fall of vision in a diabetic patient by two line warrants an OCT and an angiography, a patient with diagnosed retinopathy should go for 4-monthly screening. The best tool for of evaluation still is direct and indirect ophthalmoscopy performed by an ophthalmologist. Digital imaging of fundus has also been very helpful wherever possible in picking up early patients. With the advancement in digital technologies and transmission, telescreening is also coming up in a big way (Box 1).[16]

Box 1: Optimize glucose and blood pressure control to reduce the risk for or slow the progression of retinopathy
Screening
• Initial dilated and comprehensive eye examination by an ophthalmologist or optometrist
• Adults with type 1 diabetes: consider eye examination within 5 years after diabetes onset
• Patients with type 2 diabetes: consider eye examination shortly after diagnosis
• If no retinopathy for ≥1 eye examination, consider eye examinations every 2 years
• If retinopathy, consider eye examination annual examination
• Retinopathy progressing or sight threatening: consider more frequent eye examinations
• Fundus photographs should be considered as a screening tool, but not a substitute for comprehensive examination
Pregnant women or women planning pregnancy with preexisting diabetes
• Retinopathy counseling, eye examination in first trimester
• Close follow-up throughout pregnancy and 1 year postpartum

CONCLUSION

The expected number of diabetics by 2030 is 79.4 million in India; this figure is an indication of the attention that is required in the by various government and non-governments organizations, physicians and ophthalmologists. Intravitreal anti-VEGF, steroids, laser photocoagulation and pars plana vitrectomy are the mainstay of the treatment.

REFERENCES

1. National Society to Prevent Blindness. In: Visual problems in the US data analysis definition, data sources, detailed data tables, analysis, interpretation. New York: National Society to Prevent Blindness; 1980. pp. 1-46.
2. Ramachandran A, Snehalatha C, Shetty AS, et al. Trends in prevalence of diabetes in Asian countries. World J Diabetes. 2012;3(6):110-7.
3. Delcourt C, Massin P, Rosilio M. Epidemiology of Diabetic retinopathy: expected vs reported prevalence of cases in French population. Diabetes Metab. 2009;35(6):431-8.
4. Williams R, Airey M, Baxter H. Epidemiology of diabetic retinopathy and macular edema: A systematic review. Eye. 2004;18:963-83.
5. Malone JI, Morrison AD, Pavan PR, et al. Diabetic Control and Complications Trial: Prevalence and significance of retinopathy in subjects with type 1 diabetes of less than 5 years duration screened for the diabetes control and complications trial. Diabetes Care. 2001;124:522-6.
6. Kohner EM, Aldington SJ, Stratton IM. United Kingdom Prospective Diabetes Study, 30: Diabetic retinopathy at diagnosis of non-insulin-dependent diabetes mellitus and associated risk factors. Arch Ophthalmol. 1998;116:297-303.
7. Rema M, Ponnaiya M, Mohan V. Prevalence of retinopathy in non-insulin dependent diabetes mellitus at a diabetes centre in southern India. Diab Res Clin Pract. 1996;(34)1:29-36.
8. Arden GB, Sivaprasad S. Hypoxia and oxidative stress in the causation of diabetic retinopathy. Current Diabetes Rev. 2011;7(5):291-304.
9. Kanter Y, Bessman SP, Bessman A. Red cell 2, 3-diphosphoglycerate levels among diabetic patients with and without vascular complications. Diabetes 1975 Aug; 24(8):724-9
10. Speiser PP, Gittelsohn AM, Patz A. Studies on diabetic retinopathy, III: Influence of diabetes on intramural pericytes. Arch Ophthalmol. 1968;80:332-7.
11. Tarr JM, Kaul K, Chopra M, et al. Pathophysiology of diabetic retinopathy. ISRN Ophthalmology. 2013.
12. Kubawara T, Cogan DG. Retinal vascular patterns VI: Mural cells of the retinal capillaries. Arch Ophthalmol. 1962;69:492-502.
13. Engerman RL. Pathogenesis of diabetic retinopathy. Diabetes. 1989;38(10);1203-6.
14. Aiello LP, Avery RL, Arrigg PG, et al. Vascular endothelial growth factor in ocular fluid of patients with diabetic retinopathy and other retinal disorders. N Engl J Med. 1994;331:1480-7.
15. Early treatment diabetic retinopathy study research group. Fundus photographic risk factors for progression of diabetic retinopathy: ETDRS report number 12. Ophthalmology. 1991;98:823-33.
16. American Diabetes Association Guidelines. 2015.
17. Diabetic retinopathy study research group. Preliminary report on effects of photo-coagulation therapy. Am J Ophthalmol. 1976;81:383-96.
18. Rosenblatt BJ, Benson WE. Diabetic retinopathy. In: Yanoff M, Duker JS, (Eds). Ophthalmology. 2nd edition. vol 2. Spain: Mosby; 2004. pp. 877-86.
19. Early treatment diabetic retinopathy study design and baseline patient characteristics. ETDRS report no. 7. Ophthalmology. 1991;98(Suppl 5):741-56.
20. Panozzo G, Gusson E, Parolini B, Mercanti A. Role of OCT in the diagnosis and follow up of diabetic macular edema. Semin Ophthalmol. 2003;18:74-81.

14
CHAPTER

Management of Diabetic Neuropathy

SK Singh, S Singh, RK Singh

INTRODUCTION

Diabetic neuropathy is one of the most common complications associated with significant morbidity and mortality.[1,2] It is an outcome of metabolic derangements due to prolonged hyperglycemia in diabetes.

Diabetic neuropathy has common risk factor for all microvascular complications such as age, duration of diabetes, glycemic variability, HbA_{1c}, smoking and alcohol consumption. Strict glycemic control is important for prevention and treatment of diabetic neuropathy.[3,4] The true prevalence is not defined as it depends on criteria and methods used in assessment of neuropathy but studies have reported it to be 33% amongst diabetic patients and 10% in newly diagnosed diabetics.[5,6]

With non-specific, insidious and slowly progressive course, it can remain obscured or can mimic other neuropathic disorders of nondiabetic origin like peripheral vascular disease, arthritis, malignancy, alcohol abuse, vitamin B12 deficiency, leprosy, etc. Symptoms include decreased sensation, positive neuropathic sensory symptoms of numbness, prickling, stabbing, burning, or aching pain predominantly in toes, feet, or legs. Signs of symmetrical decrease in distal sensation or absent ankle reflex can be often seen. Major morbidity associated is foot ulceration leading to diabetic foot infection, gangrene and foot loss. Overall it increases risk of amputation by 1.7-fold[7] accounts for 50–75% of nontrauma amputation.[8]

Diabetic neuropathy has subclinical and clinical manifestations depending upon class of nerve fiber involved. Different clinical manifestations include large fiber neuropathy, small fiber neuropathy, proximal motor neuropathy, acute mononeuropathy and entrapments of nerve fibers.

Some of them progresses with duration of diabetes like sensory and autonomic neuropathies while other are short lived and remits completely like mononeuropathy, radiculopathy and acute painful neuropathy.[9]

CLINICAL MANIFESTATIONS

Diabetic neuropathy cannot be accounted for mere presence of one sign, symptom or test alone. Its diagnosis requires more elaboration and generally, a minimum of two abnormalities from symptoms and signs, nerve conduction abnormalities, quantitative sensory tests and quantitative autonomic tests are recommended.[10]

Because of variable presentation and anatomic involvement, various classifications were proposed by the clinicians, but the one of the most convenient and acceptable is described below.

FOCAL NEUROPATHY

Mononeuropathy

Mononeuropathy that mostly occur in elderly, have acute onset and associated with pain which is self-limiting and resolves in 6–8 weeks.

Entrapment Syndromes

Unlike mononeuropathies, entrapment syndromes are slowly progressive and persistent without intervention. Median, ulnar and radial nerves are commonly involved in entrapment syndromes. Carpal tunnel syndrome involving median nerve is three times more common in diabetics than normal individuals.[11,12] Diabetic cheiroarthropathy[13] repeated undetected trauma, metabolic changes and accumulation of fluid in carpal tunnel[14] is responsible for increased prevalence in diabetics.

DIFFUSE NEUROPATHY

Among diffuse neuropathy, proximal motor neuropathy and distal symmetrical polyneuropathy are well known.

Proximal Motor Neuropathy

Proximal motor neuropathy usually affects elderly, with gradual or abrupt onset. It begins with pain in thighs and hips or buttocks with remarkable weakness of proximal muscles of lower limbs. In beginning as unilateral involvement, it spreads bilaterally coexisting with spontaneous muscle fasciculation. There is prevailing weakness of iliopsoas, obturator and adductor muscles with preserved action of gluteus maximus and gluteus minimus and hamstrings. It can be secondary a variety of causes that are unrelated to diabetes but have a greater incidence in patients with diabetes than in general population. These include chronic inflammatory demyelinating polyneuropathy, monoclonal gammopathy, circulating monosialoganglioside (GM1) antibodies and antibodies to neuronal cells, and inflammatory vasculitis.[15,16] These features are to be distinguished from spinal stenosis syndromes.

Distal Symmetrical Polyneuropathy

Distal symmetrical polyneuropathy is most common form of neuropathy in diabetes. Typically, patients experience burning, tingling, and electrical pain, but sometimes they may experience simple numbness. In patients who experience pain, which is usually worse at nights. Patient with simple numbness can present with painless foot ulceration.

AUTONOMIC NEUROPATHY

Diabetic autonomic neuropathy (DAN) may present in isolation or in combination with DPN. Mostly, it manifests by gastroparesis, constipation, diarrhea, anhidrosis, bladder dysfunction, erectile dysfunction, exercise intolerance, resting tachycardia, silent ischemia and even sudden cardiac death. Cardiovascular autonomic neuropathy is most prominent amongst all because it can herald complications with life threatening events. At the time of diagnosis of type 2 diabetes mellitus and within 5 years of diagnosis of type 1 diabetes mellitus (unless individual has symptoms suggestive of autonomic dysfunction earlier), patient should be screened for cardiac autonomic neuropathy.

PAINFUL DIABETIC NEUROPATHY

Complexity of pathophysiology of pain in diabetic neuropathy has led to understanding of the concept of pain in diabetic neuropathy and its management. Neuroplasticity, or the physical remodeling of neuronal cytoarchitecture, occurs shortly after the onset of persistent acute pain and leads to the transition from acute pain into a chronic pain state. As a result of a peripheral lesion that persistently generates pain impulses to the spinal cord, inhibitory interneurons responsible for modulating painful nerve transmission impulses eventually die. It results into glial cells remodeling of neuronal synapses to intensify nociceptive transmission.

Pain syndromes lasting for 6 months are categorized as acute painful neuropathy while those lasting for more than 6 months are categorized as chronic painful neuropathy.[17]

ACUTE PAINFUL NEUROPATHY

Patients tend to develop small-fiber neuropathy with pain and paresthesia early in course of disease. Symptoms have nocturnal exacerbation manifesting more in feet than in hands. Lower legs are extremely tender to touch. Pain is invariably described as lancinating, stabbing, burning and sharp. Distorted sensations of pins and needles, tingling and numbness often accompany pain. Acute painful neuropathy may be associated with onset of insulin therapy, being termed as insulin neuritis.[18] Neuropathy with weight loss and depression may manifest as diabetic neuropathic cachexia[19] which is usually reversible with glycemic control.

CHRONIC PAINFUL NEUROPATHY

This condition usually occurs late in course of diabetes. It is resistant to most of interventions. Absence of pain is not from improvement of neuropathy but is rather consequence of neuronal loss. Neuropathic pain can be stimulus dependent (hyperalgesia) or stimulus independent (allodynia).

SMALL-FIBER NEUROPATHY

Pain is of C-fiber type. It is superficial, burning and associated with allodynia. Patients have decreased sweating, dry skin, impaired blood flow and cold feet due to autonomic involvement as well.

LARGE-FIBER NEUROPATHY

There can be involvement of both sensory and motor fibers. These fibers are responsible for motor functions, vibration perception, position sense and cold thermal perception. Myelinated rapid conducting fibers are first to be affected due to their long course. Wasting of small muscles of feet with hammertoes, and shortening of Achilles tendon with pes equinus may also be present. Generally, mixed variety of neuropathy with both small and large-fiber damage along with distal sensory polyneuropathy is seen in most of diabetic neuropathic patients.

DIAGNOSIS

The 2010 Toronto conference on diabetic neuropathy and the 2009 conference of the American Academy of Neurology[20] recommended that at least one parameter from each of the following five categories be measured to classify diabetic neuropathy: symptom profiles, neurologic examination, quantitative sensory tests (QST), nerve conduction study and autonomic function testing. Both sides of feet and hands must be evaluated for sensory examination.

Young et al.[21] criteria for clinical diagnosis of DPN [neuropathy symptoms score (NSS) + neuropathy disability score (NDS) >8] can be used as bedside tool. NSS is burning, numbness or tingling, fatigue, cramping, aching or nocturnal exacerbation, and NDS is calculated by ankle reflex, pinprick sensation, temperature sensation, vibration sense tested with tuning fork and monofilament test.

Some other symptom scoring systems are also counted like Michigan neuropathy screening instrument (MNSI)[22] and nerve impairment score of the lower limbs (NIS-LL).[23]

Quantitative autonomic function tests (QAFT) and QST have objective indices. Based on measurement of heart rate and blood pressure responses to series of maneuvers for detection of cardiovascular autonomic neuropathy, QAFT is simple and noninvasive test.[24,25]

Dyck's clinical staging[26] described in Table 1 is used for not only clinical practice but in controlled clinical trials and epidemiological studies.

Table 1: Dyck's clinical staging

Dyck's staging	*Clinical designation*
N0	No neuropathy (no objective evidence of diabetic neuropathy)
N1a	No symptoms or signs but neuropathic test abnormalities
N1b	Clinical neuropathy (test abnormalities plus neuropathic impairment on neurologic examination)
N2a	Symptoms, signs, and test abnormalities
N2b	N2a plus significant ankle dorsiflexor weakness
N3	Late complications (disabling polyneuropathy)

Biopsy of nerve tissue may be helpful to exclude other causes of neuropathy. Sural nerve is most common site for nerve tissue sample.

The importance of the skin biopsy as a diagnostic tool for diabetic peripheral neuropathy is increasingly being recognized.[27,28] This technique quantitates small epidermal nerve fibers through antibody staining of protein gene product 9.5.

Corneal confocal microscopy is newer tool to help in detecting[4] and stratifying the severity[29] of DPN with good diagnostic utility (85% sensitivity, 84% specificity)[4] and repeatability.[30,31] It can be used to assess the recovery of DPN following intervention such as continuous subcutaneous insulin therapy, pancreas-kidney transplantation or reduction of risk factors.

MANAGEMENT

Upon diagnosis of neuropathy, therapy with goal to mitigate symptoms and preventing progression of neuropathy should be instituted. Since high level of blood glucose is responsible for multidimensional complications of diabetes mellitus, control of blood glucose level with remark on fluctuation in glycemic variability proves to be mainstay of treatment.

Control of Hyperglycemia

DCCT data[32] and data from epidemiological studies have proved that optimal blood glucose helps in prevention of distal symmetrical polyneuropathy and autonomic neuropathy in both types 1 and 2 diabetes mellitus. Furthermore, in UK prospective diabetes study, control of blood glucose level provided improvement in vibration perceptions.[33-35] For prevention of other complications, improvement in lipid and blood pressure indices, avoidance of cigarette smoking and consumption of excessive alcohol are already recommended.

PHARMACOLOGICAL THERAPY

Aldose Reductase Inhibitor

Aldose reductase inhibitors (ARIs) reduce the flux of glucose through the polyol pathway, inhibiting tissue accumulation of sorbitol and fructose and preventing reduction of redox potentials. Combinations of therapy with ARIs and antioxidants may become critical to curb the relentless progression of diabetic neuropathy. But it is also clear that aldose reductase inhibition may be insufficient to achieve the desirable degree of metabolic enhancement in patients with a multitude of biochemical abnormalities.

α-Lipoic Acid

Lipoic acid (1,2-dithiolane-3-pentanoic acid), a derivative of octanoic acid, is present in food and is also synthesized by the liver. It is a natural cofactor in the pyruvate dehydrogenase complex, where it binds acyl groups and transfers them from one part of the complex to another α-lipoic acid, which is also known as thioctic acid. This replenishment of thiol made lipoic acid, a redox modulating agent. It is undergoing extensive trials in the United States and Europe, and promising results for treating diabetes and diabetic neuropathy are still to come.

γ-Linolenic Acid

It is derived from linolenic acid, an essential fatty acid. It serves as an important constituent of neuronal membrane phospholipids and as a substrate for the formation of PGE, which is important for preserving nerve blood flow. In diabetes mellitus, this conversion is impaired leading to pathogenesis of diabetic neuropathy.[36] In some trials, administration of γ-linolenic acid showed improvements in clinical measures and on electrophysiologic testing. But, its role as essential drug therapy is still inconclusive.

Protein Kinase C-β Inhibition

Insufficient blood flow to neural tissue has been proposed as a contributing factor to development of diabetic neuropathy.[37] Protein kinase C-β inhibition (PKC) is hyperactivated by hyperglycemia and disordered fatty acid metabolism. Activated PKC results in increased production of vasoconstrictive, angiogenic and chemotactic cytokines including TGF-β, VEGF, endothelin and intercellular adhesion molecules (ICAMs). Nonselective PKC inhibitors normalize hyperglycemia-induced decrease in endoneurial blood flow. This drug was well tolerated, but there were few adverse events.

Aminoguanidine

In animal studies, aminoguanidine stands as an inhibitor of the formation of AGEs and also shows improvement in nerve conduction studies, but controlled clinical trials to determine the efficacy of aminoguanidine in humans[38,39] were discontinued because of toxicity.

Human Intravenous Immunoglobulin

Patients of diabetic neuropathy associated with signs of antineuronal autoimmunity, and autonomic neuropathy may benefit from intravenous immunoglobulin.[40,41] Major toxicity is anaphylactic reactions, but some may experience severe headache due to aseptic meningitis which resolves spontaneously. Sometimes it may be necessary to combine treatment with prednisone or azathioprine.

Neurotrophic Therapy

Decreased expression of nerve growth factor (NGF) and its receptors, TrkA and p75, reduces retrograde axonal transport of NGF. Growth support of small unmyelinated neurons and their neuropeptides, such as substance P and calcitonin gene-related peptide (CGRP) is consequently reduced, and both neuropeptides are potent vasodilators. Administration of recombinant human NGF (rhNGF) restores these neuropeptide levels toward normal and prevents the manifestations of sensory neuropathy in animals. But, small trial of neurotrophin 3 (NT3) for safety was interpreted as negative for efficacy, and IGF1 and IGF11 have not been considered to be safe for administration to humans. A more promising therapy may be found with the proinsulin C-peptide.[42]

Pain Control

Different types of pain respond to different therapy according to its derivation from different types of nerve fibers (C-fiber or Aδ-fiber), from spinal cord or from cerebral cortex.

C-fiber Pain

C-fibers are modulated by sympathetic input with spontaneous firings of different neurotransmitters to the dorsal root ganglion, spinal cord and cerebral cortex. Any interruption in these modulating pathways can ameliorate pain symptoms.

Capsaicin

Capsaicin is extracted from chili peppers, and a simple, cheap mixture can be made by adding 1–3 teaspoons (15–45 mL) of cayenne pepper to a jar of cold cream. Prolonged application of capsaicin depletes stores of substance P, and possibly other neurotransmitters, from sensory nerve endings. This reduces or abolishes the transmission of painful stimuli.[43]

Clonidine

Because the peripheral sympathetic nerve fibers are also small, unmyelinated C-fibers, sympathetic blocking agents (clonidine) can improve the pain.

Aδ-fiber Pain

Aδ-fiber pain is a more deep-seated, dull and gnawing ache that often does not respond to above described drugs. A number of different agents have been used for the pain associated with these fibers.

Insulin

Aδ-fiber use Na^+ channels for conduction. Insulin inhibits Na^+ exchange. Continuous intravenous insulin infusion reduces pain usually in 48 hours[44] and then infusion can be discontinued.

Nerve Blockers

These compounds target the pain caused by hyperexcitability of superficial free nerve endings.[45] Lidocaine by continuous infusion with oral Mexiletine can relieve most intractable pain. But because of reported cardiac toxicity upon systemic use, topical use is mostly preferred nowadays.

Tramadol and Dextromethorphan

Tramadol is central opioid analgesic for moderate to severe pain. Side effects of opioid drugs are common. Dextromethorphan is NMDA (N-methyl D-aspartate) receptor blocker.[46] It targets NMDA receptors of spinal cord.

Antidepressants

Imipramine, amitriptyline and clomipramine induce a balanced reuptake inhibition of both norepinephrine and serotonin, whereas desipramine is a relatively selective norepinephrine reuptake inhibitor. This central action accentuates the effects of these neurotransmitters in activation of endogenous pain-inhibitory systems in the brain. Amitriptyline is frequently used as first choice. Anticholinergic side effects, sexual side effects and orthostatic hypotension are limiting their use. Dosages must be titrated based on positive responses, treatment adherence, and adverse events.

Selective serotonin reuptake inhibitors (SSRIs) that have been used for neuropathic pain are paroxetine, fluoxetine, sertraline and citalopram. Paroxetine appears to be associated with greater pain relief.[47] Fluoxetine failed a placebo-controlled trial.[48]

Antiepileptic Drugs

Principal mechanisms of action include sodium channel blockade (felbamate, lamotrigine, oxcarbazepine, topiramate, zonisamide), potentiation of γ-aminobutyric acid (GABA) activity (pregabalin, tiagabine, topiramate), calcium-channel blockade (felbamate, lamotrigine, topiramate, zonisamide), and antagonism of glutamate at NMDA receptors (felbamate). Carbamazepine is useful for patients with shooting or electric shock-like pain.[49] Phenytoin has long been used in the treatment of painful neuropathies.[50]

Gabapentin has been found reduce the release of neurotransmitters that are involved in nociceptive pain signaling such as glutamate, CGRP and substance P. Topical application of gabapentin overcomes the occurrence of systemic side effects like sedation and dizziness. Gabapentin penetrates in the layer of skin and retained in skin for longer time so that impulse generation from neuron is blocked. Pregabalin (Lyrica) is a GABA analog with similar structure and actions to gabapentin, but it is a more specific.

Adjunct Management and Treatment of Complications

Analgesics

They are not of much use in treatment of diabetic neuropathy but for short term, they are instituted for diabetic third nerve palsy. Other drugs used for treatment of diabetic painful neuropathy are described in Table 2.

Table 2: Analgesics which have potential to treat painful diabetic neuropathy

Class of drug	*Dosage*	*Side effects*	*Comments*
Acetaminophen	15–20 mg/kg every 4–6 h; daily maximum of 4 g	Gastrointestinal problems	Underused for acute pain
NSAIDs	400 mg Ibuprofen safest inexpensive choice; decreases some adverse GI events with misoprostol 800 mg, H 2 blockers, and PPI	Gastrointestinal problems, platelet function inhibition, renal dysfunction	No evidence that any one agent is more efficient than other
Selective COX-2 inhibitors	Once or twice per day, only advantage over most traditional NSAIDs for acute pain	Renal dysfunction; hypertension; thrombotic event	Only effective for treating acute pain
Opioids	No ceiling dose; greater analgesia can be obtained by increasing the dosage with no limit except those imposed by side effects	Sedation, nausea, vomiting, constipation	Recommended: Oxycodone, hydrocodone. Not recommended for acute pain: Codeine, propoxyphene, pentazocine

Calcitonin

In a placebo-controlled study, 10 patients with painful diabetic neuropathy were treated with 100 IU of calcitonin per day. About 39% of patients had near-complete relief of symptom. The improvement was seen after only 2 weeks of treatment.[51]

MANAGEMENT OF SMALL-FIBER NEUROPATHIES

Inspection of foot on routine basis is advised to patients of diabetic neuropathy. All diabetic patients should wear padded socks. Shoes must fit well and have adequate support, and they must be inspected for the presence of foreign bodies. Emollient creams should be used for drying and cracking. Nails should be cut transversely, preferably by a podiatrist.

Table 3: Management of autonomic neuropathy

Symptoms	*Tests*	*Treatment*
Cardiac		
1. Exercise intolerance, early fatigue and weakness with exercise	MUGA thallium scan, MIBG scan	Graded supervised exercise, ACE inhibitors, beta blockers
2. Postural hypotension	Blood pressure measure in standing and supine position, catecholamine measure	Mechanical measures, clonidine, midodrine, octreotide
Gastrointestinal		
1. Gastroparesis	Gastric emptying study, barium study	Frequent small meals, prokinetic agents (metoclopramide, domperidone)
2. Abdominal pain, nausea, vomiting, belching, bloating	Endoscopy, manometry, electrogastrogram endoscopy	Antiemetics, bulking agents, TCA, pancreatic extracts, gastric pacing
3. Constipation, diarrhea		High fiber diets and bulking agents, anticholinergic agents
Sexual dysfunction		
1. Erectile dysfunction	History and clinical examination	Psychological counseling, sildenafil, PGE1 injection, device and prosthesis
2. Vaginal dryness *Bladder dysfunction*	Cystometrogram, postvoiding sonography	Vaginal lubricants Bethanechol, intermittent catheterization
Sudomotor dysfunction	Sweat test, skin blood flow, quantitative sudomotor axon reflex	Emollients and skin lubricants, scopolamine, glycopyrrolate, vasodilators, botulinum toxins

Abbreviations: MUGA, multi gated acquisition scan; MIBG, meta-iodo-benzyl-guanidine; PGE1, prostaglandin E1; TCA, tricyclic antidepressants

MANAGEMENT OF LARGE-FIBER NEUROPATHIES

Patients with large-fiber neuropathies are uncoordinated atypia and autonomic dysfunction management of autonomic dysfunction method (Table 3). As a result, they are more likely to fall than non-neuropathic age-matched persons.[52] Therefore, it is vital for the patient to embark on a program of strength training and improvement of balance to include gait and strength training, tendon lengthening for Achilles tendon shortening, orthotics and proper shoes for the deformities, bisphosphonates for osteopenia, and surgical reconstruction and full-length casting as required.

REFERENCES

1. Vinik AI, Mitchell BD, Leichter SB, et al. Epidemiology of the complications of diabetes. In: Leslie RDG, Robbins DC (Eds). Diabetes: Clinical Science in Practice. Cambridge, UK: Cambridge University Press; 1995. pp 221-87.
2. Vinik A, Mehrabyan A. Diabetic neuropathies. Med Clin North Am. 2004;88:947-99.
3. Candrilli SD, Davis KL, Kan HJ, et al. Prevalence and the associated burden of illness of symptoms of diabetic peripheral neuropathy and diabetic retinopathy. J Diabetes Complicat. 2007;21:306-14.
4. Won JC, Kwon HS, Kim CH, et al. Prevalence and clinical characteristics of diabetic peripheral neuropathy in hospital patients with type 2 diabetes in Korea. Diabet Med. 2012;29:e290-6.
5. Young MJ, Boulton AJM, MacLeod AF, et al. A multicentre study of the prevalence of diabetic peripheral neuropathy in the United Kingdom hospital clinic population. Diabetologia. 1993;36:1-5.
6. Dyck PJ, Kratz KM, Karnes JL, et al. The prevalence by staged severity of various types of diabetic neuropathy, retinopathy, and nephropathy in a population-based cohort: the Rochester Diabetic Neuropathy Study. Neurology. 1993;43:817-24.
7. Armstrong DG, Lavery LA, Harkless LB. Validation of a diabetic wound classification system: the contribution of depth, infection, and ischemia to risk of amputation. Diabetes Care. 1998;21:855-9.
8. Holzer SE, Camerota A, Martens L, et al. Costs and duration of care for lower extremity ulcers in patients with diabetes. Clin Ther. 1998;20:169-81.
9. Watkins PJ. Progression of diabetic autonomic neuropathy. Diabet Med. 1993;10(Suppl. 2):77S-8S.
10. Dyck PJ. Severity and staging of diabetic polyneuropathy. In: Gries FA, Cameron NE, Low PA (Eds). Textbook of Diabetic Neuropathy. Stuttgart, Germany: Thieme; 2003:170-5.
11. Karpitskaya Y, Novak CB, Mackinnon SE. Prevalence of smoking, obesity, diabetes mellitus and thyroid disease in patients with carpal tunnel syndrome. Am Plast Surg. 2002;48:269-73.
12. Perkins B, Olaleye D, Bril V. Carpal tunnel syndrome in patients with diabetic polyneuropathy. Diabetes Care. 2002;25:565-9.
13. Chaudhuri KR, Davidson AR, Morris IM. Limited joint mobility and carpal tunnel syndrome in insulin dependent diabetes. Br J Rheumatol. 1989;28:191-4.
14. Vinik AI, Holland MT, LeBeau JM, et al. Diabetic neuropathies. Diabetes Care. 1992;15:1926-75.
15. Vinik AI, Pittenger GL, Milicevic Z, et al. Autoimmune mechanisms in the pathogenesis of diabetic neuropathy. In: Eisenbarth RG (Ed). Molecular Mechanisms of Endocrine and Organ Specific Autoimmunity. Georgetown, TX: Landes; 1998. pp 217-51.
16. Steck AJ, Kappos L. Gangliosides and autoimmune neuropathies: classification and clinical aspects of autoimmune neuropathies. J Neurol Neurosurg Psychiatry. 1994;57(Suppl.):26-8.
17. Vinik AI, Park TS, Stansberry KB, et al. Diabetic neuropathies. Diabetologia. 2000;43:957-73.
18. Tesfaye S, Malik R, Harris N, et al. Arterio-venous shunting and proliferating new vessels in acute painful neuropathy of rapid glycaemic control (insulin neuritis). Diabetologia. 1996;39:329-35.
19. Van Heel DA, Levitt NS, Winter TA. Diabetic neuropathic cachexia: the importance of positive recognition and early nutritional support. Int J Clin Pract. 1998;52:591-2.
20. Ebara T, Conde K, Kako Y, et al. Delayed catabolism of apoB-48 lipoproteins due to decreased heparan sulfate proteoglycan production in diabetic mice. J Clin Invest. 2000;105:1807-18.
21. Young MJ, Breddy JL, Veves A, et al. The prediction of diabetic neuropathic foot ulceration using vibration perception thresholds. A prospective study. Diabetes Care. 1994;17(6):557-60.

22. Feldman EL, Stevens MJ, Thomas PK, et al. A practical two-step quantitative clinical and electrophysiological assessment for the diagnosis and staging of diabetic neuropathy. Diabetes Care. 1994;17:1281-9.
23. Bril V. NIS-LL: the primary measurement scale for clinical trial endpoints in diabetic peripheral neuropathy. Eur Neurol. 1999;41(Suppl. 1):8-13.
24. Hanson PH, Schumaker P, Debugne TH, et al. Evaluation of somatic and autonomic small fibers neuropathy in diabetes. Am J Phys Med Rehabil. 1992;71:44-7.
25. Ducher M, Thivolet C, Cerutti C, et al. Noninvasive exploration of cardiac autonomic neuropathy. Diabetes Care. 1999;22:388-93.
26. Dyck PJ. Severity and staging of diabetic polyneuropathy. In: Gries FA, Cameron NE, Low PA (Eds). Textbook of Diabetic Neuropathy. Stuttgart, Germany: Thieme; 2003. pp. 170-5.
27. Pittenger GL, Ray M, Burcus NI, et al. Intraepidermal nerve fibers are indicators of small-fiber neuropathy in both diabetic and nondiabetic patients. Diabetes Care. 2004; 27:1974-9.
28. Kennedy WR, Wendelschafer-Crabb G, Johnson T. Quantitation of epidermal nerves in diabetic neuropathy. Neurology. 1996;47:1042-8.
29. Ahmed A, Bril V, Orszag A, et al. Detection of diabetic sensorimotor polyneuropathy by corneal confocal microscopy in type 1 diabetes: a concurrent validity study. Diabetes Care. 2012;35:821-8.
30. Tavakoli M, Quattrini C, Abbott C, et al. Corneal confocal microscopy: a novel noninvasive test to diagnose and stratify the severity of human diabetic neuropathy. Diabetes Care. 2010;33:1792-7.
31. Pritchard N, Edwards K, Vagenas D, et al. Corneal sensitivity as an ophthalmic marker of diabetic neuropathy. Optom Vis Sci. 2010;87:1003-8.
32. DCCT Research Group. The effect of intensive treatment of diabetes on the development and progression of long-term complications in insulin-dependent diabetes mellitus. N Engl J Med. 1993;329:977-86.
33. UK Prospective Diabetes Study (UKPDS) Group. Intensive blood-glucose control with sulphonylureas or insulin compared with conventional treatment and risk of complications in patients with type 2 diabetes (UKPDS 33). Lancet. 1998;352:837-53.
34. Comper WD, Osicka TM, Clark M, et al. Earlier detection of microalbuminuria in diabetic patients using a new urinary albumin assay. Kidney Int. 2004;65:1850-5.
35. Hirai A, Yasuda H, Joko M, et al. Evaluation of diabetic neuropathy through the quantitation of cutaneous nerves. J Neurol Sci. 2000;172:55-62.
36. Jamal GA. The use of gamma linolenic acid in the prevention and treatment of diabetic neuropathy. Diabet Med. 1994;11:145-9.
37. Dyck PJ. Hypoxic neuropathy: does hypoxia play a role in diabetic neuropathy? The 1988 Robert Wartenberg lecture. Neurology. 1989;39:111-8.
38. Miyauchi Y, Shikama H, Takasu T, et al. Slowing of peripheral motor nerve conduction was ameliorated by aminoguanidine in streptozocin-induced diabetic rats. Eur J Endocrinol. 1996;134:467-73.
39. Schmidt RE, Dorsey DA, Beaudet LN, et al. Effect of aminoguanidine on the frequency of neuroaxonal dystrophy in the superior mesenteric sympathetic autonomic ganglia of rats with streptozotocin-induced diabetes. Diabetes. 1996;45:284-90.
40. Sander HW, Chokroverty S. Diabetic amyotrophy: current concepts. Semin Neurol. 1996;16:173-8.
41. Barada A, Reljanovic M, Milicevic Z, et al. Proximal diabetic neuropathy-response to immunotherapy (Abstract). Diabetes. 1999;48(Suppl. 1):A148.
42. Wahren J, Ekberg K, Samnegard B, et al. C-peptide: a new potential in the treatment of diabetic nephropathy. Curr Diab Rep. 2001;1:261-6.
43. Rains C, Bryson HM. Topical capsaicin: a review of its pharmacological properties and therapeutic potential in post-herpetic neuralgia, diabetic neuropathy and osteoarthritis. Drugs Aging. 1995;7:317-28.

44. Said G, Bigo A, Ameri A, et al. Uncommon early-onset neuropathy in diabetic patients. J Neurol. 1998;245:61-8.
45. Jarvis B, Coukell AJ. Mexiletine: a review of its therapeutic use in painful diabetic neuropathy. Drugs. 1998;56:691-707.
46. Nelson KA, Park KM, Robinovitz E, et al. High-dose oral dextromethorphan versus placebo in painful diabetic neuropathy and postherpetic neuralgia. Neurology. 1997;48:1212-8.
47. Sindrup S, Gram L, Brosen K, et al. The selective serotonin reuptake inhibitor paroxetine is effective in treatment of diabetic neuropathy symptoms. Pain. 1990;42:135-44.
48. Max M, Lynch S, Muir J. Effects of desipramine, amitryptiline and fluoxetine on pain in diabetic neuropathy. N Engl J Med. 1992;326:1250-6.
49. Jensen TS. Anticonvulsants in neuropathic pain: rationale and clinical evidence. Eur J Pain. 2002;6(Suppl. A):61-8.
50. McQuay H, Carroll D, Jadad AR, et al. Anticonvulsant drugs for management of pain: a systematic review. BMJ. 1995;311:1047-52.
51. Zieleniewski W. Calcitonin nasal spray for painful diabetic neuropathy. Lancet. 1990;336:449.
52. Cavanagh PR, Derr JA, Ulbrecht JS, et al. Problems with gait and posture in neuropathic patients with insulin-dependent diabetes mellitus. Diabet Med. 1992;9:469-74.

15
CHAPTER

Management of Cardiovascular Disorders in Diabetes

Anuj Maheshwari

INTRODUCTION

Diabetic patients remain a high-risk group for myocardial infarction (MI), with poorer outcomes, whilst having a sound pathophysiological basis for aggressive treatment and intervention with greater benefits than nondiabetic patients. Thrombolysis benefits diabetic more than nondiabetic patients, but very few diabetics avail it and mostly not in time. Increased platelet activation, increased expression of coagulation factors and reduced intrinsic thrombolytic activity, are mainly responsible for cardiovascular adverse outcomes in diabetics. The glycoprotein IIb/IIIa antagonists, tirofiban and eptifibatide, have been used in the setting of unstable angina/non-Q-wave MI and shown to improve both short and medium-term outcomes in diabetics. Studies have demonstrated a benefit from direct angioplasty compared to thrombolysis in MI, high-risk patients in general and diabetic patients. Stenting provides improved outcomes in diabetic patients though it has higher restenosis rate than percutaneous transluminal coronary angioplasty (PTCA) in MI. Overall myocardial (including microvascular) perfusion is also impaired in diabetes. Higher incidence of early death prior to angiography in the diabetic group remains. The metabolic derangement that occurs at the time of MI leads to anaerobic glucose metabolism and a shift toward free fatty acid utilization, this being exacerbated by insulin deficiency or resistance. Careful modulation of glucose metabolism in the acute and follow-up phase of an infarct may favorably influence outcome. Metabolic manipulation has now established itself in mainstream treatment, although the exact regimen will continue to be refined.

Hypertension is a common diabetes comorbidity, and it is a major risk factor for both cardiovascular disease (CVD) and microvascular complications. The effects of lifestyle therapy on cardiovascular events have not been established. In people with diabetes, inhibitors of the renin-angiotensin system (RAS) may have unique advantages for initial or early treatment of hypertension. Statins are the drugs of choice for LDL cholesterol-lowering and cardioprotection. Aspirin has been shown to be effective in reducing cardiovascular morbidity and mortality in high-risk patients with previous MI or stroke, i.e. for secondary prevention but its net benefit in primary prevention is more controversial, both for patients with and without a history of diabetes. The use of additional antiplatelet agents has been advocated, and, specifically, clopidogrel has been shown to be of benefit in addition to aspirin. With the evolution of coronary intervention, primary and early intervention in diabetes may offer favorable outcomes in appropriately selected patients.

Cardiovascular disease is the major cause of morbidity and mortality for individuals with diabetes and is the largest contributor to the direct and indirect costs of diabetes. The common conditions coexisting with type 2 diabetes (e.g. hypertension and dyslipidemia) are clear risk factors for CVD, and diabetes itself confers independent risk. Numerous studies have shown the efficacy of controlling individual cardiovascular risk factors in preventing or slowing CVD in people with diabetes.

HYPERTENSION

Hypertension is a common diabetes comorbidity that affects the majority of patients, with the prevalence depending on type of diabetes, age, obesity and ethnicity. Hypertension is a major risk factor for both CVD and microvascular complications. In type 1 diabetes, hypertension is often the result of underlying nephropathy, while in type 2 diabetes it usually coexists with other cardiometabolic risk factors.

The clear body of evidence that systolic blood pressure (SBP) more than 140 mm Hg is harmful, suggests that clinicians should promptly initiate and titrate therapy in an ongoing fashion to achieve and maintain SBP less than 140 mm Hg in virtually all patients. Similarly, the clearest evidence from randomized clinical trials supports diastolic blood pressure (DBP) targets of less than 90 mm Hg. The 2015 American Diabetes Association (ADA) Standards of Care have been revised to reflect the higher-quality evidence that exists to support a goal of DBP less than 90 mm Hg, although lower targets may be appropriate for certain individuals. This is in harmonization with a recent publication by the Eighth Joint National Committee that recommended, for individuals over 18 years of age with diabetes, a DBP threshold of less than 90 mm Hg and SBP less than 140 mm Hg.[1]

LIFESTYLE MODIFICATIONS

Although there are no well-controlled studies of diet and exercise in the treatment of elevated blood pressure or hypertension in individuals with diabetes, the DASH study evaluated the impact of healthy dietary patterns in individuals without diabetes and has shown antihypertensive effects similar to those of pharmacological monotherapy.

These lifestyle (non-pharmacological) strategies may also positively affect glycemia and lipid control and should be encouraged in those with even mildly elevated blood pressure. The effects of lifestyle therapy on cardiovascular events have not been established. Non-pharmacological therapy is reasonable in individuals with diabetes and mildly elevated blood pressure (SBP >120 mm Hg or DBP >80 mm Hg). If the blood pressure is confirmed to be more than 140 mm Hg systolic and/or more than 90 mm Hg diastolic, pharmacological therapy should be initiated along with non-pharmacological therapy.[2] To enable long-term adherence, lifestyle therapy should be adapted to suit the needs of the patient and discussed as part of diabetes management.

PHARMACOLOGICAL INTERVENTIONS

Lowering of blood pressure with regimens based on a variety of antihypertensive agents, including angiotensin-converting enzyme (ACE) inhibitors, angiotensin-receptor blockers (ARBs), β-blockers, diuretics and calcium channel blockers, has been shown to be effective in reducing cardiovascular events. Several studies have suggested that ACE inhibitors may be superior to dihydropyridine calcium channel blockers in reducing cardiovascular events. However, several studies have also shown no specific advantage to ACE inhibitors as initial treatment of hypertension in the general hypertensive population, while showing an advantage of initial therapy with low-dose thiazide diuretics on cardiovascular outcomes.[2-4] In people with diabetes, inhibitors of the RAS may have unique advantages for initial or early treatment of hypertension. In a trial of individuals at high risk for CVD, including a large subset with diabetes, an ACE inhibitor reduced CVD outcomes. In patients with congestive heart failure (CHF), including subgroups with diabetes, ARBs have been shown to reduce major CVD outcomes.[5] In type 2 diabetic patients with significant diabetic kidney disease, ARBs were superior to calcium channel blockers for reducing heart failure. The blood pressure arm of the ADVANCE trial demonstrated that routine administration of a fixed combination of the ACE inhibitor perindopril and the diuretic indapamide significantly reduced combined microvascular and macrovascular outcomes, as well as death from cardiovascular causes and total mortality. The improved outcomes could also have been due to lower achieved blood pressure in the perindopril indapamide arm. Another trial showed a decrease in morbidity and mortality in those receiving benazepril and amlodipine versus benazepril and hydrochlorothiazide (HCTZ). The compelling benefits of RAS inhibitors in diabetic patients with albuminuria or renal insufficiency provide additional rationale for these agents. If needed to achieve blood pressure targets, amlodipine, HCTZ, or chlorthalidone can be added. If eGFR is less than 30 mL/min/m^2, a loop diuretic, rather than HCTZ or chlorthalidone, should be prescribed. Titration of and/or addition of further blood pressure medications should be made in timely fashion to overcome clinical inertia in achieving blood pressure targets. An important caveat is that most patients with hypertension require multiple drug therapy to reach treatment goals.[6] Identifying and addressing barriers to medication adherence (such as cost and side effects) should routinely be done. If blood pressure remains uncontrolled despite confirmed adherence to optimal doses of at least three antihypertensive agents of different classifications, one of which should be a diuretic, clinicians should consider an evaluation for secondary forms of hypertension.

PREGNANCY AND ANTIHYPERTENSIVE MEDICATIONS

During pregnancy, treatment with ACE inhibitors and ARBs is contraindicated, since they may cause fetal damage. Antihypertensive drugs known to be effective and safe in pregnancy include methyldopa, labetalol, diltiazem, clonidine and prazosin. Chronic diuretic use during pregnancy has been associated with restricted maternal plasma volume, which may reduce uteroplacental perfusion.[7]

DYSLIPIDEMIA/LIPID MANAGEMENT

Lifestyle Intervention

Lifestyle intervention, including medical nutrition therapy, increased physical activity, weight loss and smoking cessation, may allow some patients to reduce CVD risk factors, such as by lowering LDL cholesterol. Nutrition intervention should be tailored according to each patient's age, diabetes type, pharmacological treatment, lipid levels and medical conditions. Recommendations should focus on reducing saturated fat, cholesterol and trans unsaturated fat intake and increasing omega-3 fatty acids and viscous fiber (such as in oats, legumes and citrus). Glycemic control can also beneficially modify plasma lipid levels, particularly in patients with very high triglycerides and poor glycemic control.

Initiating Statin Therapy Based on Risk

Patients with type 2 diabetes have an increased prevalence of lipid abnormalities, contributing to their high risk of CVD. Multiple clinical trials have demonstrated significant effects of pharmacological (primarily statin) therapy on CVD outcomes in individual subjects with coronary heart disease (CHD) and for primary CVD prevention.[8] Meta-analyses, including data from over 18,000 patients with diabetes from 14 randomized trials of statin therapy (mean follow-up 4.3 years), demonstrate a 9% proportional reduction in all-cause mortality and 13% reduction in vascular mortality, for each mmol/L reduction in LDL cholesterol. As in those without diabetes, absolute reductions in objective CVD outcomes (CHD death and nonfatal MI) are greatest in people with high baseline CVD risk (known CVD and/or very high LDL cholesterol levels), but the overall benefits of statin therapy in people with diabetes at moderate or high risk for CVD are convincing. Statins are the drugs of choice for LDL cholesterol-lowering and cardioprotection.

Once a patient is on a statin, testing for LDL cholesterol may be considered on an individual basis to, for example, monitor adherence and efficacy. In cases where patients are adherent, but LDL cholesterol level is not responding, clinical judgment is recommended to determine the need for and timing of lipid panels. In individual patients, the highly variable LDL cholesterol-lowering response seen with statins is poorly understood. When maximally tolerated doses of statins fail to significantly lower LDL cholesterol (<30% reduction from the patient's baseline), there is no strong evidence that combination therapy should be used to achieve additional LDL cholesterol-lowering. Although niacin, fenofibrate, ezetimibe and bile acid sequestrants all offer additional LDL cholesterol-lowering to statins alone, there is insufficient evidence that such combination therapy provides a significant increment in CVD risk reduction over statin therapy alone.

Treatment of Other Lipoprotein Fractions or Targets

Hypertriglyceridemia should be addressed with dietary and lifestyle changes. Severe hypertriglyceridemia (>1,000 mg/dL) may warrant immediate pharmacological therapy (fibric acid derivatives or fish oil) to reduce the risk of acute pancreatitis. If severe hypertriglyceridemia is absent, then therapy targeting HDL cholesterol or triglycerides lacks the strong evidence base of statin therapy. If HDL cholesterol is less than 40 mg/dL and LDL cholesterol is between

100 mg/dL and 129 mg/dL, a fibrate or niacin might be used, especially if a patient is intolerant to statins.

ANTIPLATELET AGENTS

Aspirin has been shown to be effective in reducing cardiovascular morbidity and mortality in high-risk patients with previous MI or stroke (secondary prevention). Its net benefit in primary prevention among patients with no previous cardiovascular events is more controversial, both for patients with and without a history of diabetes.[9] Two randomized controlled trials of aspirin specifically in patients with diabetes failed to show a significant reduction in CVD endpoints, raising questions about the efficacy of aspirin for primary prevention in people with diabetes.[10-12] The Antithrombotic Trialists' (ATT) collaborators published an individual patient level meta-analysis of the six large trials of aspirin for primary prevention in the general population. These trials collectively enrolled over 95,000 participants, including almost 4,000 with diabetes. Overall, they found that aspirin reduced the risk of vascular events by 12% [RR 0.88 (95% CI 0.82–0.94)]. The largest reduction was for nonfatal MI with little effect on CHD death [RR 0.95 (95% CI 0.78–1.15)] or total stroke. There was some evidences of a difference in aspirin effect by gender, i.e. aspirin significantly reduced CVD events in men, but not in women.

The main adverse effects appear to be an increased risk of gastrointestinal bleeding. The excess risk may be as high as 1–5 per 1,000 per year in real-world settings. In adults with CVD risk greater than 1% per year, the number of CVD events prevented will be similar to or greater than the number of episodes of bleeding induced, although these complications do not have equal effects on long-term health.

In 2010, a position statement of the ADA, the American Heart Association, and the American College of Cardiology Foundation recommended that low-dose (75–162 mg/day) of aspirin for primary prevention is reasonable for adults with diabetes and no previous history of vascular disease who are at increased CVD risk (10-year risk of CVD events over 10%) and who are not at increased risk for bleeding. However, aspirin is no longer recommended for those at low CVD risk (women under the age 60 years and men under the age 50 years with no major CVD risk factors; 10-year CVD risk under 5%) as the low benefit is likely to be outweighed by the risks of significant bleeding. Clinical judgment should be used for those at intermediate risk (younger patients with one or more risk factors or older patients with no risk factors; those with 10-year CVD risk of 5–10%) until further research is available. Aspirin use in patients under the age of 21 years is contraindicated due to the associated risk of Reye syndrome.

A P2Y12 receptor antagonist in combination with aspirin should be used for at least 1 year in patients following an acute coronary syndrome. Evidence supports use of either ticagrelor or clopidogrel if no percutaneous coronary intervention (PCI) was performed, and the use of clopidogrel, ticagrelor or prasugrel if PCI was performed.[13]

CORONARY HEART DISEASE

Intensive lifestyle intervention focusing on weight loss through decreased caloric intake and increased physical activity as performed in the action for health in diabetes (Look AHEAD trial) may be considered for improving glucose control, fitness and some CVD risk factors. Patients at increased CVD risk should receive aspirin and a statin, and ACE inhibitor or ARB therapy if hypertensive, unless there are contraindications to a particular drug class. While clear benefit exists for ACE inhibitor and ARB therapy in patients with nephropathy or hypertension, the benefits in patients with CVD in the absence of these conditions are less clear, especially when LDL cholesterol is concomitantly controlled.[14,15]

Diabetic subjects are more likely to have MI and worse outcomes compared to nondiabetic subjects. The prothrombotic and procoagulant state with which diabetes is associated, contributes to the higher incidence and poor prognosis of MI. Increased platelet activation, increased expression of coagulation factors and reduced intrinsic thrombolytic activity, are mainly responsible for this. Endothelial dysfunction is associated with insulin resistance, the metabolic syndrome and the chronic inflammatory state seen in diabetes.[16]

This diffuse coronary disease may limit collateralization, potentially increasing infarct size. Detrimental effect of sulfonylureas on protective ischemic preconditioning further deteriorates it.[17] Standard pharmacological approaches like ACE inhibitors, statins and thiazolidinediones are known to improve endothelial function. They may have a particular role in the peri-infarct management of people with diabetes.

Left ventricular dysfunction is more common following MI in diabetic patients. The compensatory hyperdynamic response of the remaining non-ischemic myocardium has, however, been shown to be impaired.[18] It is possibly a reflection of the diabetic systolic and diastolic myopathy induced by altered cellular calcium balance and exacerbated by accelerated ventricular hypertrophy.[19,20] Disturbed autonomic function may also contribute to this process as well as increase the risk of arrhythmic sudden death.[19] Regardless of the degree of left ventricular impairment, in the light of the HOPE Study, all diabetic subjects post-MI should be treated with an ACE inhibitor.

Thrombolysis benefits diabetic more than nondiabetic patients,[21] but very few diabetics receive it, and those that do, receive late.[22] Diabetic autonomic neuropathy reduces pain sensation. Therefore diabetic patients present approximately 15 minutes later than nondiabetic patients after the onset of symptoms. The delivery of thrombolysis is also delayed. This is being compounded by reduced sensitivity of the standard 12-lead ECG in patients taking sulfonylureas, because of changes in T-wave morphology. Many a times, diabetic patients are less likely to be considered appropriate candidates for thrombolysis, majorly due to a perceived high risk of hemorrhagic complications or the existence of comorbidities. Despite the greater relative and absolute benefits of thrombolysis in diabetic patients sustaining MI, re-occlusion rates, 30-day and 1-year mortality remains worse in diabetic than nondiabetic patients.

Enhanced platelet activation and the procoagulant state associated with diabetes increase the likelihood of a thrombotic event, encourage thrombus propagation, impair the action of thrombolytic drugs and increase the chance of re-occlusion. Overall myocardial (including microvascular) perfusion is also impaired in diabetes. Higher incidence of early death prior to angiography in the diabetic group remains. Recurrent ischemia occurs more frequently in the diabetic group.[18] However, due to delay in thrombolysis and its reduced efficacy, early vessel patency assumes even greater importance, and accelerated administration of t-PA may be of particular benefit in diabetic patients.[23] It is clear that aspirin is of equal benefit in diabetic and nondiabetic patients and meta-analyses have not demonstrated any additional risk.[23] The use of additional antiplatelet agents has been advocated, and, specifically, clopidogrel has been shown to be of benefit in addition to aspirin in the setting of unstable angina and non-Q-wave MI.[24]

Several studies have demonstrated a benefit from low-molecular-weight heparins (LMWH) over unfractionated heparin in the management of unstable angina and non-Q-wave MI. Neither the ESSENCE trial[25] nor TIMI 11B[26] demonstrated additional benefit in diabetic subjects, although the latter showed a greater advantage in a "high-risk" group, identified on the basis of raised troponin I, which had a greater proportion of diabetic patients. The GUSTO IIb study suggested a marginal additional benefit from the use or hirudin, a direct thrombin inhibitor in diabetic subjects.[27]

The glycoprotein IIb/IIIa antagonists, tirofiban and eptifibatide, have been used in the setting of unstable angina/non-Q-wave MI and shown to improve both short- and medium-term outcomes. The risks of death and MI were more significantly reduced in diabetic patients in both PRISM-PLUS[28] and PURSUIT[29] studies, although this benefit was limited to insulin-requiring diabetic patients in PURSUIT.[23] A meta-analysis of the major glycoprotein IIb/IIIa studies in unstable coronary syndromes suggests that the absolute benefit in diabetic patients is twice that of nondiabetic patients.[30] In resistant unstable angina, and possibly as a bridging measure to definitive revascularization procedures, the glycoprotein IIb/IIIa antagonists may have a particularly important role in diabetes.

Difficulties of re-establishing vascular patency by thrombolytic or mechanical means contribute to the high morbidity and mortality. The diffuse nature of arterial disease with accompanying metabolic derangement contribute to impaired compensatory mechanisms, increased infarct size and a disproportionately more substantial impairment of left ventricular function. The newer adjuvant antithrombotic and anticoagulant agents have particular roles in management, therefore. The metabolic derangement that occurs at the time of MI leads to anaerobic glucose metabolism and a shift toward free fatty acid utilization; this being exacerbated by insulin deficiency or resistance. This shift increases oxygen demand, worsens ischemia, increases superoxide production, promotes sympathetic activity and reduces myocardial contractility.[31] This change affects both ischemic and nonischemic territories, increasing infarct size and reducing the compensatory response of viable myocardial tissue. Insulin therapy in the setting of MI promotes glucose oxidation, and the enhanced availability of glycolytic substrate counters these adverse effects, particularly in the diabetic patient, where it may also improve the prothrombotic state.[32] The DIGAMI study demonstrated benefits from a glucose and insulin infusion, to achieve early improved metabolic control,[33] careful modulation of glucose metabolism in the acute and follow-up phase of an infarct may favorably influence outcome.

In patients with a prior MI, β-blockers should be continued for at least 2 years after the event.[48] β-blockers have consistently been under-prescribed in diabetes.[34] β-blockers not only reduce myocardial oxygen demand, but they may also shift energy production from fatty acids to glucose usage.[35] Their effect is in proportion to the magnitude of the reduction in heart rate,[36] which in diabetic patients is higher following MI, possibly through a free fatty acid-mediated increase in sympathetic drive. The benefit of β-blockers may therefore be more marked in this group of patients.[37]

Studies have demonstrated a benefit from direct angioplasty compared to thrombolysis in MI, high-risk patients in general and diabetic patients.[20,38] Although complication and restenosis rates are higher in diabetic patients in both the elective and acute setting,[39,40] Stent deployment in nondiabetic patients has been shown to be feasible and is associated with a lower restenosis rate than PTCA in MI. Stenting is also associated with improved outcomes in diabetic patients.[41]

The debate regarding the role of an early invasive strategy in the management of post-MI patients remains active[42,43] and has evolved in parallel with the development in interventional strategies and adjuvant therapies. A further shift in favor of mechanical reperfusion in acute MI has been prompted by a series of trials examining the role of adjunctive therapy with the glycoprotein IIb/IIIa inhibitor, abciximab.[44,45]

These have demonstrated improved achievement of TIMI grade III flow following intervention, evidence of better microcirculatory perfusion, an associated improvement in echocardiographic left ventricular wall-motion scores and better clinical outcome at 30 days and 6 months. Given the concerns regarding distal embolization of platelet thrombi and microcirculatory dysfunction such benefits may be of particular importance in the diabetic patient. This has been borne out by the findings of subgroup analysis of the ADMIRAL study[46,47] which showed a reduction in the primary endpoint of death (0 vs 16.7% $p = 0.02$) and the combined endpoint of death, re-infarction or revascularization (20.7 vs 50.0% $p = 0.02$) at 6 months in diabetic subjects treated with abciximab.

A number of pathophysiological factors adversely affect the incidence and outcomes of acute MI in diabetic patients. The failure of delivery of well-established therapies may add to this. Thrombolytic therapy is as appropriate to diabetic as nondiabetic patients and may carry greater benefit. Antiplatelet treatment with aspirin should be instituted early and may be augmented with clopidogrel. With the prothrombotic state associated with diabetes, additional benefit may be gained from LMWH and glycoprotein IIb/IIIa inhibition. Metabolic manipulation has now established itself in mainstream treatment, although the exact regimen will continue to be refined. With the evolution of coronary intervention, primary and early intervention in diabetes may offer favorable outcomes in appropriately selected patients.

Diabetic patients remain a high-risk group for MI, with poorer outcomes, whilst having a sound pathophysiological basis for aggressive treatment and intervention with greater benefits than nondiabetic patients. An increased awareness and appropriate delivery of established therapies to this group is essential in the face of a rising diabetic population worldwide.

A systematic review of 34,000 patients showed that metformin is as safe as other glucose-lowering treatments in patients with diabetes and CHF, even in those with reduced left ventricular ejection fraction or concomitant chronic kidney disease; however, metformin should be avoided in hospitalized patients.[49]

REFERENCES

1. James PA, Oparil S, Carter BL, et al. Evidence-based guideline for the management of high blood pressure in adults: report from the panel members appointed to the Eighth Joint National Committee (JNC 8). JAMA. 2014;311:507-20.
2. Chobanian AV, Bakris GL, Black HR, et al. National Heart, Lung, and Blood Institute Joint National Committee on Prevention, Detection, Evaluation, and Treatment of High Blood Pressure; National

High Blood Pressure Education Program Coordinating Committee. The Seventh Report of the Joint National Committee on Prevention, Detection, Evaluation, and Treatment of High Blood Pressure: the JNC 7 report. JAMA. 2003;289:2560-72.

3. ALLHAT Officers and Coordinators for the ALLHAT Collaborative Research Group. Major outcomes in high-risk hypertensive patients randomized to angiotensin-converting enzyme inhibitor or calcium channel blocker vs diuretic: the Antihypertensive and Lipid-Lowering Treatment to Prevent Heart Attack Trial (ALLHAT). JAMA. 2002;288:2981-97.
4. Psaty BM, Smith NL, Siscovick DS, et al. Health outcomes associated with anti-hypertensive therapies used as first-line agents. A systematic review and meta-analysis. JAMA. 1997;277:739-45.
5. McMurray JJV, Ostergren J, Swedberg K, et al. Effects of candesartan in patients with chronic heart failure and reduced left-ventricular systolic function taking angiotensin-converting enzyme inhibitors: the CHARM-Added trial. Lancet. 2003;362:767-71.
6. Sacks FM, Svetkey LP, Vollmer WM, et al. Effects on blood pressure of reduced dietary sodium and the Dietary Approaches to Stop Hypertension (DASH) diet. N Engl J Med. 2001;344:3-10.
7. Sibai BM. Treatment of hypertension in pregnant women. N Engl J Med. 1996;335:257-65.
8. Kearney PM, Blackwell L, Collins R, et al. Efficacy of cholesterol-lowering therapy in 18,686 people with diabetes in 14 randomized trials of statins: a meta-analysis. Lancet. 2008;371:117-25.
9. Baigent C, Blackwell L, Collins R, et al. Aspirin in the primary and secondary prevention of vascular disease: collaborative meta-analysis of individual participant data from randomised trials. Lancet. 2009;373:1849-60.
10. Perk J, De Backer G, Gohlke H, et al. European Association for Cardiovascular Prevention & Rehabilitation (EACPR); ESC Committee for Practice Guidelines (CPG). European Guidelines on cardiovascular disease prevention in clinical practice (version 2012). The Fifth Joint Task Force of the European Society of Cardiology and Other Societies on Cardiovascular Disease Prevention in Clinical Practice (constituted by representatives of nine societies and by invited experts). Eur Heart J. 2012;33:1635-701.
11. Ogawa H, Nakayama M, Morimoto T, et al. Japanese Primary Prevention of Atherosclerosis With Aspirin for Diabetes (JPAD) Trial Investigators. Low-dose aspirin for primary prevention of atherosclerotic events in patients with type 2 diabetes: a randomized controlled trial. JAMA. 2008;300:2134-41.
12. Belch J, MacCuish A, Campbell I, et al. The prevention of progression of arterial disease and diabetes (POPADAD) trial: factorial randomized placebo controlled trial of aspirin and antioxidants in patients with diabetes and asymptomatic peripheral arterial disease. BMJ. 2008;337:a1840.
13. Vandvik PO, Lincoff AM, Gore JM, et al. American College of Chest Physicians. Primary and secondary prevention of cardiovascular disease: antithrombotic therapy and prevention of thrombosis, 9th edition: American College of Chest Physicians Evidence-Based Clinical Practice Guidelines. Chest. 2012;141(Suppl.):e637S-e668S.
14. Braunwald E, Domanski MJ, Fowler SE, et al. PEACE Trial Investigators. Angiotensin converting-enzyme inhibition in stable coronary artery disease. N Engl J Med. 2004;351:2058-68.
15. Telmisartan Randomised Assessment Study in ACEiN tolerant subjects with cardiovascular Disease (TRANSCEND) Investigators; Yusuf S, Teo K, et al. Effects of the angiotensin-receptor blocker telmisartan on cardiovascular events in high-risk patients intolerant to angiotensin converting enzyme inhibitors: a randomised controlled trial. Lancet. 2008;372:1174-83.
16. Kip KE, Faxon DP, Detre KM, et al. Coronary angioplasty in diabetic patients. The National Heart, Lung, and Blood Institute Percutaneous Transluminal Coronary Angioplasty Registry. Circulation. 1996;94:1818-25.
17. Cleveland JC Jr, Meldrum DR, Cain BS, et al. Oral sulfonylurea hypoglycemic agents prevent ischemic preconditioning in human myocardium. Two paradoxes revisited. Circulation. 1997;96:29-32.

18. Woodfield SL, Lundergan CF, Reiner JS et al. Angiographic findings and outcome in diabetic patients treated with thrombolytic therapy for acute myocardial infarction: the GUSTO-I experience. J Am Coll Cardiol. 1996;28:1661-9.
19. Mahgoub MA, Abd-Elfattah AS. Diabetes mellitus and cardiac function. Mol Cell Biochem. 1998;180:59-64.
20. Mak KH, Topol EJ. Emerging concepts in the management of acute myocardial infarction in patients with diabetes mellitus. J Am Coll Cardiol. 2000;35:563-8.
21. Indications for fibrinolytic therapy in suspected acute myocardial infarction: collaborative overview of early mortality and major morbidity results from all randomised trials of more than 1000 patients. Fibrinolytic Therapy Trialists' (FTT) Collaborative Group. Lancet. 1994;343:311-22.
22. Mak KH, Moliterno DJ, Granger CB, et al. Influence of diabetes mellitus on clinical outcome in the thrombolytic era of acute myocardial infarction. GUSTO-I Investigators. Global Utilization of Streptokinase and Tissue Plasminogen Activator for Occluded Coronary Arteries. J Am Coll Cardiol. 1997;30:171-9.
23. Hammoud T, Tanguay JF, Bourassa MG. Management of coronary artery disease: therapeutic options in patients with diabetes. J Am Coll Cardiol. 2000;36:355-65.
24. Yusuf S, Zhao F, Mehta SR, et al. Effects of clopidogrel in addition to aspirin in patients with acute coronary syndromes without ST-segment elevation. N Engl J Med. 2001;345:494-502.
25. Cohen M, Demers C, Gurfinkel EP, et al. Low-molecular-weight heparins in non-ST-segment elevation ischemia: the ESSENCE trial. Efficacy and Safety of Subcutaneous Enoxaparin versus intravenous unfractionated heparin, in non-Q-wave Coronary Events. Am J Cardiol. 1998;82:19L-24L.
26. Morrow DA, Antman EM, Tanasijevic M, et al. Cardiac troponin I for stratification of early outcomes and the efficacy of enoxaparin in unstable angina: a TIMI-11B substudy. J Am Coll Cardiol. 2000;36:1812-7.
27. McGuire DK, Emanuelsson H, Granger CB, et al. Influence of diabetes mellitus on clinical outcomes across the spectrum of acute coronary syndromes. Findings from the GUSTO-IIb study. GUSTO IIb Investigators. Eur Heart J. 2000;21:1750-8.
28. Inhibition of the platelet glycoprotein IIb/IIIa receptor with tirofiban in unstable angina and non-Q-wave myocardial infarction. Platelet Receptor Inhibition in Ischemic Syndrome Management in Patients Limited by Unstable Signs and Symptoms (PRISM-PLUS) Study Investigators. N Engl J Med. 1998;338:1488-97.
29. Inhibition of platelet glycoprotein IIb/IIIa with eptifibatide in patients with acute coronary syndromes. The PURSUIT Trial Investigators. Platelet Glycoprotein IIb/IIIa in Unstable Angina: Receptor Suppression Using Integrilin Therapy. N Engl J Med. 1998;339:436-43.
30. Roffi M, Chew DP, Mukherjee D, et al. Platelet glycoprotein IIb/IIIa inhibitors reduce mortality in diabetic patients with non-ST-segment-elevation acute coronary syndromes. Circulation. 2001;104:2767-71.
31. Oliver MF, Opie LH. Effects of glucose and fatty acids on myocardial ischaemia and arrhythmias. Lancet. 1994;343:155-8.
32. Malmberg K, McGuire DK. Diabetes and acute myocardial infarction: the role of insulin therapy. Am Heart J. 1999;138:S381-6.
33. Malmberg K, Ryden L, Efendic S, et al. Randomized trial of insulin-glucose infusion followed by subcutaneous insulin treatment in diabetic patients with acute myocardial infarction (DIGAMI study): effects on mortality at 1 year. J Am Coll Cardiol. 1995;26:57-65.
34. Younis N, Burnham P, Patwala A, et al. Beta blocker prescribing differences in patients with and without diabetes following a first myocardial infarction. Diabet Med. 2001;18:159-61.
35. Opie LH, Thomas M. Propranolol and experimental myocardial infarction: substrate effects. Postgrad Med J. 1976;52(Suppl. 4):124-32.

36. Kjekshus J. Heart rate reduction--a mechanism of benefit? Eur Heart J. 1987;8(Suppl. L):115-22.
37. Malmberg K, Norhammar A, Wedel H, et al. Glycometabolic state at admission: important risk marker of mortality in conventionally treated patients with diabetes mellitus and acute myocardial infarction: long-term results from the diabetes and Insulin-Glucose Infusion in Acute Myocardial Infarction (DIGAMI) study. Circulation. 1999;99:2626-32.
38. Thomas K, Ottervanger JP, de Boer MJ, et al. Primary angioplasty compared with thrombolysis in acute myocardial infarction in diabetic patients. Diabetes Care. 1999;22:647-9.
39. Elezi S, Kastrati A, Pache J, et al. Diabetes mellitus and the clinical and angiographic outcome after coronary stent placement. J Am Coll Cardiol. 1998;32:1866-73.
40. Van Belle E, Abolmaali K, Bauters C, et al. Restenosis, late vessel occlusion and left ventricular function six months after balloon angioplasty in diabetic patients. J Am Coll Cardiol. 1999;34: 476-85.
41. Silva JA, Ramee SR, White CJ, et al. Primary stenting in acute myocardial infarction: influence of diabetes mellitus in angiographic results and clinical outcome. Am Heart J. 1999;138:446-55.
42. Wallentin L, Lagerqvist B, Husted S, et al. Outcome at 1 year after an invasive compared with a non-invasive strategy in unstable coronary-artery disease: the FRISC II invasive randomised trial. FRISC II Investigators. Fast Revascularisation during Instability in Coronary artery disease. Lancet. 2000;356:9-16.
43. Boden WE, O'Rourke RA, Crawford MH, et al. Outcomes in patients with acute non-Q-wave myocardial infarction randomly assigned to an invasive as compared with a conservative management strategy. Veterans Affairs Non-Q-Wave Infarction Strategies in Hospital (VANQWISH) Trial Investigators. N Engl J Med. 1998;338:1785-92.
44. Stone GW, Grines CL, Cox DA, et al. Comparison of angioplasty with stenting, with or without abciximab, in acute myocardial infarction. N Engl J Med. 2002;346:957-66.
45. Chan AW, Moliterno DJ. Defining the role of abciximab for acute coronary syndromes: lessons from CADILLAC, ADMIRAL, GUSTO IV, GUSTO V, and TARGET. Curr Opin Cardiol. 2001;16:375-83.
46. Montalescot G, Barragan P, Wittenberg O, et al. Platelet glycoprotein IIb/IIIa inhibition with coronary stenting for acute myocardial infarction. N Engl J Med. 2001;344:1895-903.
47. Montalescot G, Barragan P, Wittenberg O, et al. Abciximab reduces clinical restenosis in diabetic patients undergoing primary stenting for acute myocardial infarction (The ADMIRAL study). Circulation. 2001;104:386.
48. Kezerashvili A, Marzo K, De Leon J. Beta blocker use after acute myocardial infarction in the patient with normal systolic function: when is it "ok" to discontinue? Curr Cardiol Rev. 2012;8:77-84.
49. Eurich DT, Weir DL, Majumdar SR, et al. Comparative safety and effectiveness of metformin in patients with diabetes mellitus and heart failure: systematic review of observational studies involving 34,000 patients. Circ Heart Fail. 2013;6:395-402.

16
CHAPTER

Oral Complications of Diabetes Mellitus and Their Management

Richik Tripathi

INTRODUCTION

Oral cavity is affected by diabetes likewise other organs/organ system in body. Etiopathogenesis of oral complications of diabetes are similar to other systemic complications of diabetes; these are disturbance of oral microbial flora, altered immune response, microangiopathy of blood vessels leading to poor vascularity of oral organs and altered bone metabolism.

Oral health in diabetic patient depends upon following factors:

- Status of oral hygiene
- Status of periodontal tissues
- Presence of dental prosthesis or dental implants. Poor oral hygiene leads to plaque accumulation on tooth surface or on the dental prosthesis which predispose diabetic patients toward various periodontal diseases.

In diabetic patients, there is significant change in oral microflora.[1] Bacterial population and number of bacterial species are much higher in diabetics compared to nondiabetics.[1] Gram-negative bacteria population is also high in diabetics compared to nondiabetics.

ORAL CANDIDIASIS

Candida species which are present in low concentration in oral cavity in healthy individuals appear to increase during hyperglycemic state[2] in diabetics while poor immune resistance and decreased salivary flow rate is responsible for the most common oral complication of diabetes 'oral candidiasis'.[2]

Causative organisms are mainly *Candida* spp or *Aspergillus* spp. Denture stomatitis is another common complication. Main reason behind its occurrence is frequent irritation from denture which in turn alters mucosal resistance to infection while altered neutrophil function and hyperglycemia plays secondary role in causing denture stomatitis. *Candida albicans* infection of oral cavity in diabetics can be present in following four forms:

Pseudomembranous Candidiasis

- Pseudomembranous candidiasis, commonly known as "thrush," is the most common form of candidiasis seen in diabetics and HIV infected patients. It can also be seen in patients receiving topical corticosteroid therapy or immune suppressants.
- Pseudomembranous candidiasis presents as multiple white plaques of material resembling cottage cheese (Fig. 1) that can easily be wiped away (Fig. 2).

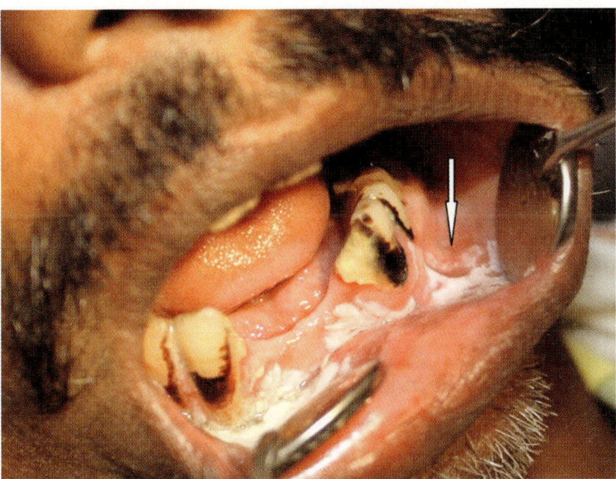

Fig. 1: Extensive candida infection in 45-year-old diabetic patient

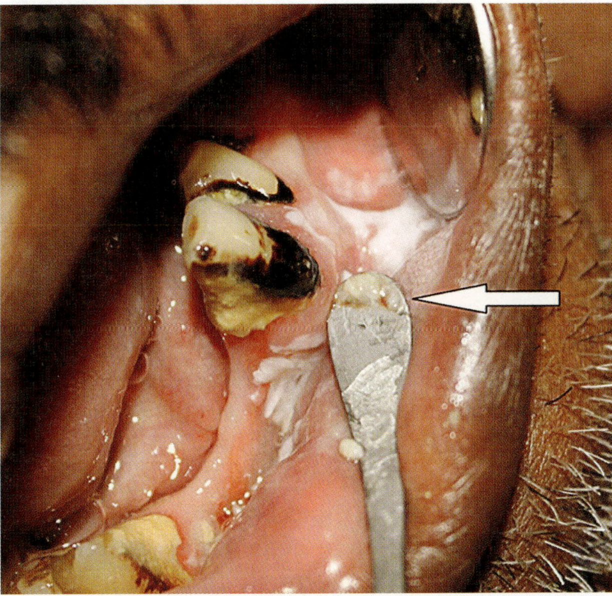

Fig. 2: White plaque can be easily scrapped from oral mucosa

- These plaques consist of tangled aggregates of hyphae. The underlying mucosa may be erythematous, but ulceration may or may not be present. Diagnosis is by clinical examination and by medical history of patient. To confirm diagnosis the scrapings from oral mucosa can be sent for fungal culture test.

Atrophic Candidiasis

- Atrophic candidiasis exhibits a diffusely reddened, often relatively dry mucosa.
- The red areas are often confined to mucosa underlying dental appliances such as partial dentures or orthodontic retainers. Approximately 26% of patients with complete dentures have atrophic candidiasis.

Hyperplastic Candidiasis

This form can be referred to as "candidal leukoplakia". Like leukoplakia, hyperplastic candidiasis will present as a white plaque that cannot be wiped away by the clinician. It resolves completely with routine antifungal therapy.

Erythematous Candidiasis

It clinically appears as red or erythematous patch on oral mucosa. Any mucosal site may be affected, it commonly involves the tongue and palate.

Angular Cheilitis

This form presents as cracking, peeling, or ulceration involving the corners of the mouth. It is due to the increased folding of the soft tissue at the corners of the mouth creating a furrow which is non-self-cleansing area and favors growth of microbial organisms.

Management

Most important step of management is restoration of glycemic level to normal state otherwise it is very difficult to treat oral complications. Oral candidal infections respond readily to tropical clotrimazole solution which is available in oral base form. Vitamin B12 and lycopene can be added to promote early recovery. In severe or recurrent candidiasis oral fluconazole therapy is started as 50 mg once daily for 7–14 days depending on severity.[3] Fluconazole can cause renal impairment and it is not uncommon to have renal disorders in diabetes. In such patients either dosage reduction or increase in dose interval is recommended.[3] Itraconazole owing to its lipid solubility and better bioavailability is good alternative to fluconazole.[4] It is given in dose of 100–200 mg daily for 7 days.[4] Nephrotoxic effects of itraconazole has not been proven, however there are reports of its interaction with tacrolimus.[5] To manage burning sensation and pain due to atrophic or ulcerative candidiasis local antiseptics containing chlorhexidine and benzocaine can be used effectively. Tropical or oral steroids in acute stage of candidal infection are not recommended. For denture-induced stomatitis, patient should be advised not to wear denture till symptoms subside and are referred to dentist to check the fit and finish of denture. Poor fitting dentures cause mucosal irritation which is major contributing factor toward denture-induced stomatitis.

PERIODONTITIS

Periodontitis is a common chronic inflammatory disease characterized by destruction of the supporting structures of the teeth (Fig. 3). Patients complain of swollen gums, halitosis and loosening of teeth. Diagnosis and estimation of severity of periodontitis is done by probing around tooth. Loss of attachment of gingiva to tooth confirms presence of periodontitis while severity is graded by level of attachment loss. Periodontitis is not necessarily a complication of diabetes but progression of gingivitis to periodontitis is rapid in diabetics compared to nondiabetics.[6] Studies have suggested that prevalence of periodontitis is much higher in diabetics compared to nondiabetics.[7] Altered immune response, poor salivary flow rate plus hyperglycemia provide favorable environment for rapid progression of gingivitis to periodontitis. Intracrestal and crestal bone loss incidence is also higher in diabetics. Microangiopathy of bone blood vessels and disturbed bone metabolism due to altered insulin function are responsible factors for rapid crestal/intracrestal bone loss in diabetics. Diabetics with periodontitis are at higher risk of developing coronary artery disease (CAD) and renal impairment.[8,9] A number of studies done in past has clearly shown high prevalence of renal disorders and CAD in diabetics.[8,9] In periodontitis the inflammatory response is characterized by dysregulated secretion of host-derived mediators of inflammation and tissue breakdown. The most extensively studied include interleukin (IL)-1β, IL-6, prostaglandin E_2 (PGE_2), tumor necrosis factor (TNF)-α, receptor activator of nuclear factor κB ligand (RANKL), and the matrix metalloproteinases (MMPs); particularly MMP-8, MMP-9 and MMP-13, as well as T cell regulatory cytokines (e.g. IL-12, IL-18) and the chemokine. These circulating inflammatory mediators produce an elevated inflammatory state in diabetes which contributes to micro- and macrovascular complications like CAD and renal disorders.

Management

Most important aspect of periodontitis management is to improve oral hygiene. Next step in management is smoothening of rough surface on crown or root of tooth or on dental prosthesis to reduce plaque accumulation. Doxycycline and metronidazole are very effective in reducing microbial population from periodontium.[10,11]

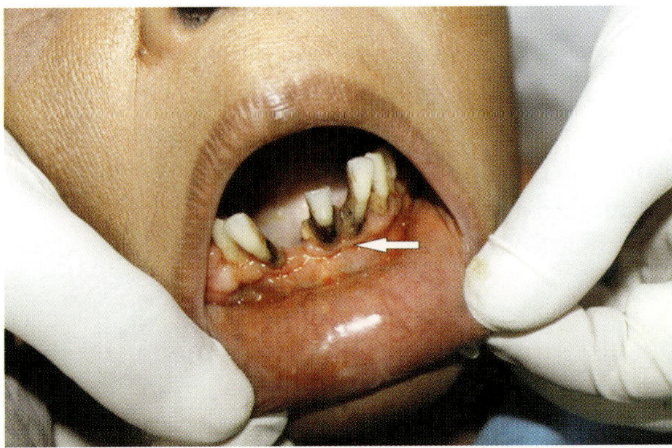

Fig. 3: Periodontitis in 54-year-old female diabetic patient. Note the level of bone loss and bleeding gums

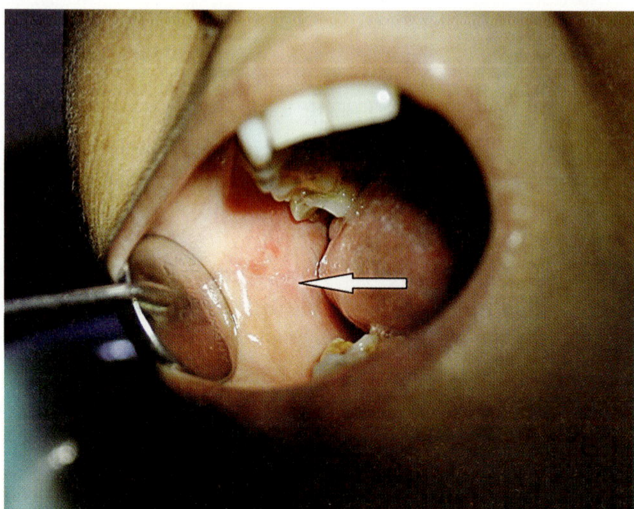

Fig. 4: Xerostomia in 48-year-old female diabetic patient. Note the shiny appearance of oral mucosa and absence of wetting by saliva

Chlorhexidine mouthwash and toothpaste containing chlorhexidine are advised to reduce bacterial population in plaque biofilm. Patients are regularly followed every 3 months. All these management modalities are within expertise of general dentist. For physicians, it is prudent to refer the patient to dentist if he complains of foul breath, bleeding gums or loose teeth.

XEROSTOMIA

Xerostomia is excessive dryness in oral cavity. There may be hyposalivation or absent salivation in diabetic patient. Oral mucosa in such patient appears very shiny (Fig. 4) and tongue may lose filiform papillae (Fig. 5). Patient complaints of frequent oral ulceration (Fig. 4) and burning sensation in oral cavity. All these symptoms are due to increased friction from food stuffs as lubricating action of saliva is missing. Burning sensation is due to prolonged retention of irritant spices or food stuffs in oral cavity because of reduced salivary flow rate. Exact mechanism of occurrence of xerostomia in diabetes mellitus is not clear, however studies suggest that it might be due to overall dehydration associated with hyperglycemia decreasing the volume of secreted saliva. Microangiopathy of blood vessels supplying salivary gland and reduced autonomic innervations of salivary glands owing to neuropathy are also responsible for decreased saliva production and xerostomia.

Management

Apart from restoring blood glucose to normal level measures are taken to provide symptomatic relief from dryness of mouth. Patients are asked to take lemon juice in lukewarm water before meals to stimulate saliva secretion. Artificial salivary substitutes which contain sorbitol and glycerin are advised to keep mouth wet.[12] Sugar free lozenges can also be prescribed to stimulate saliva secretion. Oral parasympathomimetic (pilocarpine) can be given as 30 mg

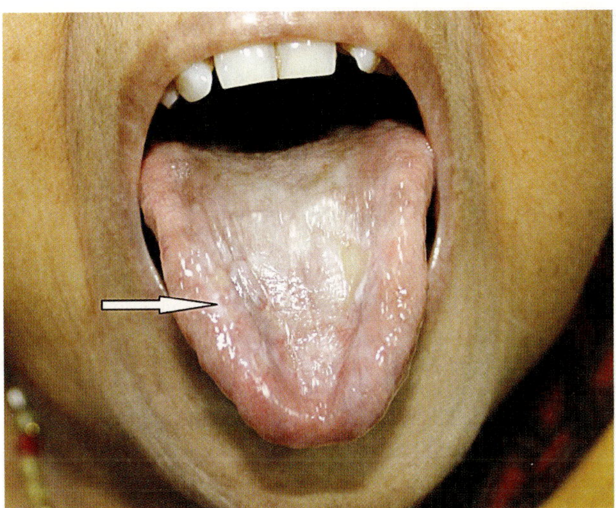

Fig. 5: Smooth and shiny tongue in patient having xerostomia

thrice daily for at least 3 months.[13] But it must be used with caution in diabetic patients as it has significant side effects on cardiovascular system and respiratory system.

DENTAL IMPLANT FAILURE

Dental implant failure in uncontrolled diabetes is due to poor healing of wound at implant placement site and poor bone formation around dental implant which causes poor osseointegration of implant to alveolar bone.[14] In patients already having dental implant uncontrolled diabetes causes loss of alveolar bone height and loss of attachment of oral epithelium around dental implant leading to its early failure.[14] Preventive measures include routine dental check-up by dentist and avoidance of dental implant until optimal glycemic control has been achieved.

NONHEALING ORAL WOUNDS

Nonhealing oral wounds respond well to oral antibiotics like amoxicillin and fluoroquinolones once good glycemic control is achieved. Local antiseptics containing chlorhexidine and metronidazole has promising role in reducing healing time of oral wounds. Role of epidermal growth factor and its clinical safety in management of oral wounds has not been widely studied.

DENTAL CARIES

Dental caries develop secondary to reduce salivary flow rate and increased microbial population in oral cavity. Their management includes restoration of carious tooth or dental extraction after optimal glycemic control has been achieved.

REFERENCES

1. Sharma M, Tiwari SC, Singh K, et al. Occurrence of bacterial flora in oral infections of diabetic and nondiabetic patients. Life Sci Med Res. 2011;32:1-6.
2. Budtz-Jørgensen E. Ecology of Candida-associated denture stomatitis. Microb Ecol Health Dis. 2000;12:170-85.
3. Anil Kumar D, Muralidhar S, Biswas K, et al. Species diversity, antifungal susceptibility, and virulence attributes of candida colonising the oral cavities of adult diabetic patients. J Mycol. 2014;1-19.
4. Pallavan B, Ramesh V, Dhanasekaran BP, et al. Comparison and correlation of candidal colonization in diabetic patients and normal individuals. J Diabetes Metab Disord. 2014;13:66.
5. Martin MV. The use of fluconazole and itraconazole in the treatment of *Candida albicans* infections: a review. J Antimicrob Chemother. 1999;44(4):429-37.
6. Preshaw PM, Alba AL, Herrera D, et al. Periodontitis and diabetes: a two-way relationship. Diabetologia. 2012;55(1):21-31.
7. Apoorva SM, Sridhar N, Suchetha A. Prevalence and severity of periodontal disease in type 2 diabetes mellitus (non-insulin-dependent diabetes mellitus) patients in Bangalore city: an epidemiological study. J Indian Soc Periodontol. 2013;17(1):25-9.
8. Shultis WA, Weil EJ, Looker HC, et al. Effect of periodontitis on overt nephropathy and end-stage renal disease in type 2 diabetes. Diabetes Care. 2007;30(2):306-11.
9. Saremi A, Nelson RG, Tulloch-Reid M, et al. Periodontal disease and mortality in type 2 diabetes. Diabetes Care. 2005;28(1):27-32.
10. Preshaw PM, Hefti AF, Jepsen S, et al. Subantimicrobial dose doxycycline as adjunctive treatment for periodontitis: a review. J Clin Periodontol. 2004;31(9):697-707.
11. Loesche WJ, Schmidt E, Smith BA, et al. Effects of metronidazole on periodontal treatment needs. J Periodontol. 1991;62(4):247-57.
12. Villa A, Connell CL, Abati S. Diagnosis and management of xerostomia and hyposalivation. Ther Clin Risk Manag. 2014;11:45-51.
13. Aframian DJ, Helcer M, Livni D, et al. Pilocarpine treatment in a mixed cohort of xerostomic patients. Oral Dis. 2007;13(1):88-92.
14. Javed F, Romanos GE. Impact of diabetes mellitus and glycemic control on the osseointegration of dental implants: a systematic literature review. J Periodontol. 2009;80(11):1719-30.

17 CHAPTER

Imaging of Macrovascular Complications and Comorbid Conditions in Diabetic Patients

Amit Nandan Dwivedi, Shivi Jain

INTRODUCTION

Diabetes mellitus (DM) is a global health issue affecting people of all ages. According to the World Health Organization, approximately 180 million people worldwide currently have type 2 DM (formerly called adult-onset diabetes); over 95% of people with diabetes have this form. The number of people with type 2 DM (T2DM) is estimated to double by 2030.[1] In the year 2000, death from diabetes-associated complications accounted for approximately 6% of worldwide mortality.[2]

Diabetes is associated with both microvascular and macrovascular complications, including retinopathy, nephropathy and neuropathy (microvascular) and ischemic heart disease, peripheral vascular disease, and cerebrovascular disease (macrovascular) resulting in multiorgan dysfunction.[3]

MACROVASCULAR COMPLICATIONS AND NEED FOR IMAGING

Cardiovascular Disease

Cardiovascular disease (CVD) is the leading cause (~70%) of death in people with T2DM.[4] People with diabetes have a 4-fold-greater risk for having a CVD event than people without diabetes after controlling for traditional risk factors for CVD, such as age, obesity, tobacco use, dyslipidemia and hypertension. Also, diabetes itself is an independent risk factor for CVD. People with diabetes also have a fivefold-greater risk for a first myocardial infarction (MI) and a twofold-greater risk for a recurrent MI than people who previously had an MI but do not have diabetes.

Cerebrovascular Disease

Diabetes is also an independent risk factor for stroke across all ages,[5] the risk in people with diabetes is up to twofold to fourfold greater, more so in women. Diabetes is also a risk factor for sudden and eventual death from stroke, and people who have diabetes and who have a stroke have more severe neurological deficits and disability, a poorer long-term prognosis and a higher incidence of stroke recurrence than people without diabetes. As in CVD, the presence of diabetes adversely affects the cerebrovascular circulation by increasing the risk of intracranial and extracranial (e.g. carotid artery) atherosclerosis.

Peripheral Artery Disease

Peripheral artery disease is characterized by occlusion of the lower-extremity arteries,[6] which can cause intermittent claudication and pain, especially upon exercise and activity, and which can result in functional impairments and disability. Peripheral artery disease, like the aforementioned vascular diseases, is also related to the duration and severity of diabetes.

IMAGING IN CARDIOVASCULAR DISEASE: CORONARY ARTERY DISEASE

Coronary artery disease (CAD) increases with advancing age but often occurs at a younger age in patients with diabetes. Occult CAD among asymptomatic diabetics is common, ranging from 20 to more than 50%.[7]

If the resting ECG shows previously unrecognized MI (i.e. abnormal Q waves or deep T wave inversions, left bundle branch block, nonspecific ST-T changes), this triggers need for evaluation for CAD and inducible ischemia.[8]

Atherosclerotic vascular disease involving the lower extremities, cerebral, renal or mesenteric arteries, can predict the future chance of a cardiac event.[9] Patients with T2DM with chronic kidney disease (CKD) due to diabetic nephropathy have a very high risk for MI and cardiac death, with 40% experiencing a cardiac complication over a 5-year period.[10]

Coronary Calcium Score

Coronary calcium score (CCS) on CT can be highly correlated with total coronary atherosclerotic burden and it identifies asymptomatic diabetics at higher risk for inducible ischemia.[11] Coronary calcium score is quantified by calculating the Agatston score and the volume score. The Agatston score for each lesion in each segment of coronary artery is computed as the product of the area of each lesion with a weighting factor assigned according to the maximum attenuation value of the lesion.[12] The sum of the scores for all lesions in all coronary artery segments yields the total Agatston score. The volume score for each lesion is estimated as the product of the number of vowels containing calcium and the volume of one voxel.[13] The scores for all lesions in all coronary arteries is summed to obtain the total volume score.

If the CCS is zero, it is associated with a high level of confidence that an individual has no obstructive CAD with a very low rate of death or MI over 3–5 years.[14] It is well established that the detection of coronary calcium indicates an increased risk of incident coronary artery disease above that predicted by standard risk factors, from twofold for scores of up to 100 and increasing to elevenfold for scores above 1,000.[15]

The drawback of CCS lies in the fact that it is an anatomical study and not a functional one. Hence, it may be considered only as a second-line testing modality or for patients who are unable to exercise. However, CCS can confirm or reclassify individual risk derived from the initial risk assessment and hence is preferred as the initial mode of screening for CAD in patients who do not achieve therapeutic targets with medical treatment.[16] CCS when combined with coronary CT angiography (CCTA) helps in assessing type and location of plaque (Figs 1 and 2), percent stenosis and detects presence of any benign/malignant coronary anomaly and myocardial bridging.

Cardiac Magnetic Resonance Imaging

Over the past 20 years, cardiac magnetic resonance (CMR) has evolved from imaging of myocardial function and morphology to perfusion, edema, energetics and fibrosis.[17] High spatial and temporal resolution that rivals echocardiography can be achieved in most patients.

Cardiac magnetic resonance is able to quantify cardiac function and structure with relatively low restrictions from operator-dependency, echocardiographic windows, and is free from the use of ionizing radiation, thus providing important benefits in certain emerging at-risk populations, including obesity—the primary comorbid illness. Besides volumetric ventricular function, CMR "tagging" technique labels the myocardium with grids or lines to track intramyocardial motion. Such method has provided important insights into myocardial strain in diabetic cardiomyopathy and the determinants of subclinical systolic and diastolic function in T2DM.[18]

With the advent of contrast-enhanced imaging via gadolinium chelates, CMR can measure the presence, extent and location of fibrosis and perfusion deficits within the heart, providing prognostically important evidence on otherwise clinically unrecognized MI or ischemia.

Cardiac magnetic resonance provides the ability to visualize first-pass myocardial perfusion during administration of stress vasodilator (e.g. regadenoson or adenosine) or adrenergic (e.g. dobutamine and more recently exercise) agents[19] across short- and long-axis views of the LV with high spatial resolution. The advent of gadolinium administration also can detect and quantify areas of myocardial scar.

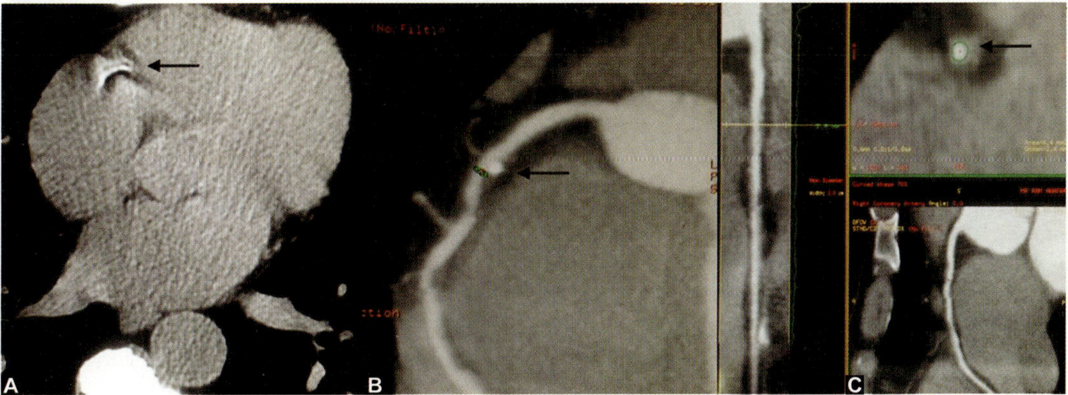

Figs 1A to C: Coronary CT angiography. (A) Axial noncontrast CT shows focal calcific plaque (arrow) in segment one of right coronary artery. (B and C) Curved and stretched multiplanar reformatted CT angiography images show presence of less than 50% luminal stenosis (arrows) by plaque, so hemodynamically insignificant. Coronary calcium score in this patient was 15

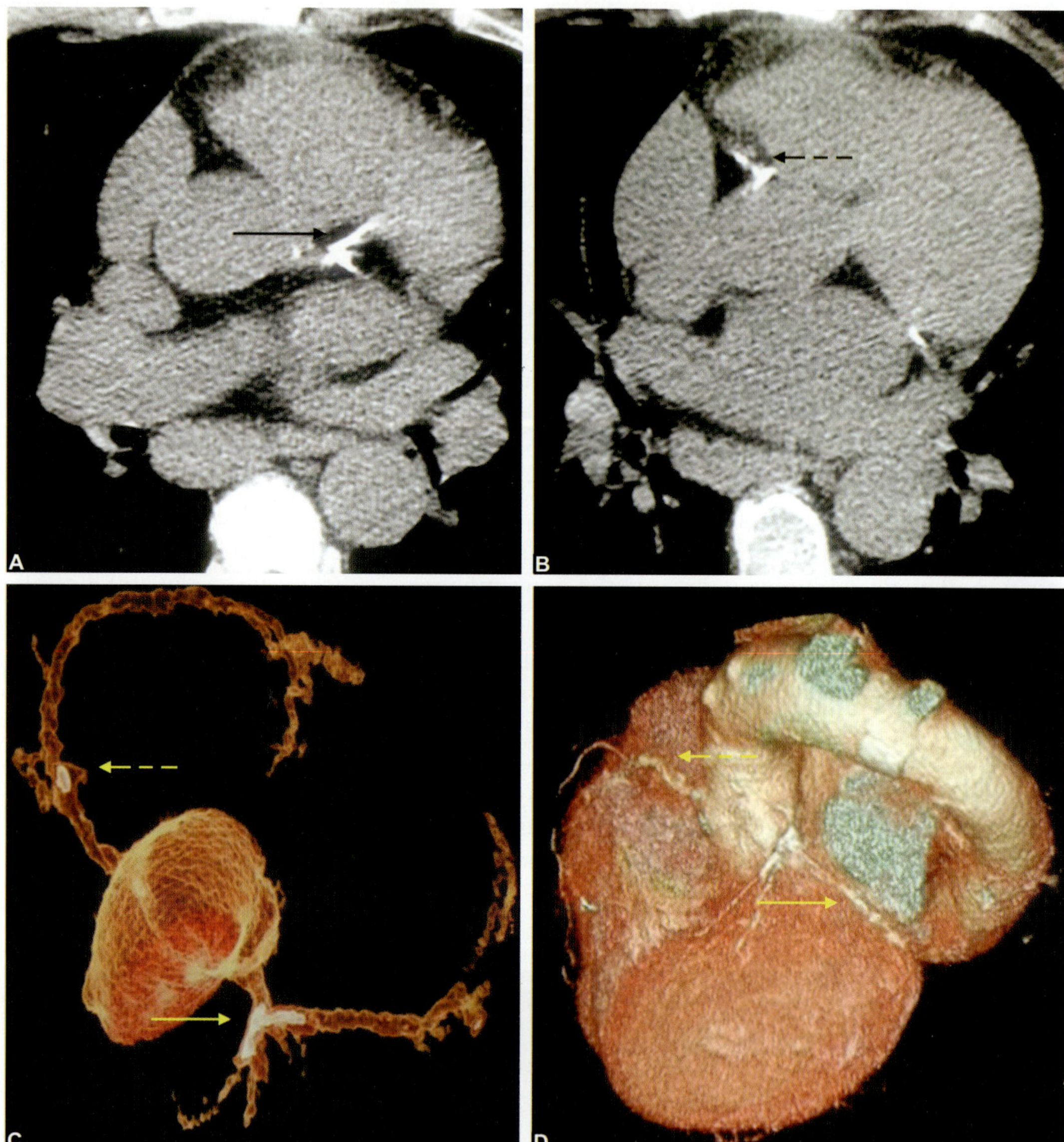

Figs 2A to D: Coronary CT angiography. (A) Axial noncontrast CT shows calcific plaque involving distal left main coronary artery (LMA), bifurcation of LMA and proximal left anterior descending and left circumflex (LCX) arteries; (segments 5, 6 and 11 shown by arrow). (B) Axial noncontrast CT shows calcific plaque involving segment 1 (dashed arrow) of right coronary artery. (C and D) Volume-rendered 3D CT images showing the same and depicting hemodynamically significant luminal stenosis

IMAGING IN CEREBROVASCULAR DISEASE

Ruling Out Intracranial Hemorrhage

The initial step in the evaluation of patients with symptoms of acute stroke is to differentiate between hemorrhagic and ischemic stroke. Since intracranial hemorrhage is an absolute contraindication for reperfusion therapies;[20] most stroke protocols begin with noncontrast head CT (NCHCT). Although CT is the standard method, gradient T2*-weighted MRI sequences [including gradient-recalled echo (GRE) and susceptibility-weighted imaging (SWI) sequences] are equally—if not more—sensitive for the detection of acute intracranial hemorrhage.[21]

Diagnosing Ischemic Stroke

Early ischemic changes in NCHCT include loss of gray-white distinction, indistinct insular cortex and obscured basal ganglia, and hyperattenuated clot in the proximal vessels. The hyperdense vessel sign is most specific but has low sensitivity.[22] Abnormalities on NCHCT are present in 40–50% of acute ischemic strokes. Diffusion-weighted imaging (DWI) is approximately 4–5 times more sensitive in detecting acute stroke than NCHCT. About 95% of hyperacute infarcts are positive on DWI.[23] DWI can detect acute brain infarction within 1–2 hours, while NCHCT may be negative for the first 24–36 hours. DWI can distinguish acute from chronic ischemia, thereby delineating new lesions even when located in proximity to prior ischemic injury. Obscure lesions indiscernible on CT scans, such as lacunar infarcts, particularly those located in the posterior fossa, are better visualized on DWI. Restricted diffusion is not exclusively observed in acute ischemic stroke, but can also be noted in nonischemic entities like seizure, encephalitis, abscesses, metabolic derangement (hypoglycemia), etc.

Determining Large Artery Occlusion

Imaging of the intracranial and extracranial vessels is needed to determine whether an embolus/thrombus is present and whether it is amenable to endovascular revascularization.

Digital subtraction angiography (DSA) is considered the reference standard for detection of vascular occlusions and stenoses. CT angiography (CTA) has reportedly high sensitivity (97–100%) and specificity (98–100%) for detecting intracranial occlusions and stenoses.[24] CTA also performs well in characterizing extracranial occlusions and stenoses with high sensitivity (95 97%) and specificity (90–99%). In addition to evaluating the degree of stenosis in the extracranial arteries, CTA provides valuable information of the plaque—such as morphology and composition.[25]

Magnetic resonance angiography (MRA) can also be used to detect and localize the occlusion.[26] Three-dimensional time-of-flight (TOF) MRA is the standard magnetic resonance technique for the examination of intracranial vessels. TOF MRA is, however, especially susceptible to motion artifact and tends to overestimate the degree of stenosis. Traditional contrast-enhanced MRA (bolus-chase MRA) is the magnetic resonance technique of choice for the study of the extracranial arteries. It is relatively independent of flow dynamics and is less susceptible to motion artifacts. Peak arterial enhancement is obtained by estimating the arrival of the contrast bolus.

Assessing Viable Ischemic Brain Tissue

Following an arterial occlusion, brain tissue that cannot sustain the sudden drop in perfusion rapidly undergoes infarction. The surrounding hypoperfused tissue that can autoregulate to sustain metabolic needs remains viable.[27] The former is labeled "ischemic infarct core," and the injury to this tissue is irreversible. The latter is known as "ischemic penumbra." The penumbra is in danger of proceeding to infarction, but represents potentially salvageable tissue if recanalization is achieved quickly.[28]

Magnetic resonance imaging delineation of the ischemic core and penumbra relies on DWI and perfusion-weighted imaging (PWI) techniques.[29] Characterization of the ischemic core and penumbra on MRI is based on the assumption that the DWI abnormality reflects the ischemic core, whereas the PWI abnormality reflects the overall area of ischemia. The PWI/DWI-mismatch is often thought to represent the ischemic penumbra.

IMAGING IN LOWER-EXTREMITY ARTERIAL DISEASE

Lower-extremity arterial disease (LEAD) is clinically identified by intermittent claudication and/or absence of peripheral pulses in the distal legs and feet. LEAD is defined as arterial disease involving the aorta, iliacs and infrainguinal arteries.

An ankle-brachial index (ABI) less than 0.90 diagnoses significant lower-extremity peripheral arterial disease (PAD) (>50% stenosis) with a sensitivity and specificity of 79% and 96%, respectively.[30] An ABI between 0.90 and 1.0 is considered borderline. For patients with suspected PAD and a normal ABI at rest, it is valuable to obtain post-exercise ABI measurements, which if less than 0.85 are consistent with PAD and is an independent predictor of mortality. Imaging is then needed to confirm the location and degree of stenosis before revascularization or if the diagnosis of PAD is uncertain.

Characterization of PAD can be performed with noninvasive angiography using computed tomography (CTA) or MRA, as well as with duplex ultrasonography. Invasive DSA has been the accepted standard for evaluation of lower-extremity atherosclerosis. Although DSA is a robust technique for diagnosing significant arterial stenosis or obstruction, it provides a 2D view of the vessels, which may underestimate the degree of stenosis for tortuous vessels.[31] Furthermore, there are inherent risks with arterial access, ionizing radiation and the use of iodinated contrast media.

Duplex Ultrasonography

Duplex ultrasonography uses the combination of gray scale (B-mode) for vessel morphology and color pulsed wave Doppler techniques. It is safe, inexpensive, and can provide functional information about vessel stenosis. A peak systolic velocity (PSV) ratio of more than 2.5 suggests a stenosis of 50–74% and if the end-diastolic velocity is more than 60 cm/s, this suggests a tighter stenosis, in the range of 75–99%.[32]

However, the most commonly used criteria is PSV ratio more than 2.0, along with PSV more than 200 cm/s, and aliasing and spectral broadening seen with color Doppler to diagnose a stenosis >50%.[30] The addition of color flow imaging improves the diagnostic performance of duplex ultrasonography for aortoiliac and femoropopliteal arteries.[33] If no color Doppler signal is visible in the vessel, arterial occlusion is suggested. The evaluation of infrapopliteal vessels although feasible by ultrasonography is time consuming and may be technically challenging. Thus, a complete evaluation of the native lower-extremity arterial system may not be feasible in many patients. For evaluation with duplex ultrasonography, patient body habitus may limit evaluation of the aortoiliac vessels because of abdominal girth or intestinal gas.

Computed Tomography Angiography

With the advent of multidetector row CT, images of inflow and runoff vessels became possible using a single acquisition and contrast injection. It resulted in increased speed of scanning and greater longitudinal field of view while maintaining near-isotropic imaging voxels.

Image interpretation is aided by the use of advanced postprocessing techniques. Volume-rendered 3D reconstruction of the arterial tree provides a global overview for the rapid identification of pathology. Maximum intensity projection (MIP) images provide similar views to traditional angiography and are useful for qualitatively assessing the degree of stenosis. The usefulness of both volume-rendered and MIP are limited by obscuration of the vessels by bones. Thus, automated software techniques for bone removal have been implemented (Figs 3 and 4).

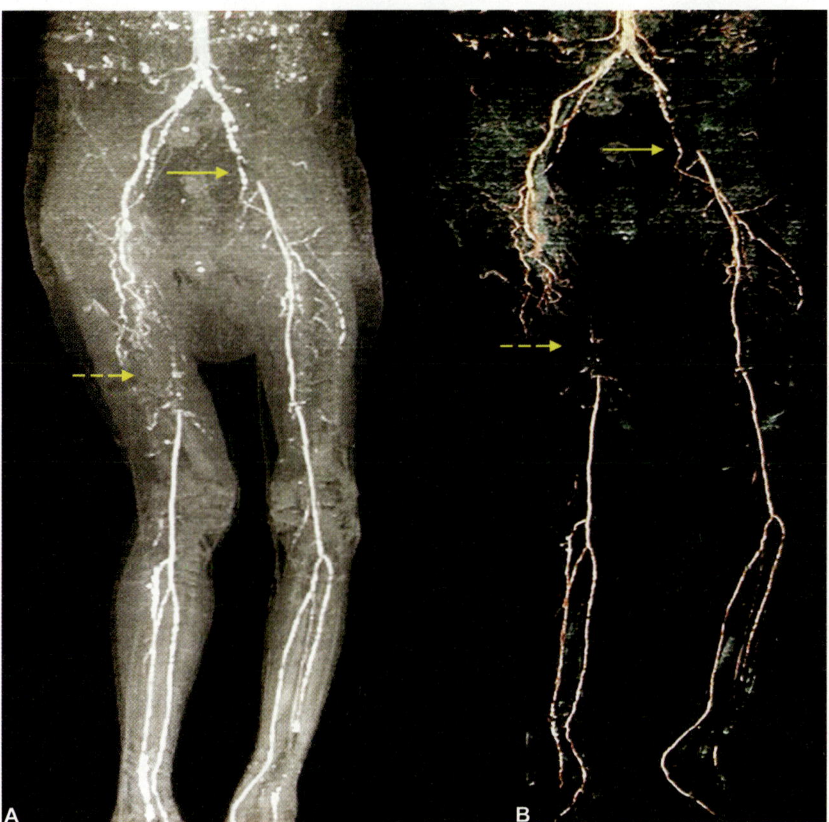

Figs 3A and B: CT angiography of lower limbs. (A) Maximum intensity projection image and (B) three-dimensional volume-rendered image. Occlusion of right common and deep femoral arteries (dashed arrows) and left external iliac and common femoral arteries (arrows) is present. Reconstitution of runoff flow is seen bilaterally by collateral formation

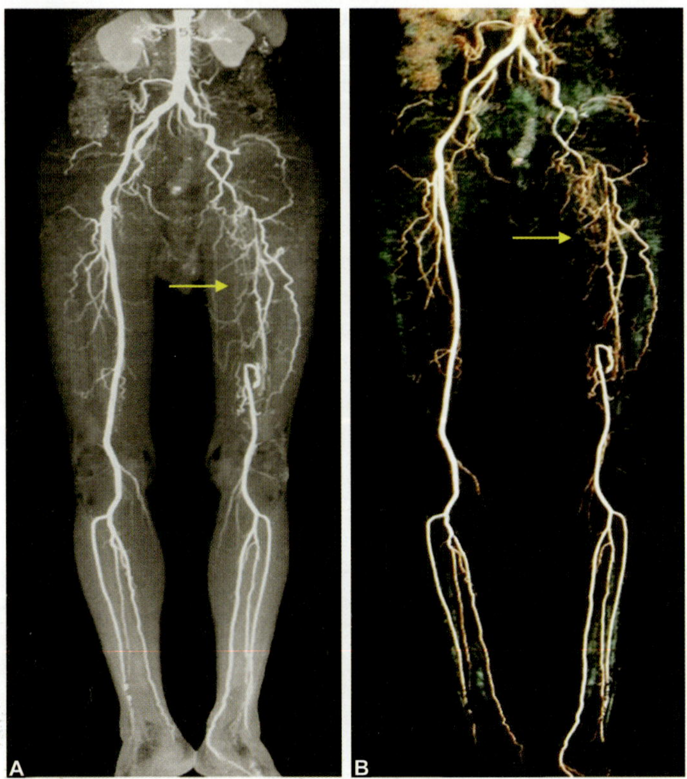

Figs 4A and B: CT Angiography of lower limbs. (A) Maximum intensity projection image and (B) three-dimensional volume-rendered image. Long segment occlusion of left common, superficial and deep femoral arteries (arrows) is present. Reconstitution of runoff flow is seen at distal deep femoral artery by collateral formation

Magnetic Resonance Angiography

Magnetic resonance angiography has several advantages for visualizing the peripheral arterial tree. There is no ionizing radiation exposure to the patient, and the gadolinium-based contrast agent is less nephrotoxic than the iodinated contrast agents used for CTA and DSA.[34] The sensitivity and specificity of arterial stenoses using contrast-enhanced MRA compared with DSA are in the 80–90% range, respectively.[35] 2D time-of-flight MRA can be performed without the use of contrast, but generally suffers from poorer resolution and longer imaging times with increased risk of patient motion artifact.

The major limitations to contrast-enhanced MRA remain the cost, length of the examination and inability of the patient to tolerate the examination. Severely claustrophobic patients frequently cannot tolerate the 60 minutes examination even with pre-medication. Patients with pacemakers, automated implantable cardioverter–defibrillators, certain types of stent grafts and brain aneurysm clips are excluded from receiving the examination. In the newer, more powerful magnet machines (3T), the manufacturers recommend against studying patients with several other types of intravascular stents (including some coronary stents). MRA is also limited in most centers to patients with glomerular filtration rates more than 30–35 mL/min secondary to reports of nephrogenic systemic fibrosis developing in patients with either end-stage renal disease or declining renal function exposed to gadolinium. The risk is likely greater with certain formulations of gadolinium,[36] although newer ferrous-based contrast agents may eventually prevent this problem. Last, metallic artifacts from prior intra-arterial stents preclude evaluation of the stented area.[37]

Venous contamination of the tibial level images can be a problem for MRA, especially in patients with critical limb ischemia and diabetic foot ulcers.[38] However, newer time-resolved contrast-enhanced MRA repeatedly acquires images of a volume during the passage of the contrast material. Differentiation of arterial vasculature from venous is more accurate.

SPECIAL IMAGING CONCERNS IN DIABETICS

Atherosclerosis

Patients with DM often have heavily calcified vessels, which presents a diagnostic challenge in terms of using duplex ultrasonography or CTA. With duplex ultrasonography, heavily calcified vessels may result in an obscured arterial lumen and inability to diagnose the degree of PAD reliably. CE-MRA is not subject to image artifact generated by heavily calcified vessels. Interobserver agreement for degree of stenosis or occlusion is higher with CE-MRA than CTA, in the presence of arterial calcifications. MRA should be considered the test of choice because of calcified vessels and concomitant renal insufficiency.

Renal Function Impairment

The use of contrast media may lead to kidney dysfunction, especially in patients with pre-existing renal impairment and in those with diabetes. Contrast-induced nephropathy (CIN) is defined as acute renal failure occurring within 24–72 hours of exposure to intravascular radiographic contrast media that cannot be attributed to other causes. It is commonly a nonoliguric and asymptomatic transient decline in renal function, generally occurring within 24 hours of contrast administration, usually peaking on the third to fifth day, and returning to baseline within 10–14 days. The impairment of renal function is usually mirrored by an absolute (0.5 mg/dL or greater) or relative (by 25% or greater) increase in serum creatinine from baseline.[39] The estimated glomerular infiltration rate (eGFR) is more accurate and significantly easier to obtain, using the modification of diet in renal disease calculation[40] or the very simple Cockcroft-Gault formula: (140 – number years of age) × kg of body weight/72/mg% of serum creatinine; in females the result × 0.85.[41] Moderately decreased renal function is defined as eGFR 30–60 mL/min (renal insufficiency). An eGFR of 60 mL/min/1.73 m^2 is a reliable cutoff point for identifying patients at high risk for the development of CIN.

Diabetes mellitus particularly when associated with renal insufficiency predisposes to CIN. At any given degree of baseline GFR, diabetes doubles the risk of developing CIN compared with nondiabetic patients. It has been demonstrated that, in patients with diabetes, hypercholesterolemia is the strongest predictor of CIN.[42] An established observation is that the coupling of CKD and diabetes dramatically increases the risk for CIN compared with that observed for CKD alone.[43] It has been observed, in fact, that diabetic patients with advanced chronic renal failure (serum creatinine >3.5 mg/dL) due to causes other than diabetic nephropathy are at significantly higher risk for CIN.[44]

As discussed previously, because of concerns regarding nephrogenic systemic fibrosis with gadolinium-based contrast agents, the current recommendation is to avoid them[45] in patients with advanced renal failure with an estimated glomerular filtration rate <30 mL/min per 1.73 m^2 unless the information provided by the CE-MRI is not obtainable by another means. Patients with any degree of renal insufficiency can be safely imaged with duplex ultrasonography and noncontrast MRA.

Implanted Metal Devices

For patients with implanted metal devices, it is important to determine compatibility with exposure to magnetic fields. Newer pacemakers are being developed that are MRI-compatible. Patients who are pacemaker-dependent or have certain types of brain aneurysm clips, neurostimulator devices, or retained ocular ferromagnetic foreign bodies are best imaged with another modality because of potential risk. In addition, even if an implanted medical device is considered compatible with the MRI environment; there may be significant susceptibility artifact generated during the scan.

SUMMARY

Imaging of macrovascular complications in diabetes is important both for screening and diagnosis. Various imaging modalities are available and choice in a particular case is affected by multiple factors. Moreover, patients should be screened for presence of any absolute/ relative contraindication to a particular modality and accordingly, adequate precautions should be taken.

REFERENCES

1. World Health Organization. Diabetes facts. Available from http://www.who.int/mediacentre/factsheets/fs312/en/index.html [accessed December, 2007].
2. World Health Organization. Diabetes action now booklet: a life-threatening condition. Available from www.who.int/diabetes/Booklet_HTML/en/index3 [accessed December, 2007].
3. Rahman S, Rahman T, Ismail AA, et al. Diabetes-associated macrovasculopathy: pathophysiology and pathogenesis. Diabetes Obes Metab. 2007;9:767-80.
4. Laakso M. Hyperglycemia and cardiovascular disease in type 2 diabetes. Diabetes. 1999;48:937-42.
5. Abbott RD, Curb JD, Rodriguez BL, et al. Age-related changes in risk factor effects on the incidence of thromboembolic and hemorrhagic stroke. J Clin Epidemiol. 2003;56:479-86.
6. Kullo IJ, Bailey KR, Kardia SL et al. Ethnic differences in peripheral arterial disease in the NHLBI Genetic Epidemiology Network of Arteriopathy (GENOA) Study. Vasc Med. 2003;8:237-42.
7. Di Carli MF, Hachamovitch R. Should we screen for occult coronary artery disease among asymptomatic patients with diabetes? J Am Coll Cardiol. 2005;45:50-3.
8. Rajagopalan N, Miller TD, Hodge DO, et al. Identifying high risk asymptomatic diabetic patients who are candidates for screening stress single photon emission computed tomography imaging. J Am Coll Cardiol. 2005;45:43-9.
9. Golomb BA, Dang TT, Criqui MH. Peripheral arterial disease: Morbidity and mortality implications. Circulation. 2006;114:688-99.
10. Mann JF, Gerstein HC, Pogue J, et al. Renal insufficiency as a predictor of cardiovascular outcomes and the impact of ramipril: the HOPE randomized trial. Ann Intern Med. 2001;134:629-36.

11. Anand DV, Lim E, Hopkins D, et al. Risk stratification in uncomplicated type 2 diabetes: Prospective evaluation of the combined use of coronary artery calcium imaging and selective myocardial perfusion scintigraphy. Eur Heart J. 2006;27:713-2.
12. Agatston AS, Janowitz WR, Hildner FJ, et al. Quantification of coronary artery calcium using ultrafast computed tomography. J Am Coll Cardiol. 1990;15:827-32.
13. Callister TQ, Cooil B, Raya SP, et al. Coronary artery disease: Improved reproducibility of calcium scoring with an electron-beam CT volumetric method. Radiology. 1998;208:807-14.
14. Erbel R, Mohlenkamp S, Kerkhoff G, et al. Non-invasive screening for coronary artery disease: Calcium scoring. Heart. 2007;93:1620-9.
15. Greenland P, Bonow RO, Brundage BH, et al. ACCF/AHA 2007 clinical expert consensus document on coronary artery calcium scoring by computed tomography in global cardio-vascular risk assessment and in evaluation of patients with chest pain. J Am Coll Cardiol. 2007;49:378-402.
16. Bax JJ, Young LH, Frye RL, et al. Screening for coronary artery disease in patients with diabetes. Diabetes Care. 2007;30:2729-36.
17. Raman SV, Simonetti OP, Winner MW 3rd, et al. Cardiac magnetic resonance with edema imaging identifies myocardium at risk and predicts worse outcome in patients with non-ST-segment elevation acute coronary syndrome. J Am Coll Cardiol. 2010;55:2480-8.
18. Rosen BD, Saad MF, Shea S, et al. Hypertension and smoking are associated with reduced regional left ventricular function in asymptomatic: individuals the multi-ethnic study of atherosclerosis. J Am Coll Cardiol. 2006;47:1150-8.
19. Paetsch I, Jahnke C, Wahl A, et al. Comparison of dobutamine stress magnetic resonance, adenosine stress magnetic resonance, and adenosine stress magnetic resonance perfusion. Circulation. 2004;110:835-42.
20. Jauch EC, Saver JL, Adams HP Jr, et al. Guidelines for the early management of patients with acute ischemic stroke: a guideline for healthcare professionals from the American Heart Association/American Stroke Association. Stroke. 2013;44:870-947.
21. Kidwell CS, Chalela JA, Saver JL, et al. Comparison of MRI and CT for detection of acute intracerebral hemorrhage. JAMA. 2004;292:1823-30.
22. Leys D, Pruvo JP, Godefroy O, et al. Prevalence and significance of hyperdense middle cerebral artery in acute stroke. Stroke. 1992;23:317-24.
23. Engelter ST, Wetzel SG, Bonati LH, et al. The clinical significance of diffusion-weighted MR imaging in stroke and TIA patients. Swiss Med Wkly. 2008;138:729-40.
24. Wildermuth S, Knauth M, Brandt T, et al. Role of CT angiography in patient selection for thrombolytic therapy in acute hemispheric stroke. Stroke. 1998;29:935-8.
25. Wintermark M, Jawadi SS, Rapp JH, et al. High-resolution CT imaging of carotid artery atherosclerotic plaques. AJNR Am J Neuroradiol. 2008;29:875-82.
26. Jauch EC, Saver JL, Adams HP Jr, et al. Guidelines for the early management of patients with acute ischemic stroke: a guideline for healthcare professionals from the American Heart Association/American Stroke Association. Stroke. 2013;44:870-947.
27. Wintermark M, Reichhart M, Thiran JP, et al. Prognostic accuracy of cerebral blood flow measurement by perfusion computed tomography, at the time of emergency room admission, in acute stroke patients. Ann Neurol. 2002;51:417-32.
28. Jansen O, Schellinger P, Fiebach J, et al. Early recanalisation in acute ischaemic stroke saves tissue at risk defined by MRI. Lancet. 1999;353:2036-7.
29. Grandin CB. Assessment of brain perfusion with MRI: methodology and application to acute stroke. Neuroradiology. 2003;45:755-66.
30. Lijmer JG, Hunink MG, van den Dungen JJ, et al. ROC analysis of noninvasive tests for peripheral arterial disease. Ultrasound Med Biol. 1996;22:391-8.
31. Ota H, Takase K, Rikimaru H, et al. Quantitative vascular measurements in arterial occlusive disease. Radiographics. 2005;25:1141-58.

32. de Smet AA, Ermers EJ, Kitslaar PJ. Duplex velocity characteristics of aortoiliac stenoses. J Vasc Surg. 1996;23:628-36.
33. de Vries SO, Hunink MG, Polak JF. Summary receiver operating characteristic curves as a technique for meta-analysis of the diagnostic performance of duplex ultrasonography in peripheral arterial disease. Acad Radiol. 1996;3:361-9.
34. Leiner T, Kessels AG, Nelemans PJ, et al. Peripheral arterial disease: comparison of color duplex US and contrast-enhanced MR angiography for diagnosis. Radiology. 2005;235(2):699-708.
35. Bui BT, Miller S, Mildenberger P, et al. Comparison of contrast-enhanced MR angiography to intraarterial digital subtraction angiography for evaluation of peripheral arterial occlusive disease: results of a Phase III multicenter trial. J Magn Reson Imaging. 2010;31(6):1402-10.
36. Wertman R, Altun E, Martin DR, et al. Risk of nephrogenic systemic fibrosis: evaluation of gadolinium chelate contrast agents at four American universities. Radiology. 2008;248(3):799-806.
37. Leiner T. Magnetic resonance angiography of abdominal and lower extremity vasculature. Top Magn Reson Imaging. 2005;16(1):21-66.
38. Dinter DJ, Neff KW, Visciani G, et al. Peripheral bolus-chase MR angiography: analysis of risk factors for nondiagnostic image quality of the calf vessels - a combined retrospective and prospective study. AJR Am J Roentgenol. 2009;193(1):234-40.
39. Mehran R, Nikolsky E. Contrast-induced nephropathy: definition, epidemiology, and patients at risk. Kidney Int Suppl. 2006;(100):S11-5.
40. Levey S, Bosch JP, Lewis JB, et al. A more accurate method to estimate glomerular filtration rate from serum creatinine: a new prediction equation," Ann Inter Med. 1999;130(6):461-70.
41. Cockcroft DW, Gault MH. Prediction of creatinine clearance from serum creatinine. Nephron. 1976;16(1):31-41.
42. Pakfetrat M, Nikoo MH, Malekmakan L, et al. Comparison of risk factors for contrast-induced acute kidney injury between patients with and without diabetes. Hemodial Int. 2010;14(4):387-92.
43. Rudnick MR, Goldfarb S, Tumlin J. Contrast-induced nephropathy: is the picture any clearer? Clin J Am Soc Nephrol. 2008;3(1):261-2.
44. Manske CL, Sprafka JM, Strony JT, et al. Contrast nephropathy in azotemic diabetic patients undergoing coronary angiography. Am J Med. 1990;89(5):615-20.
45. Kribben A, Witzke O, Hillen U, et al. Nephrogenic systemic fibrosis: pathogenesis, diagnosis, and therapy. J Am Coll Cardiol. 2009;53:1621-8.

18
CHAPTER

Dermatological Manifestations of Diabetes Mellitus

Satvik Khaddar, Amit Kumar Singh, Niti Singh, SS Pandey

INTRODUCTION

Nearly all patients with diabetes have cutaneous findings related to their condition. Some diabetes-associated skin conditions are a direct result of the related metabolic changes such as hyperglycemia and hyperlipidemia. Progressive damage to the vascular, neurologic, or immune systems also contributes significantly to skin manifestations. The mechanisms for other diabetes-associated skin conditions remain unknown.

Hyperglycemia leads to nonenzymatic glycosylation (NEG) of various structural and regulatory proteins, including collagen. Although NEG occurs normally with aging, the process is greatly accelerated in diabetes. NEG leads to the formation of advanced glycation end products (AGEs) that are responsible for decreases in both acid solubility and enzymatic digestion of cutaneous collagen.[1] Disorders such as diabetic thick skin and limited joint mobility (LJM) are thought to result directly from accumulation of AGEs. Derangements of immunoregulatory mechanisms also occur in diabetes. Hyperglycemia and ketoacidosis diminish chemotaxis, phagocytosis and bactericidal ability of white blood cells. Metabolic abnormalities, including hyperinsulinemia, as is seen in early insulin-resistant type 2 diabetes, can contribute to cutaneous manifestations as well. The action of insulin on the insulin-like growth factor 1 (IGF1) receptor appears to mediate the abnormal epidermal proliferation and resulting phenotype of acanthosis nigricans.

Dysregulated lipid metabolism occurs with diabetes-associated insulin deficiency.[2] The activity of lipoprotein lipase (LPL) is directly dependent on insulin, making insulin central to the processing of triglyceride-rich chylomicrons and very low-density lipoproteins. In insulin-deficient diabetic patients, defective lipid processing can lead to massive hypertriglyceridemia, manifesting in the skin as eruptive xanthomas. Macroangiopathy and microangiopathy contribute significantly to the cutaneous complications of diabetes. In patients with diabetes, there is increased "leakiness" or vessel wall permeability decreased vascular responsiveness to sympathetic innervation, and less ability to respond to thermal and hypoxemic stress. In combination with arteriosclerosis of large vessels, these microvascular abnormalities contribute to the formation of diabetic ulcers. In addition, a loss of cutaneous sensory innervation occurs with diabetes, predisposing patients to infection and injury. The loss of neuroinflammatory cell signaling plays a causal role in nonhealing, lower extremity ulcers.

CLASSIFICATION OF SKIN MANIFESTATIONS

Classification of skin manifestations has been shown in Table 1.[3]

Table 1: Classification of skin manifestations

Lesions associated with but not specific for diabetes mellitus (DM)	• Pruritus • Necrobiosis lipoidica diabeticorum • Granuloma annulare • Diabetic dermopathy • Scleroderma-like syndrome • Acanthosis nigricans • Diabetic bullae • Fournier gangrene
Lesions due to diabetic complications	• Diabetic foot • Cutaneous infections associated with diabetes—furunculosis, carbuncle, pyoderma, candidiasis, dermatophytosis • Erythrasma • Xanthomatosis • Xanthelasma • Phycomycetes • Malignant otitis media
Lesions associated with neurovascular complications	• Macroangiopathy • Microangiopathy • Diabetic neuropathy
Lesions due to complications of diabetes treatment	• With oral hypoglycemic • With insulin
Endocrine syndromes with skin alterations and DM	• Migratory necrolytic erythema in glucagonoma
Dermatoses more common in DM	• Perforating dermatosis • Vitiligo • Lichen planus • Eruptive xanthomas • Kaposi's sarcoma • Bullous pemphigoid • Dermatitis herpetiformis • Psoriasis

LESIONS ASSOCIATED WITH BUT NOT SPECIFIC FOR DIABETES MELLITUS

Pruritus[4]

Generalized pruritus is associated with diabetes complications of chronic renal insufficiency, occasionally neuropathy. High levels of urea in the blood cause pruritus. Candidiasis or dermatophytosis may underlie pruritus in diabetic patients. Anogenital pruritus is often

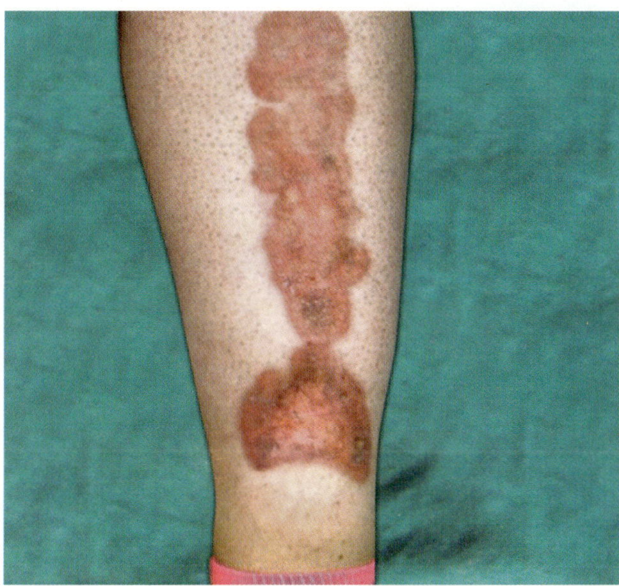

Fig. 1: Necrobiosis lipoidica diabeticorum[6]

caused by candidiasis in diabetic patients. Jock itch, athlete's foot and ringworm are among other causes.

Necrobiosis Lipoidica Diabeticorum (Fig. 1)[5,6]

It is one of the cutaneous markers of diabetes. At the time of diagnosis, 10% of the people will develop diabetes within 5 years or have abnormal glucose tolerance or history of the disease in at least one parent. The lesions are characteristically found on the anterior and lateral surface of lower legs, may also be present on the face, arms and trunk. The lesion begins as a small, dusky-red elevated nodule with a sharply circumscribed border which slowly enlarges to turn into a plaque of irregular outline, flattened, and eventually depressed as the dermis becomes more atrophic. The epidermis is smooth or slightly scaly and atrophic. The lesions may be anesthetic or have reduced sensation to pinprick and to fine touch due to destruction of cutaneous nerves.

The chronic lesions of necrobiosis lipoidica diabeticorum (NLD) are indolent, shallow often painful ulcers frequently appear in longstanding lesions. The treatment of NLD is not very satisfactory. Local therapy with topical glucocorticoids under occlusion or by intralesional injection may afford some improvement of active lesions. UV light treatment has been found to control his condition when it is flaring.

Granuloma Annulare (Fig. 2)[7]

It is a benign necrobiotic condition associated with lesions similar to NLD, the only difference being the absence of epidermal atrophy. It is occasionally associated with diabetes. Skin signs are characterized by red spots in the initial stages that expand outward and elbows are commonly affected. Mostly it is asymptomatic and resolves spontaneously.

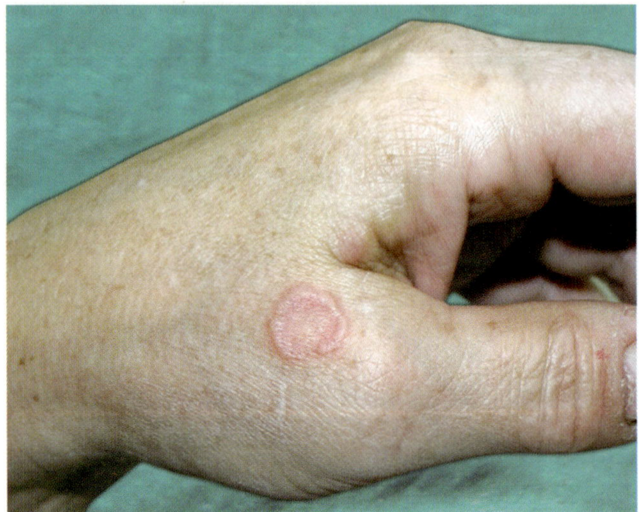

Fig. 2: Granuloma annulare[8]

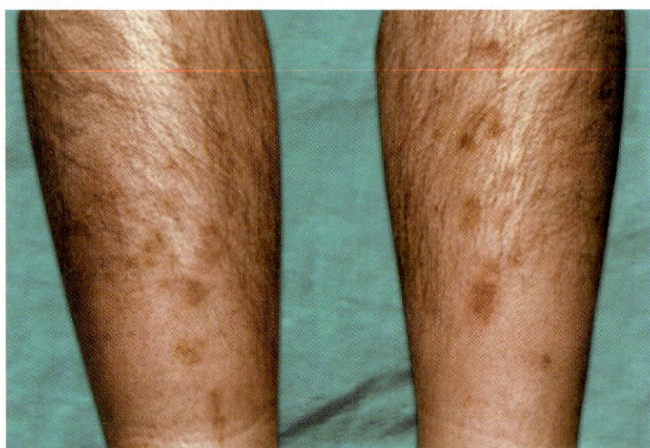

Fig. 3: Diabetic dermopathy[11]

Diabetic Dermopathy (Fig. 3)[9-11]

It presents as small (< 1 cm), atrophic, pink to brown, scar-like macules on the pretibial areas. The lesions are asymptomatic and clear within 1–2 years with slight residual atrophy or hypopigmentation.[12]

Scleroderma-like Syndrome/Waxy Skin Syndrome[13]

As many as one-third of diabetic patients have tight, thickened waxy skin over the dorsum of the hands. Reduced joint motion, first involving metacarpophalangeal (MCP) and proximal interphalangeal (PIP) joints, is seen. Clinical signs include impossible extension of the palm on the table and impossible clasping hands as in prayer (prayer sign). Skin becomes thickened, with a waxy appearance resembling sclerodermic skin. This cutaneous manifestation can

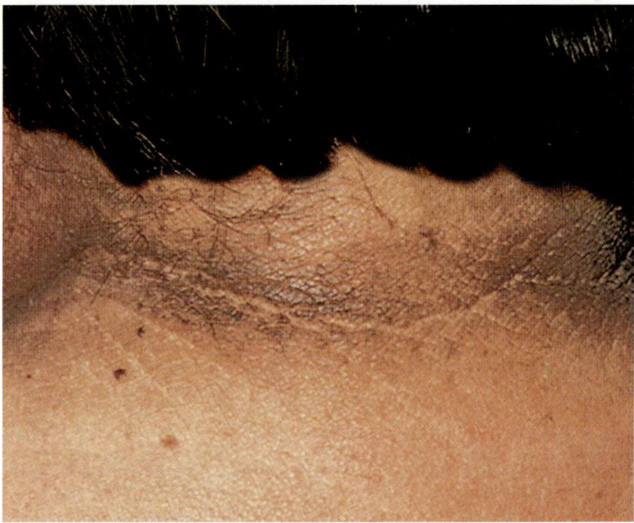

Fig. 4: Acanthosis nigricans involving nape of neck[11]

accompany maturity onset diabetes of young (MODY) and is considered to be associated with poor prognosis in terms of prediction of retinopathy and nephropathy.

Acanthosis Nigricans[14]

It is probably the most readily recognized skin manifestation of diabetes. Insulin resistance is the underlying cause for this disorder even in the absence of diabetes. It presents as brown to gray-black papillomatous cutaneous thickening in the flexural areas, including posterolateral neck (Fig. 4),[11] axillae, groin and abdominal folds with symmetric distribution. The affected skin has a dirty, velvety texture. The histology of clinical lesions demonstrates papillomatosis and hyperkeratosis but minimal acanthosis. Treatment is generally ineffective. Topical treatments with calcipotriol, salicylic acid, urea, systemic and topical retinoids have all been used. Medications that improve insulin sensitivity, such as metformin, have a theoretic benefit.

Diabetic Bullae

These are very rare but characteristic of diabetes mellitus. The bullae appear spontaneously, commonly in the dorsum and sides of the lower legs, especially feet. The blisters are painless, nonpruritic and contain sterile fluid. They heal spontaneously in 2–5 weeks without significant scarring. Usually they do not require any treatment apart from prevention of secondary infection which can be done by the application of bio-occlusive dressings.

Fournier Gangrene

Fournier gangrene is a type of necrotizing infection or gangrene usually affecting the perineum. In the majority of cases, it is a mixed infection caused by both aerobic and anaerobic bacteria. Studies have identified approximately one-third of patients are having underlying diabetes, alcoholism or malnutrition. Fournier gangrene is an emergency requiring intravenous antibiotics and debridement of necrotic tissue. In addition to surgery and antibiotics, hyperbaric oxygen therapy (HBOT) may be useful.

LESIONS DUE TO DIABETIC COMPLICATIONS

Diabetic Foot (Fig. 5)[11]

Peripheral neuropathy, pressure and trauma are felt to play prominent roles in the development of diabetic ulcers. Neuropathy (associated with uncontrolled hyperglycemia) is one of the major predictors of diabetic ulcers. Patients with diabetes also suffer the loss of cutaneous sensory nerves. The subsequent diminished neuroinflammatory signaling via neuropeptides to keratinocytes, fibroblasts, endothelial cells and inflammatory cells may adversely affect wound healing. Once an ulcer develops, peripheral vascular disease and intrinsic wound healing disturbances contribute to adverse outcomes. Standard therapy for neuropathic diabetic ulcers includes debridement, off-loading (often nonweight bearing), moist wound care and protective dressings.

Ulcer prevention is the most important intervention which can be provided for diabetic patients. Optimizing glycemic control, daily foot care and smoking cessation are among many of the preventive measures.

Cutaneous Infections Associated with Diabetes[15]

Furunculosis

It is caused by *Staphylococcus aureus*. It begins as a tender area, which rapidly develops into an inflammatory indurated nodule of 2–3 cm diameter. Within the next few days, the area becomes necrotic and discharges pus from a point at the follicular opening.

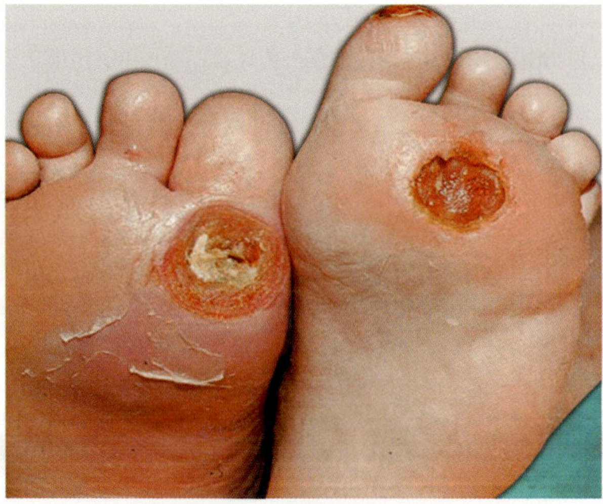

Fig. 5: Diabetic foot[11]

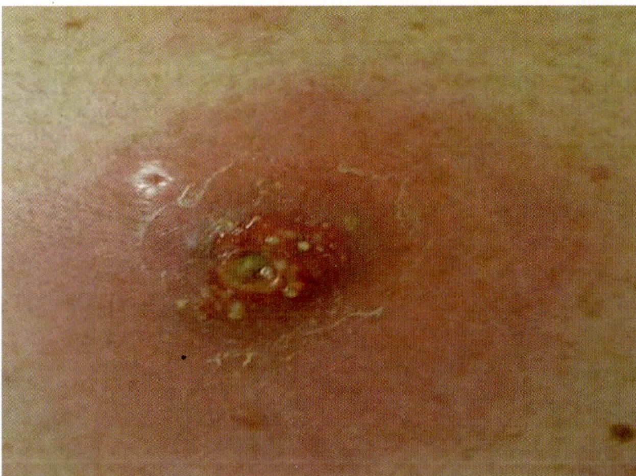

Fig. 6: Carbuncle[8]

Carbuncle (Fig. 6)[8]

It is a group of furuncles which spread from one follicle to other through subcutaneous tissue. The lesion starts as a painful, tender, firm to hard indurated lump associated with intense inflammatory changes in surrounding tissues. The common sites are the back of neck, shoulders, hips and thighs.

Candidiasis

It is a common complication in poorly controlled diabetics. Most common sites are groins, perineum, breasts and axillae. It may also involve nails and oral cavity. The yeast may be identified microscopically or by culture from swabs or scrapings from the lesions and be cultured from the blood in systemic disease. Cutaneous candidiasis is treated with topical azoles. Mucosal infection usually responds well to lozenges. Persistent and nail infections require oral fluconazole or itraconazole. Systemic infections should be treated with intravenous amphotericin or with amphotericin plus flucytosine.

Dermatophytosis (Figs 7 and 8)[6,16,17]

Tinea pedis: Most common is tinea pedis (athlete's foot) which may present as soggy interdigital scaling, diffuse powdery scaling of the soles and recurrent bouts of vesiculation of the soles. Other dermatophytoses are tinea unguium, tinea manuum, tinea cruris and tinea corporis.

Erythrasma (Fig. 9)

Erythrasma is a chronic superficial localized skin infection caused by bacteria called *Corynebacterium minutissimum*. The initial lesions are reddish-brown which later become brownish-black with irregular but well-defined borders which may be scaly. Common sites are genitocrural folds, axillae and submammary regions. The lesions fluoresce coral-red under Wood's light or UV-A light.

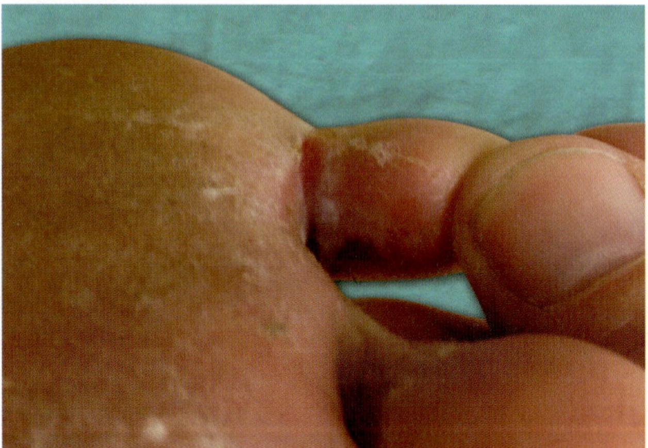

Fig. 7: Dermatophytosis[6]

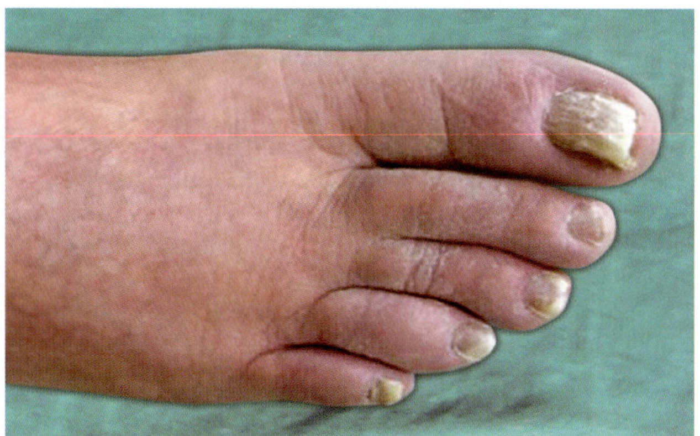

Fig. 8: Onychomycosis[6]

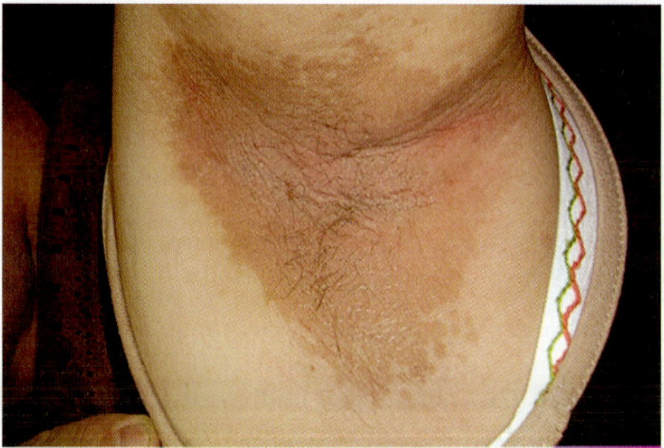

Fig. 9: Erythrasma[8]

Xanthomatosis

Eruptive xanthomas (Fig. 10)[6] are a characteristic but uncommon complication of diabetes associated with a more sustained hyperlipidemia affecting plasma triglycerides and cholesterol more than phospholipids, and hyperglycemia with glycosuria. The decreased LPL activity results in the accumulation of serum triglycerides, whose levels are occasionally highly elevated to produce eruptive xanthomas.

Eruptive xanthomas present clinically as 1–4 mm, reddish-yellow papules on the buttocks and extensor surfaces of the extremities.[16] The lesions occur in crops and may coalesce into plaques over time. Treatment of hypertriglyceridemia involves strict dietary fat restrictions and control of the underlying diabetes. LPL activity returns to normal after treatment with long-term insulin or oral glucose-lowering agents. The eruptive xanthomas respond rapidly and usually resolve completely in 6–8 weeks.

Xanthelasma (Fig. 11)

Basic underlying pathology is hyperlipidemic state. It presents as yellowish discoloration of the skin of the palms, soles, eyelids and nasolabial folds due to deposition of carotene presents in excess quantities in plasma. The contrasting feature of xanthelasma with xanthomatosis is that it does not regress with therapy for diabetes.[19]

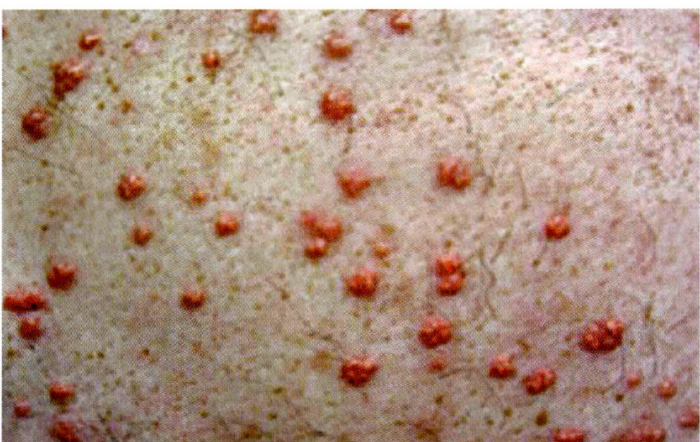

Fig. 10: Eruptive xanthomas[6]

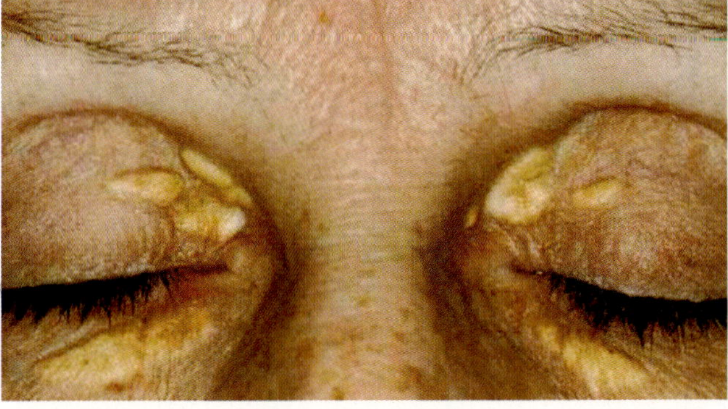

Fig. 11: Xanthelasma[8]

Phycomycetes[20]

Sometimes hyperglycemia may permit organisms that are nonpathogenic to produce infection in traumatized skin, which may lead to gangrene and loss of the limb. Many factors lead to infection such as pre-existing leg ulcers, nonhealing surgical wounds, deep-seated fungal infections, etc. Treatment must be aggressive, consisting of correcting acid-base balance, debridement of devitalized tissue and intravenous antifungal therapy.

Malignant Otitis Media

It is caused by *Pseudomonas aeruginosa*. Initially there is purulent discharge and pain in the external ear canal. It begins as a cellulitis and can progress to chondritis, osteomyelitis and infective cerebritis. It usually has a fatal outcome. Treatment includes use of antipseudomonal antibiotics and debridement of devitalized tissue if necessary.

LESIONS ASSOCIATED WITH NEUROVASCULAR COMPLICATIONS

Macroangiopathy

Atherosclerosis of the arteries of the legs results in skin atrophy, hair loss, coldness of the toes, nail dystrophy, pallor on elevation and mottling on dependence. A reliable sign of large vessel disease is dependent rubor with delayed return of color (> 15 seconds) after pressure has been applied to the skin.

Microangiopathy

The signs include diabetic dermopathy, pigmented purpura, and erysipelas such as erythema, NLD, periungal telangiectasias and diabetic foot.

Mechanism includes thickening of the vessel walls, perivascular deposition of periodic acid-Schiff (PAS)-positive increased deposition of type IV collagen within and around the vessel wall. The space between the pericytes and endothelial cells is wider resulting in increased permeability. The capillary leakage leads to the loss of albumin and water, and the platelets have a higher tendency to aggregate which creates a sluggish microcirculation.

Diabetic rubeosis is a peculiar rosy reddening of the face, sometimes of the hands and feet, which may be observed in longstanding diabetics. It has been attributed to diabetic microangiopathy or a decreased vascular tone.

Diabetic Neuropathy[21]

A common neuropathy in diabetes mellitus is a distal, symmetric, mixed polyneuropathy involving both motor and sensory nerves. The skin manifestations of autonomic neuropathy are disturbances in sweating and peripheral hyperemia with erythema, edema and atrophy. Motor neuropathy of the feet leads to imbalance between flexor and extensor muscles, displacement of fat pads and subluxation of digits.

Typical signs of sensory neuropathy in diabetes are paresthesias with loss of temperature and pain sensation, as well as aching and burning legs that are worse at night. The combination of neuropathy and microangiopathy along with mechanical factors plays a major role in development of diabetic foot.

DERMATOLOGICAL MANIFESTATIONS DUE TO TREATMENT OF DIABETES

Oral Hypoglycemic Drugs

There are few cutaneous complications of oral hypoglycemic agents. They are more common with first generation sulfonylureas such as chlorpropamide and tolbutamide. Manifestations usually develop within first 2 months of treatment. They may be either phototoxic or allergic in nature. Phototoxic reactions presenting as excessive sunburn after exposure to sunlight occur in a few patients. Allergic reactions are uncommon and are similar to all sulfonylureas. They are usually mild and self-limited. Other manifestations may be urticaria, erythema multiforme which may progress to Stevens-Johnson syndrome. Other rare manifestations include erythema nodosum, exacerbation of porphyria cutanea tarda and generalized hypersensitivity reaction. Some patients develop chlorpropamide alcohol flush which usually begins within 15 minutes after ingestion of drug. It causes flushing, headache, tachycardia and dyspnea that gradually subside within an hour.

Insulin

Cutaneous complications due to insulin therapy are rare these days after introduction of newer insulins.

Lipoatrophy: It presents as circumscribed atrophic plaques showing atrophy of the subcutaneous fat at the site of injection and rarely shows complete resolution.

Lipohypertrophy: It presents as soft dermal nodule. The overlying skin appears normal at injection. It may be due to the lipogenic action of insulin.

Insulin edema: Edema of the abdomen and legs is a more common and usually a self-limiting complication which appears shortly after starting or increasing the dose of insulin. It is more common in females and unrelated to the cardiac or renal disease. It has unknown etiology and drug of choice is ephedrine.

ENDOCRINE SYNDROMES WITH SKIN ALTERATIONS AND DIABETES MELLITUS

Glucagonoma

It is the most characteristic endocrine syndrome manifesting with skin alterations and diabetes mellitus. The syndrome is caused by tumors of the alpha-cell. It has four components:

1. Hyper secretion of glucagon
2. Diabetes that is usually mild
3. Weight loss
4. Necrolytic migratory erythema (Fig. 12).[8]

The chronic, fluctuating dermatosis is characterized by an annular and figurative erythema that forms bullae and erosions with peripheral vesiculopustules and coalesce before healing only to be replaced by new ones. They commonly occur in the intertriginous areas, perioral regions and on extremities. Necrolytic migratory erythema resolves after extirpation of the pancreatic tumor.

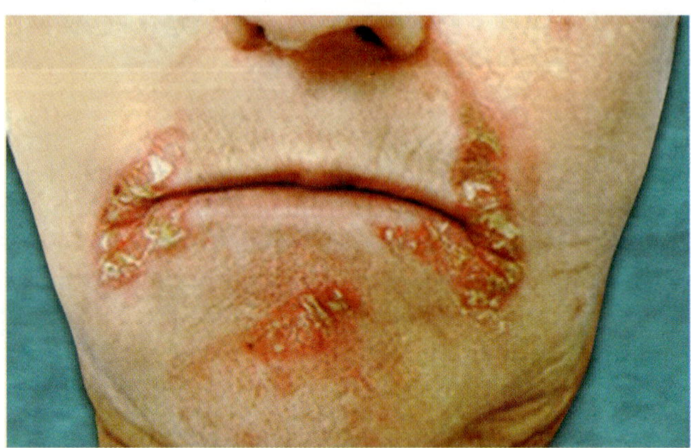

Fig. 12: Necrolytic migratory erythema[8]

DERMATOSIS REPORTED TO BE MORE COMMON IN DIABETICS THAN NONDIABETICS

Perforating Dermatosis

Acquired perforating dermatitis (APD), also known as Kyrle disease, has a prevalence of approximately 10% in dialysis populations and occurs predominantly in African Americans and patients with diabetes mellitus. APD is also associated with other entities such as hepatic disease, thyroid illnesses, malignancies, scabies and acquired immunodeficiency syndrome (AIDS).

Acquired perforating dermatitis is usually characterized by a linear confluence of papules with a central, oyster shell-like keratotic plug on the trunk, proximal extremities, scalp and face. Lesions are red or pink in white patients, and hyperpigmented in black patients. APD can initiate intense pruritus with secondary development of scratch marks (Koebner phenomenon). The origin of APD lesions is not known; suspected causes include an inflammatory skin reaction secondary to the presence of uremic toxins, uric acid deposits or scratching-induced trauma. Histological changes include the presence of epidermal invaginations with a central, basophilic, keratotic plug, uric acid and calcium hydroxyapatite deposits and chronic inflammatory granulomas.

Vitiligo (Fig. 13)[8]

It is a disease with diminished or absent function of melanocytes resulting in macular depigmentation. Mostly found in periorificial regions and also on the extensor aspect of extremities. It is asymptomatic but emotionally stressful, particularly in people with dark skin. It occurs with greater incidence than expected in patient with maturity onset diabetes.

Lichen Planus (Fig. 14)[8]

The most common presentation is as a well-defined area of purple-colored, itchy, flat-topped papules with interspersed lacy white lines (Wickham's striae). Patients with diabetes and abnormal insulin response to glucose challenge test are found to have higher incidence of lichen planus. This seems to be more particularly in adult, especially those with erosive oral forms.

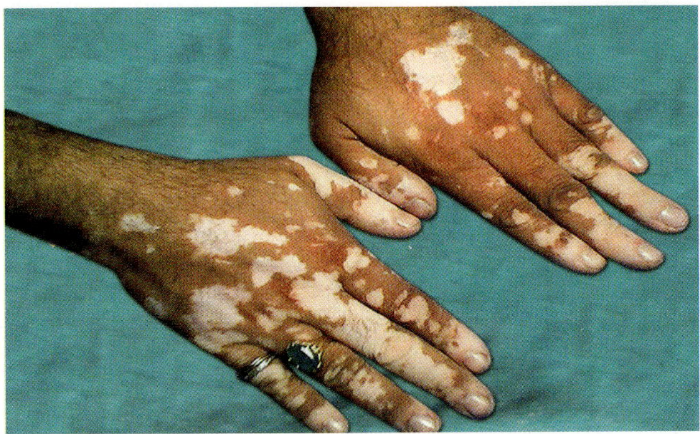

Fig. 13: Vitiligo[8]

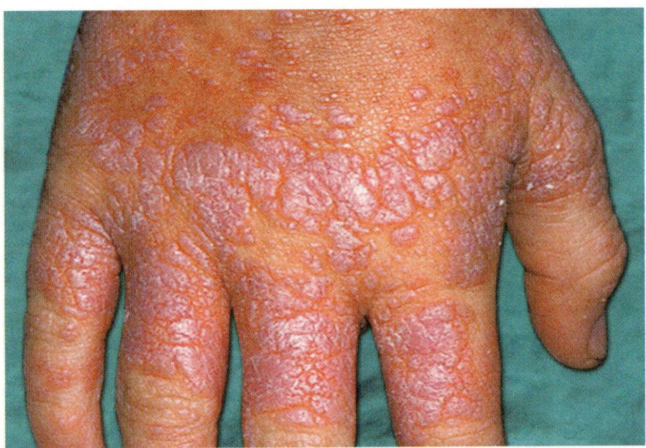

Fig. 14: Lichen planus[8]

Kaposi's Sarcoma (Fig. 15)[8]

It is a multiple idiopathic hemorrhagic sarcoma, which manifests as multiple vascular nodules in the skin and other organs. Predominantly occurs in males and usually begin in the legs as multiple, purple macules, nodules or plaques. Later on other areas of skin, mucous membranes and internal organs may be involved. Histologic picture reveals accumulation of spindle cells forming vascular slits containing erythrocytes.

Bullous Pemphigoid

There are few studies relating these two. But, theoretically their association may be due to lower threshold of diabetes in traumatically induced blisters or on the basis of antigenic changes at the level of lamina lucida because of enzymatic glycosylation.

Dermatitis Herpetiformis

The HLA association of dermatitis herpetiformis and diabetes may be a possible explanation for the disease to appear more frequently together than expected.

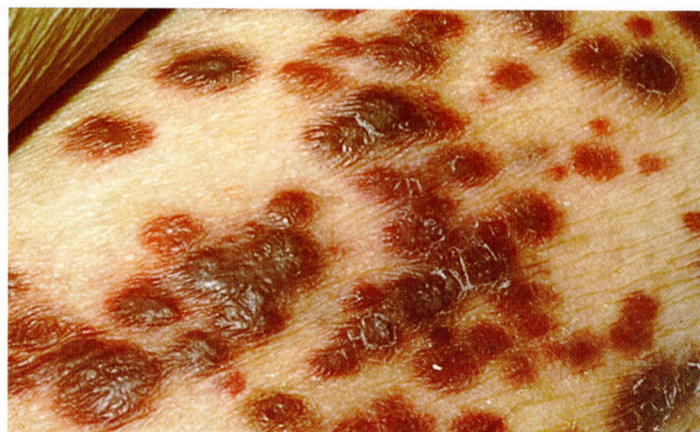

Fig. 15: Kaposi's sarcoma[8]

REFERENCES

1. Beisswenger PJ, Moore LL, Curphey TJ. Relationship between glycemic control and collagen-linked advanced glycosylation end products in type I diabetes. Diabetes Care. 1993;16:689-94.
2. Buckingham B, Perejda AJ, Sandborg C, et al. Skin, joint, and pulmonary changes in type I diabetes mellitus. Am J Dis Child. 1986;140:420-3.
3. Sreedevi C, Car N, Pavlic-Renar I. Dermatologic lesions in diabetes mellitus. Diabetologia Croatica. 2002;31:147-59.
4. Romano G, Moretti G, Di Benedetto A, et al. Skin lesions in diabetes mellitus: prevalence and clinical correlations. Diabetes Res Clin Pract. 1998;39:101-6.
5. Muller SA, Winkelmann RK. Necrobiosis lipoidica diabeticorum. A clinical and pathological investigation of 171 cases. Arch Dermatol. 1966;93:272-81.
6. Duff M, Demidova O, Blackburn S, Shubrook J. Cutaneous manifestation.
7. Dabski K, Winkelmann RK. Generalized granuloma annulare: clinical and laboratory findings in 100 patients. J Am Acad Dermatol. 1989;20:39-47.
8. Google Images: Various webpages
9. Binkley GW. Dermopathy in diabetes mellitus. Arch Dermatol. 1965;92:106-7.
10. Shemer A, Bergman R, Linn S, et al. Diabetic dermopathy and internal complications in diabetes mellitus. Int J Dermatol. 1998;37:113-5.
11. Kalus AA, Chien AJ, Olerud JE. Diabetes mellitus and other endocrine diseases. In: Goldsmith LA, Katz SI, Gilchrest BA, Paller AS, Leffell DJ, Wolff K (Eds). Fitzpatrick's Dermatology in General Medicine, 8th edition. New York: McGraw-Hill; 2012.
12. Danowski TS, Sabeh G, Sarver ME, et al. Shin spots and diabetes mellitus. Am J Med Sci. 1966;251:570-5.
13. Cole GW, Headley J, Skowsky R. Scleredema diabeticorum: a common and distinct cutaneous manifestation of diabetes mellitus. Diabetes Care. 1983;6:189-92.
14. Schwartz RA. Acanthosis nigricans. J Am Acad Dermatol. 1994;31:1-19.
15. Joshi N, Caputo GM, Weitekamp MR, et al. Infections in patients with diabetes mellitus. N Engl J Med. 1999;341:1906-12.
16. Higa M. Clinical epidemiology of fungal infection in diabetes. Nihon Rinsho. 2008;66:2239-44.
17. Romano C, Massai L, Asta F, et al. Prevalence of dermatophytic skin and nail infections in diabetic patients. Mycoses. 2001;44:83-6.
18. Parker F. Xanthomas and hyperlipidemias. J Am Acad Dermatol. 1985;13:1-30.
19. Puri N. A study on cutaneous manifestations of diabetes mellitus. Our Dermatology Online. 2012;3:87.
20. Goyal A, Raina S, Kaushal SS, et al. Pattern of cutaneous manifestations in diabetes mellitus. Indian J Dermatol. 2010;55:39-41.
21. Van Hattem S, Bootsma AH, Thio HB. Skin manifestations of diabetes. Cleve Clin J Med. 2008;75:772, 774, 776-7 passim.

19
CHAPTER

Oral Hypoglycemic Agents: Drug Interaction and Toxicity

Banshi Saboo

INTRODUCTION

Type 2 diabetes mellitus (T2DM) is the most common type of diabetes in adults and is characterized by hyperglycemia and insulin deficiency and resistance. There are several categories of medications used in the treatment of diabetes as oral hypoglycemic agents (OHAs) including sulfonylureas (SUs), thiazolidinediones (TZDS), biguanides, alpha-glucosidase inhibitors (AGIs), dipeptidyl peptidase-4 (DPP-4) inhibitors and sodium-glucose cotransporter 2 (SGLT2) inhibitors.[1] Oral antidiabetic (OAD) agents are FDA-approved for use in type 2 diabetics as monotherapy or in combination with other OAD agents or insulin, when the single agent alone, in addition to diet and exercise, does not provide sufficient glycemic control.[2]

Each of these agents has been shown in various experimental and clinical settings to be efficacious in T2DM, but each is also associated with a number of adverse effects. The increasing number of drugs, together with numerous combination options in polypharmacy, presents with the clinician an increasing complexity of therapeutic options and chances of drug interactions. The likely pathogenetic mechanism of diabetes operating in the patient, as well as the mode of action, efficacy and safety of the drugs are some of the major considerations in the choice of any given agent or its combinations.[3]

All of the oral hypoglycemic drugs have the potential to interact with other medications and if the result is hypoglycemia or hyperglycemia the consequences can be serious.

The interactions may be pharmacodynamic (another drug independently raises or lowers blood glucose) or pharmacokinetic (another drug alters the absorption, metabolism or excretion of the hypoglycemic drug). Both mechanisms may have the effect of changing the apparent efficacy of the hypoglycemic drugs. Pharmacokinetic interactions may also exacerbate other adverse effects of oral hypoglycemic drugs.[4] This review focuses on the current role of only OHAs in T2DM in terms of dug-drug interaction and its toxicity.

METFORMIN

Metformin is the only biguanide available in a class since phenformin and buformin have been withdrawn from the market because of toxicity. It decreases hepatic glucose production, decreases intestinal glucose absorption and increases glucose uptake and utilization.

It is not metabolized at all but is completely excreted in urine. Metformin may therefore accumulate and cause lactic acidosis if other medications have induced renal failure. Examples include contrast media, cyclosporine and aminoglycosides.[4] Metformin should therefore be stopped before, and for 48 hours after, contrast radiography. Metformin should not be initiated when serum creatinine is raised (120–150 µmol/L) and should be withdrawn when serum creatinine exceeds 150–200 µmol/L. Common causes of increased lactic acid production include alcoholism (due to depletion of NAD^+ stores), heart failure and respiratory disease (due to inadequate oxygenation of tissues); the most common cause of impaired lactic acid excretion is kidney disease.

Metformin is excreted by the renal tubules and this process can be inhibited by cimetidine, but not the other H2 receptor antagonists. This interaction causes retention of metformin and increases the risk of lactic acidosis. Other side effects associated with metformin therapy are gastrointestinal, including diarrhea, nausea, abdominal discomfort and anorexia, which improve with dose reduction and can be minimized by slow dose titration. Long-term use of metformin may interfere with absorption of vitamin B_{12} and folic 265 acid; this may produce deficiency of these vitamins.[3]

SULFONYLUREAS

Sulfonylureas mainly work by stimulating the release of insulin (secretagogue) from the remaining functional—cell mass of the pancreas, by decreasing the potassium ion efflux at a "SU receptor site". Hypoglycemia is the most troublesome side effect, but less likely if a low dose is started, and uptitration is at 2-week intervals at least. Hypoglycemia is more likely in the presence of impaired renal function and in the underweight elderly patient. SUs may be used in combination with all other classes except the meglitinides, which are also insulin secretagogues. Difficulty losing weight, or weight gain, and hyponatremia may also occur.[5]

All drugs in this class are partially or totally metabolized by the liver. It is excreted much more rapidly in alkaline urine so its half-life and duration of action are reduced with excessive ingestion of alkalis. Antacids may increase the absorption of all the SUs and hence produce higher peak concentrations of the drugs and a risk of temporary hypoglycemia. SUs are highly protein bound drugs and may be displaced from blood protein binding sites by drugs such as the nonsteroidal anti-inflammatory drugs. This can cause a short-term increase in free (unbound) SU and hence temporary hypoglycemia. The majority of significant interactions with SUs are due to the induction or inhibition of cytochrome P450 enzymes in the liver.[4]

Increase in area under plasma concentration-time curve (AUC) due to CYP2C9 inhibition could be seen with clarithromycin since it can increase glyburide concentration to the extent of 35% same as fluconazole can also increase glimepiride concentration 138% likewise. Decrease in AUC due to CYP2C9 inducement could be seen with rifampin since it can decrease gliclazide concentration 70%, glimepiride concentration 34% and glyburide concentration to the extent of 39%.[6]

THIAZOLIDINEDIONES

These are also known as the "glitazones". There were total three drugs belong to this class (1) troglitazone, (2) rosiglitazone and (3) pioglitazone. Troglitazone was introduced in the market in 1997 and withdrawn in 2000 due to an increased incidence of drug-induced hepatitis. Rosiglitazone was first released in 1999, but sales declined after the drug was found to increase risk of heart attack. The drug was withdrawn from the market in Europe (September, 2010) and New Zealand (April, 2011), banned in India (2010) and was put underselling restrictions in the United States.[3]

Pioglitazones appear to truly reduce insulin resistance, also being called "insulin sensitizers". They, therefore, are in theory most useful in insulin resistance states, as may occur in most T2DM patients and especially in obese (> BMI > 30 kg/m^2) T2DM patients. Unfortunately, weight gain appears commonly on TZDs, sometimes due to fluid retention (edema), which must be distinguished from cardiac failure. This is more likely in the patient with ischemic heart disease (IHD) and high blood pressure (BP).

Thiazolidinediones have their action through intranuclear enzyme systems involved in transcription of insulin sensitive genes. These results from binding to the peroxisome proliferator-activated receptors, in particular the gamma type (PPAR-γ). This process is slow and clinical and biochemical benefits may take 2–3 months, so initiation as monotherapy particularly in symptomatic new type 2 patients may be an issue. These drugs are indicated in monotherapy only when metformin is contraindicated or not tolerated. TZDs are usually withdrawn if serum alanine transaminase (ALT) levels exceed 2.5 times normal. TZDs are better tolerated in cases of impaired renal function than metformin. There are studies showing an increased risk of bone fractures in women. TZDs are not indicated in patients with coronary disease or heart failure, and there is currently increasing concern about their use in this context.[5] Pioglitazone was the highest selling drug in the class since its cardiovascular (CV) safety profile compares favorably with rosiglitazone which has been banned. France and Germany have suspended the sale of pioglitazone and it has been withdrawn in some countries after a study suggested the drug could raise the risk of bladder cancer.

DIPEPTIDYL PEPTIDASE-4 INHIBITORS

These are the inhibitors of dipeptidyl peptidase were approved by FDA in 2006. This class includes various gliptins such as vildagliptin, sitagliptin, saxagliptin, linagliptin and alogliptin. They act by competitively inhibiting the enzyme DPP-4. This enzyme is responsible for breakdown of the incretins, glucagon-like peptide-1 (GLP-1) and glucose-dependent insulinotropic peptide (GIP), which are gastrointestinal hormones released in response to a meal. These hormones have insulinotropic effect. By preventing GLP-1 and GIP inactivation, they tend to increase and prolong the incretins, especially the GLP-1, in T2DM patients. This increases the secretion of insulin and suppresses the release of glucagon by the pancreas, thereby reducing blood glucose levels in the diabetic patients.[3]

Potential advantages of DPP-4 inhibitors include a neutral effect on weight and a relatively low incidence of adverse effects and drug-drug interactions. There have been several post-marketing reports of pancreatitis which are fatal in some cases in people treated with sitagliptin and other DPP-4 inhibitors. The US package insert carries a warning to this effect and this is under investigation by the FDA and the European Medicines Agency (EMA).

Dosage adjustments are recommended in patients with renal insufficiency for both sitagliptin and saxagliptin but not with linagliptin; alogliptin is contraindicated in patients with renal impairment.[1] With Saxagliptin and alogliptin, the chances of heart failure and hospitalization will be on higher side comparatively as per the Saxagliptin Assessment of Vascular Outcomes Recorded in Patients with Diabetes Mellitus—Thrombolysis in Myocardial Infarction 53 (SAVOR-TIMI 53) and examine trial results. However, the Trial Evaluating Cardiovascular Outcomes with Sitagliptin (TECOS) Trial has provided reassurance that sitagliptin did not increase risk of CV events. Other adverse effects reported include rare cases of nausea and common cold-like symptoms, including photosensitivity which was noted during clinical trial of sitagliptin. Spontaneously-reported adverse events of saxagliptin include anaphylaxis, angioedema. In clinical trials, the most frequently reported adverse events with linagliptin were headache, influenza-like illness and nausea.

Increase in AUC due to CYP3A4 inhibition could be seen with diltiazem to the extent of 109% and with ketoconazole 145% so consider reducing dose of saxagliptin by 50% (to 2.5 mg daily) likewise same. Decrease in AUC due to CYP3A4 inducement could be seen with rifampin to the extent of 76% while in case of other gliptins, such as linagliptin, alogliptin, sitagliptin and vildagliptin, there is no significant metabolic drug interactions.[6]

ALPHA-GLUCOSIDASE INHIBITORS

Alpha-glucosidase inhibitors are oral antidiabetic drugs used for T2DM that work by preventing or delaying the digestion of carbohydrates to simple sugars in the intestine. Apha-glucosidases are saccharides that act as competitive inhibitors of the small intestines. The drugs in this class include acarbose, miglitol and voglibose. Unlike SUs and glinides, AGIs do not cause hypoglycemia, hyperinsulinemia or weight gain. They do have the potential to cause weight loss by lowering the amount of sugar metabolized. Voglibose scores over both acarbose and miglitol in terms of side effect profile but acarbose has an edge over voglibose in terms of efficacy.

Gastrointestinal disturbances in the form of flatulence, abdominal discomfort, and, to a lesser extent, diarrhea are common side effects of therapy with AGIs. Higher doses of acarbose (100 mg or greater) have been associated with a low incidence of elevated serum ALT levels, most often in patients weighing less than 60 kg. Hepatitis has been reported with acarbose use. It usually goes away when the medicine is stopped. Therefore, liver enzymes should be checked before and during use of this medicine.[3]

SODIUM-GLUCOSE COTRANSPORTER 2 INHIBITORS

The SGLT2 is expressed in the proximal tubule and mediates reabsorption of approximately 90% of the filtered glucose load. SGLT2 inhibitors promote the renal excretion of glucose and thereby modestly lower elevated blood glucose levels in patients with T2DM. The ability to lower blood glucose and A1c levels is limited by the filtered load of glucose and the osmotic diuresis caused by this therapy, and therefore is independent of insulin (beta-cell function and insulin sensitivity).

All the gliflozins means dapagliflozin, canagliflozin and empagliflozin, which all are US FDA-approved are once daily oral treatments, and the most common adverse effects include genital mycotic infections and urinary tract infections. Since the drugs lead to heavy glycosuria (sometimes up to about 70 g/day) as part of their action, this can lead to polyurea, rapid weight loss, dehydration and tiredness; glucose acts as an osmotic diuretic leading to dehydration. There has been concern about the risk of bone fracture with canagliflozin but this has not been proved by dual-energy X-ray absorptiometry (DEXA) results.[3] An abnormally high number of trial participants who used dapagliflozin developed bladder cancer, so dapagliflozin is not recommended for people with active bladder cancer.[1]

SUMMARY

Oral hypoglycemic agents are by definition the starting point of pharmacological treatment of T2DM. The modes of action of the different classes described are different, and offer an opportunity to "tailor treatment" to the likely pathogenetic mechanism or mechanisms in what is probably a heterogeneous condition. "Failure" of one level of treatment should be monitored for at all times by appropriate checks on well-being, weight, fasting and postprandial blood glucose (self-monitoring) and hemoglobin A1c (HbA1c).[5] Interactions with OHAs are important because the outcomes, particularly hypoglycemia, are serious. As with all interactions the times of high risk are when a second drug is started or stopped or has its dose changed. Regular coprescription of the same dose of another drug is not likely to cause major problems.[4]

REFERENCES

1. BMC Health Net Plan. (2015). Clinical coverage guidelines: antidiabetic agents. [online] Available from www.bmchp.org. [Accessed August, 2015].
2. Medicaid drug use review criteria for outpatient use: oral antidiabetic agents, October 2012.
3. Osadebe PO, Odoh EU, Uzor PF. Oral antidiabetic agents—review and updates. Department of Pharmaceutical and Medicinal Chemistry, Faculty of Pharmaceutical Sciences, University of Nigeria. 2014.
4. Shenfield GM. Drug interactions with oral hypoglycaemic drugs, Australian Prescriber. 2001; 24(4):83-5.
5. Fsadni D. The use of oral hypoglycemic agents. DESG Teaching Letter Number 37. November 2007.
6. Antihyperglycemic agents comparison chart: 2012 August; Bill Cornish, Drug Information, Sunnybrook Health Sciences Centre.

20
CHAPTER

Chronic Kidney Disease and Diabetes

Vinay Kumar BR, Dheeraj Kishore, Amita Diwaker, Madhukar Rai

INTRODUCTION

Chronic kidney disease (CKD) is a spectrum of different pathophysiologic processes associated with abnormal kidney function and a progressive decline in glomerular filtration rate (GFR). CKD, regardless of its etiology, can be defined as either kidney damage or decreased kidney function for 3 months, which can present as a range of complex deleterious alterations in physiological and metabolic function, causing worsening and eventual failure of kidney function.[1,2]

These metabolic dysfunction can be accumulation of uremic toxins (uremia), metabolic acidosis, abnormalities in lipid, amino acid, mineral, bone and homocysteine metabolism, malnutrition, insulin resistance, inflammatory and oxidative stress, anemia, vitamin D deficiency, skeletal muscle dysfunction with a reduction in exercise tolerance, and lean body mass (LBM).[3,4]

CLINICAL DEFINITION

Diabetes is often associated with CKD, according to studies, among 45% of patients who receive dialysis therapy, diabetes is the primary cause of their kidney failure. And also studies say that moderate to severe CKD is estimated to be found in 15–23% of patients with diabetes.[5] Diabetic nephropathy is characterized by increased urinary albumin excretion (UAE). Persistent albuminuria starts with microalbuminuria (UAE $\geq$ 20 μg/min and $\leq$ 199 μg/min) and progresses to macroalbuminuria (> 300 mg/24 h or $\geq$ 200 μg/min). Later, referred as "overt proteinuria or dipstick positive" heralds the beginning of decline in renal function.

However, microalbuminuria besides being a marker of nephropathy is a marker of increased risk for cardiovascular disease (CVD). Clinically, diabetic nephropathy is suspected in presence of increased UAE and the presence of diabetic retinopathy in absence of clinical or laboratory evidence of other kidney or renal tract disease; it holds good for both type 1 diabetes mellitus (T1DM) and T2DM.[6-8]

PATHOLOGICAL FINDINGS

Development of diabetes-associated renal changes starts with glomerular hyperperfusion leading to increased GFR. This causes increased intraglomerular hypertension and thickening of the glomerular basement membrane (GBM), which is the first change that can be identified. Thickening of tubular basement membranes (TBMs) parallels this GBM thickening, then afferent and efferent glomerular arteriolar hyalinosis can also be detected within 3–5 years after onset of diabetes or following transplantation of a normal kidney into the diabetic patient.

During the course of the disease, a waxy, homogeneous, translucent-appearing material that is positive for the periodic acid-Schiff reaction which usually consists of immunoglobulins, complement, fibrinogen, albumin, and other plasma proteins[9] are deposited in smooth muscle cells of these small vessels. As disease progress, there appears arteriolar hyalinosis, glomerular capillary subendothelial hyaline (hyaline caps) and capsular drops along the parietal surface of Bowman's capsule forming exudative lesions of diabetic nephropathy, then mesangial cell starts proliferating. When these changes are diffuse and there is generalized process of mesangial expansion, it is termed as diffuse diabetic glomerulosclerosis. However, the characteristic nodular glomerulosclerosis (Kimmelstiel-Wilson nodular lesions) of diabetic nephropathy results from glomerular capillary wall detachment from a mesangial anchoring point with consequent microaneurysm formation and subsequent filling of the increased capillary space with mesangial matrix material. Podocyte number and/or numerical density (number/volume) are also decreased. This causes albuminuria and disease progression. Podocyte detachment from GBM may be an early phenomenon in type 1 diabetes, appears to worsen with increasing albuminuria.[10]

Pathologic classification of diabetic nephropathy has been shown in Table 1.

Table 1: Pathologic classification of diabetic nephropathy

Class	*Description*	*Inclusion criteria*
I.	Mild or nonspecific changes and EM-proven GBM thickening	Biopsy does not meet any of the criteria mentioned below for class II, III, or IV
		GBM> 395nm in female and >430 nm in male individuals 9 years of age and older podocyte hypertrophy
IIa.	Mild mesangial expansion	Biopsy does not meet criteria for class III or IV
		Severe mesangial expansion in >25% of the observed mesangium
IIb	Severe mesangial expansion	Biopsy does not meet criteria for class III or IV
		Severe mesangial expansion in >25% of the observed mesangium
III	Nodular scierosis (Kimmeistiel-Wilson lesion	Biopsy does not meet criteria for class IV
		At least one convincing Kimmeistiel-Wilson lesion
IV	Advanced diabetic glomerulosclerosis	Global glomerular sclerosis in >50% of gomeruli
		Lesions from classes I through III

Source: Tervaert TW, Mooyaart AL, Amann K, et al. Pathologic classification of diabetic nephropathy. J Am Soc Nephrol. 2010;21(4):556-63.

PATHOPHYSIOLOGY

The high blood glucose levels and high levels of saturated fatty acids create an inflammatory medium, resulting in activation of the innate immune system, which results in activation of the nuclear transcription factor-kappa B (NF-κB), and release of inflammatory mediators including interleukin (IL)–1β and tumor necrosis factor-alpha (TNF-α), promoting systemic insulin resistance and β-cell damage as a result of autoimmune insulitis. Hyperglycemia and high serum levels of free fatty acids and IL-1 lead to glucotoxicity, lipotoxicity, and IL-1 toxicity, resulting in apoptotic β-cell death. Other factors such as inflammatory and oxidative stress, erythropoietin (EPO) resistance, anemia, vitamin D deficiency and vascular calcification can also be seen in these CKD patients. Some of the studies have also demonstrated the presence of the "cardiorenal syndrome", whereby dysfunction of the kidney and cardiac systems may amplify progressive failure of both systems.

The initial development of abnormalities in kidney function has been linked to chronic obesity and insulin resistant conditions, such as the metabolic syndrome (MetS), also factors like sympathetic hyperactivity, activation of the renin-angiotensin-aldosterone system (RAAS), which is related to development of hypertension are implicated in pathogenesis and excess dietary salt intake further aggravates the process[11] and adipocytokines and abnormal glucocorticoid activity also play a role.[12]

The progression of metabolic and cellular dysfunction both systemically and locally within kidney tissue is linked to many diverse and complex pathways (Fig. 1); these are enumerated below:

- The heightened production of proinflammatory cytokines IL-1β, IL-6, IL-8, TNF-α and interferon-gamma (IFN-γ)
- The oxidative stress
- Abnormalities in glucose and lipid metabolism (e.g. impaired glucose tolerance, glycemia and dyslipidemia). The dyslipidemia associated with worsening CKD and in end-stage renal disease (ESRD)
- The endothelial dysfunction which promotes or accelerates atherosclerosis
- Insulin resistance, depressed nitric oxide synthesis, adipocytokine dysfunction and hemodialysis-induced factors (in ESRD).[10]

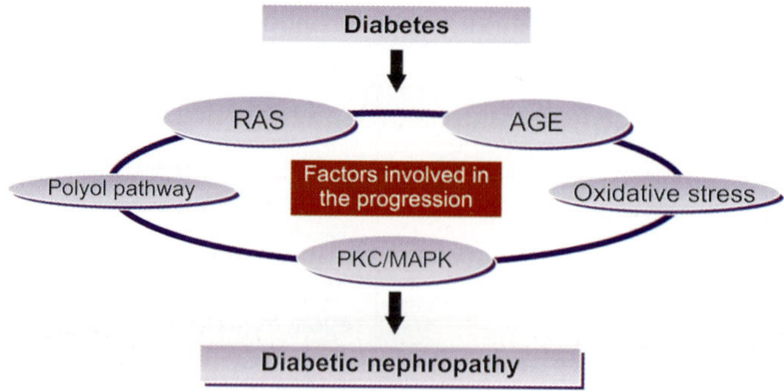

Fig. 1: Factors affecting the development of diabetic nephropathy

Flow chart 1: Unifying mechanism

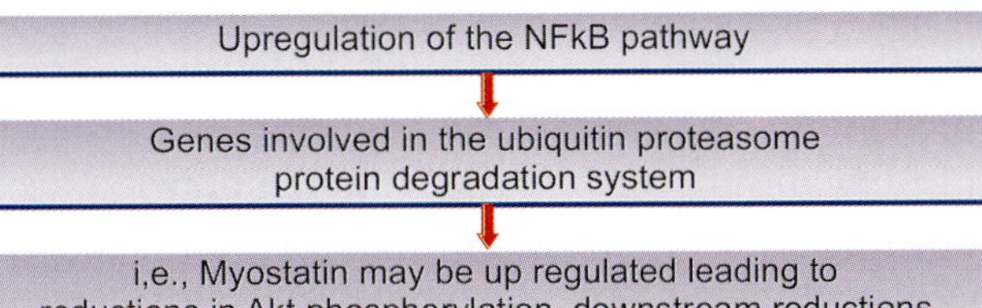

So there are multiple factors playing different role in development of diabetes-associated kidney disease, through various mechanisms affecting kidney function and causing damage, these considered separately and unifying mechanism will be discussed in Flow chart 1.

Acute Phase Response, Proinflammatory Cytokines and Metabolism

Diabetes like any chronic disease states leads to activation of typical systemic and local physiological immunologic stress response. This increase in immunologic response manifests as elevated proinflammatory cytokines, leading to heightened protein synthesis in hepatic and visceral tissues with a simultaneous depression of anabolic activities within skeletal muscle. This increased synthesis produces more acute phase proteins and reactants (APRs), causing alteration in the carbohydrate and lipid metabolism [increased glycogenolysis and lipolysis, formation of advanced glycation end products (AGEs)].

This alteration in metabolism is mainly caused by increase in glucagon, glucocorticoids, catecholamines and growth hormone (GH) release with simultaneous depression GH-insulin-like growth factor (IGF) pathway, especially within skeletal muscle, ultimately depressing the anabolic state.[13]

Various studies have shown that these cytokines IL-1β, IL-6, TNF-α and IFN-γ and others such as serum albumin (S-Alb), C-reactive protein (CRP) and fibrinogen may be helpful in the clinical assessment of patients and are potentially related with CVD risk, clinical outcome and mortality rates.[14]

Insulin/IGF-1 Resistance and Upregulation of Glucocorticoids—Cachexia

Cytokines IL-1β, IL-6, TNF-α and IFN-γ have proinflammatory actions and modulating effects on appetite induces anorexia. This ultimately increases the production of reactive oxygen species (ROS) and is regulated in a positive feedback loop via the NF-κB pathway.

Due to excessive increase in these cytokines causes characteristic reduction in food intake (anorexia) and increase in resting energy expenditure (REE), along with protein breakdown and a progressive loss of LBM and skeletal muscle, which is termed as "anorexia-cachexia" syndrome (ACS), driven by proinflammatory cytokines and their effects are both peripheral and central, they primarily act on peripheral skeletal muscle pathways affecting the protein turnover and centrally in hypothalamic neurons regulating appetite.[9]

The levels/activities of leptin (an anorexigenic peptide reducing food intake) and ghrelin (orexigenic peptide increasing food intake) may be disturbed causing persistent activation of the anorexigenic pro-opiomelanocortin/cocaine- and amphetamine-regulated transcript (POMC/CART) neuronal systems, and reduced activation of neuropeptide Y/agouti-related peptide (NPY/AgRP) with subsequent effects of reducing appetite.[10]

GH-IGF-1 Axis

The GH-IGF-1 axis controls the cell and tissue growth and development in human, stimulating protein synthesis in a range of tissues. GH is stimulated by the exercises and sleep, forms IGF-1 in liver, causing protein turnover and anabolic state, possesses glucose-disposal, antiapoptotic and antiproteolytic activities in muscle, and shares some cell signaling pathways with insulin.[11]

They have major effect on kidney growth and function, which is reduced in CKD causing attenuation of GH receptor-Janus kinase-2-signal transducers and activators of transcription (JAK2-STAT) signal transduction pathways. Hence accelerating the cachectic phenomena, this decreased function, increases corticosteroid production, uremia and insulin resistance. Recombinant human GH (rhGH) and recombinant human IGF-1 (rhIGF-1) in CKD patients have potential to improve muscle protein turnover and nitrogen retention.[15]

Renin-Angiotensin-Aldosterone System and Angiotensin II

The activation of RAAS system leads to increased production of renin, which ultimately results in increased production of angiotensin II (ANG II). ANG II is the main effector peptide of the RAAS, with potent hypertensive actions and has been implicated in vascular remodeling and pathogenesis in cardiac and renal tissues mediated by ANG II receptor, contributes to the development and progression of insulin resistant conditions such as obesity, MetS and cachexia.

Angiotensin II and aldosterone contribute to atherogenesis through increasing oxidative stress (ROS) and the expression of proinflammatory genes via the NF-κB pathway.[16]

Inhibition of ANG II through the use of pharmacological ATII-1R blockers (ARBs) or angiotensin-converting enzyme inhibitors (ACEIs) is used even in CKD patients, delaying the progression to stage 5 kidney diseases, hence having a "renoprotective" type action.

Adipocytokines

Adipose tissue is highly active endocrine organ regulates appetite, body equilibrium. Altered function might produce lipodystrophy, ectopic lipid accumulation in hepatic and skeletal muscle tissues, lipotoxicity and insulin resistance.

Adipocytokines with autocrine, paracrine and endocrine activities include leptin, adiponectin, resistin. Many studies link these dysfunctional adipose tissue (e.g. as in obesity) and/or raised proinflammatory adipocytokine patterns and systemic inflammation, with insulin resistance and cellular dysfunction.[13]

Leptin

Leptin levels rise in response to increased energy deposition as fat mass and in obesity, to decrease energy intake and increase energy expenditure, causing the rise in sympathetic activity and peripheral activating AMP-activated protein kinase (AMPK).

In obesity, there is severe resistance to leptin due to reduced renal clearance of leptin, since leptin has control over immune regulatory mechanism. During CKD disease progression, research shows that hyperleptinemia is observed in humans, and that this is associated with concomitant inflammation and loss of LBM.[15]

Adiponectin

Adiponectin is reported to modulate lipid and glucose metabolism and insulin sensitivity, exhibits antidiabetic, anti-inflammatory and antiatherogenic effects. The decreased function results in insulin resistance. Thiazolidinediones (TZDs) act as insulin sensitizers and act through the activation of the peroxisome proliferator-activated receptor-γ (PPAR-γ) and through the upregulation of mediators such as adiponectin.

Ghrelin

Ghrelin is an endogenous ligand for the growth hormone secretagogue receptor (GHSR), stimulating GH release, and it is a 28-amino acid peptide synthesized and secreted principally in the stomach.

Ghrelin stimulates appetite through activation of NPY neurons in the hypothalamus. Elevated ghrelin levels in advanced kidney failure which also correlated well with levels of fat mass, plasma insulin and serum leptin levels can be of great potential benefits as a pharmacological treatment in improving appetite, body composition (anticachectic therapy) and potentially decreasing inflammation.[10]

Vitamin D

Chronic kidney disease is associated with a host of disorders of mineral and bone metabolism termed CKD-metabolic bone disease (MBD), characterized by hyperphosphatemia, hypocalcemia, secondary hyperparathyroidism and decreased synthesis of active vitamin (vit) D [1,25(OH)D/1, 25-vit D] and helps in the maintenance of skeletal muscle function, proliferation and differentiation and immune function.[17] Hence treating this becomes important in managing the CKD patients.[18]

Glucocorticoids

Glucocorticoid activities are increased during obesity states and may be due to increased hypothalamic-pituitary-adrenal activity (and sympathoadrenal stress) and adipose tissue-derived cortisol which have important role in the pathogenesis in CKD.[19] And also it plays an important role in the development of hypertension, insulin resistance, glucose intolerance and dyslipidemia.

APPROACH TO MANAGE DIABETES IN CKD

Diabetes-associated kidney disease has a preclinical phase of diabetic nephropathy consisting of a normoalbuminuric and a microalbuminuric stage and a clinical phase characterized by albuminuria which are well documented in both type 1 and type 2 diabetic patients.

Natural progression of diabetic nephropathy has been shown in Table 2.

Table 2: Natural progression of diabetic nephropathy[31]

	Designation	*Characteristics*	*GFR (min)*	*Albumin excretion*	*Blood pressure*	*Chronology*
Stage 1	Hyperfunction, hypertrophy	Glomerular hyperfiltration	Increased	May be increased	Type 1: Normal Type 2: Normal/ hypertension	Present at diagnosis
Stage 2	Silent stage	Thickened basement membrane, expanded mesangium	Normal	Type 1: normal Type 2: <30:300 mg/day	Type 1: Normal Type 2: Normal/ hypertension	First 5 years
Stage 3	Incipient stage	Micro-albuminuria	Begins to decrease	30-300 mg/day	Type 1: Elevated Type 2: Normal/ hypertension	6–15 years
Stage 4	Overt diabetic nephropathy	Macro-albuminuria	Below normal	>380 mg/day	Hypertension	15–25 years
Stage 5	Uremic	End-stage renal disease	0–10	Decreasing	Hypertension	25–30 years

Screening is done using "untimed urine checks" for the presence of proteinuria, by measuring the total protein creatinine (> 300 mg/g) and/or albumin-creatinine ratio (ACR) (> 30 mg/g as designated cutoff point).[8]

Kidney function can be measured either using directly measured GFR (mGFR); measuring the clearance of specific exogenous compounds, such as inulin or most frequently through the estimation of GFR (eGFR) via serum creatinine levels. Many formulas including the Cockroft-Gault and "modification of diet in renal disease (MDRD)" study equations which use factors such as age, sex, body size and race can be used to calculate eGFR, a potentially more precise formula has been presented as the CKD Epidemiology Collaboration (CKD-EPI) study equation.[20]

DIAGNOSIS OF CHRONIC KIDNEY DISEASE

Chronic kidney disease (CKD) believed to result from diabetes has been termed "diabetic nephropathy". The diagnosis of CKD presumed to be caused by diabetes should be referred to as "diabetic kidney disease (DKD)" and the term "diabetic nephropathy" should be reserved for kidney disease attributed to diabetes with histopathological injury demonstrated by renal biopsy. Renal biopsy is only recommended in special situations.[3]

The clinical diagnosis of DKD is primarily identified by detection of proteinuria

- Microalbuminuria is defined as an ACR of 30–300 mg/g from a spot urine collection, 30–300 mg/24 hours in a 24-hour urine collection, or 20–200 μg/min in a timed urine collection[3]
- Macroalbuminuria is defined as greater than 300 mg/g, greater than 300 mg/24 hours, and greater than 200 μg/min in the same tests, respectively.

The ACR by spot urine sample has demonstrated excellent correlation with the 24-hour urine protein measurements.[21] If protein is detected, then conditions such as infection, congestive heart failure, pregnancy, severe hypertension, or hematuria must be excluded. Due to wide intraindividual variation of urinary albumin measurement, three tests should be performed and found to be positive over a 3- to 6-month period before making a definitive diagnosis of persistent proteinuria.

If retinopathy is present in patients with type 2 diabetes and microalbuminuria, this is strongly suggestive of DKD, with a sensitivity of 100% and specificities of 46–62%, but microalbuminuria in patients with type 1 diabetes appears to be associated with less severe pathological lesions. Hence, macroalbuminuria or microalbuminuria in combination with diabetic retinopathy, DKD is suspected.[3,19]

Measurement of Glycemic Control

Hemoglobin A1c (HbA1c) levels are frequently monitored to determine glycemic control for patients with diabetes. There is concern that the measurement of A1c may be affected by the severity of kidney dysfunction or the hematological complications of kidney disease, such as iron deficiency, hemolysis, shorter red blood cell life span, or acidosis.

In patients with CKD who are not on dialysis, there was no difference in the magnitude of the correlations between A1c and blood glucose compared to diabetes patient without nephropathy. Therefore, a target goal of less than 7.0% may be applied to this patient group, but the correlation between A1c and blood glucose in hemodialysis patients was unclear. But overall it has been seen in various study that lower A1c levels reduce mortality.[22]

Similarly, serum fructosamine measures failed to show a significant correlation with blood glucose measures in patients receiving dialysis or in those with severe CKD. Fructosamine does not appear to most accurately reflect glycemic control in patients with CKD. So ultimately, the "gold standard" remains serum blood glucose, so one can use continuous glucose monitoring, to guide the therapy.[22] Management of diabetes includes many areas that may be influenced by the severity of a patient's kidney dysfunction.

GOALS OF TREATMENT

- Needs strict glucose control and optimization of HbA1c levels.
- Management of comorbid conditions such as hypertension and hyperlipidemia.
- Evaluation for the development of conditions associated with CKD such as anemia, hyperphosphatemia and hyperparathyroidism.

When the goal is to achieve a lower A1c and tighter glycemic control, the risk of hypoglycemic episodes increases. In the Diabetes Control and Complications Trial (DCCT) and ADVANCE trial showed that who received intensive diabetes therapy had greater mortality and morbidity. It was shown that greater than three times the risk of having a severe hypoglycemic episode than those receiving conventional therapy.[23] A1c levels (7%) are associated with decreased risk for clinical and structural manifestations of diabetic nephropathy in type 1 and type 2 diabetic patients, DCCT trial and the United Kingdom Prospective Diabetes Study (UKPDS) demonstrated that glycemic control had a long-lasting reduction of 40% in the risk for development of microalbuminuria and hypertension 7–8 years after the end of the DCCT. In the UKPDS, a 30% risk reduction for the development of microalbuminuria was observed in the group intensively treated for. Hence approach should be to have good glycemic control, but also to have less episodes of hypoglycemia.

PHARMACOLOGICAL TREATMENT OF HYPERGLYCEMIA

Insulin

Insulin is normally metabolized in kidney, so when kidney function is reduced causes increased insulin levels, thus increasing chances of hypoglycemia, as much as five times that of patients without kidney disease. There are no evidence-based guidelines or recommendations about which types of insulin to use or avoid depending on severity of CKD. Some studies suggest avoiding long-acting insulin, whereas others support its use. The clearance is reduced for both regular insulin and insulin lispro.[24] Hence it is advised to reduce the total dose. But in some patients, there is also increased incidence of insulin resistance, hence requiring more insulin dose in some patients. Frequent blood glucose monitoring may be used to adjust dosing and prevent hypoglycemia.

Oral Agents

Similar to insulin metabolism of oral hypoglycemic agent (OHA) also depends on the kidney, hence more chances of hypoglycemia. The greatest risk for this to occur is with patients with moderate to severe CKD (stages 3–5). Kidney disease warrants a re-evaluation of drug therapies chosen for treatment of diabetes and possible adjustments to their dosing to achieve glycemic control while minimizing adverse effects.

Sulfonylurea

The clearance of both sulfonylureas and its metabolites is highly dependent on kidney function, and severe prolonged episodes of hypoglycemia ensue as a result of sulfonylurea use has been described in dialysis patients. In patients with stages 3–5 CKD, first-generation sulfonylureas should be avoided. Of the second-generation sulfonylureas, glipizide is recommended because its metabolites are not active, with much lower potential for development of hypoglycemia.[25]

- **Alpha-glucosidase inhibitors**: *Alpha*-glucosidase inhibitors and its metabolites may cause cumulative dose effects and result in possible hepatic damage. Therefore, this class of medications is not recommended for patients with a serum creatinine greater than 2 mg/dL.
- **Metformin**: Metformin does not exhibit the high risk of hypoglycemia associated with other drug classes used to treat diabetes. However, special care must be taken when it is used in patients with CKD. Metformin is contraindicated in male patients with a serum creatinine

greater than 1.5 mg/dL and in female patients with serum creatinine greater than 1.4 mg/dL/ or CrCl less than 30.

- **Thiazolidinediones**: Thiazolidinediones may have a protective effect to either prevent or slow the progression of DKD independent from glycemic control. Several small studies have reported a greater reduction in albuminuria in patients administered TZDs. It has been demonstrated to be effective without increasing the risk of hypoglycemic episodes in patients with CKD, including those receiving dialysis, and in patients who require therapy for glycemic control after kidney transplant. But should be carefully used in patients with heart failure. *No adjustment in dosing of TZDs is required for these patient groups.* The known TZD side effect of fluid retention may be accentuated in patients with CKD.[26]
- **Gliptins/dipeptidase 4 inhibitor**: It is widely used as an add-on therapy to ongoing management or as monotherapy where it is deemed necessary. It has been found to be beneficial in improving β-cell function and glycemic control, and also is used in special circumstances like CKD, with appropriate dose reductions. Gliptins, in general, predominately have renal excretion profile. The exception is linagliptin which primarily excreted via bile and gut.[27]
- **Sitagliptin**:
  - Mild renal impairment (CrCl ≥ 50 mL/min), no dose adjustment is required
  - Moderate renal impairment (CrCl ≥ 30 and CrCl < 50 mL/min), the dose of sitagliptin is 50 mg once daily
  - Severe renal impairment (CrCl < 30 mL/min) or with ESRD requiring hemodialysis or peritoneal dialysis, the dose of sitagliptin is 25 mg once daily.
- **Saxagliptin**:
  - No dose adjustment is recommended for patients with mild renal impairment, the dose of saxagliptin should be reduced to 2.5 mg once daily in patients with moderate or severe renal impairment, but it is not recommended for patients with ESRD requiring hemodialysis.
- **Vildagliptin**:
  - No dose adjustment is required in patients with mild renal impairment (CrCl > 50 mL/min), with moderate or severe renal impairment or with ESRD, the recommended dose of vildagliptin is 50 mg once daily.
- **Linagliptin**:
  - No dose adjustment is required in patients with renal disease.

However, exenatide is eliminated by renal mechanisms and should not be given in patients with severe CKD. Liraglutide is not eliminated by the kidney, but it should be used with caution because of the limited experience in patients with CKD. Only limited pharmacokinetic data are also available for lixisenatide, exenatide long-acting release (LAR) and other once-weekly GLP-1 receptor agonists are in current development. Several case reports of acute renal failure have been described with GLP-1 receptor agonists, probably triggered by dehydration resulting from gastrointestinal adverse events.

Recommendations for OHA usage in diabetic CKD have been shown in Table 3.

Table 3: Recommendations for oral hypoglycemic agent (OHA) usage in diabetic CKD

Class	Drug	CKD (Stage 3–5)	Dialysis	Complication
First-generation sulfonylurea	Acetohexamide	Avoid	Avoid	Hypoglycemia
	Chlorpropamide	GFR 50-70 mL/min/1.73 m^2; ↓ 50% GFR <50 mL/min/1.73 m^2; avoid	Avoid	Hypoglycemia
	Tolazamide	Avoid	Avoid	Hypoglycemia
	Tolbutamide	Avoid	Avoid	Hypoglycemia
Second-generation sulfonylurea	Glipizide	No dose adjustment	No dose adjustment	
	Glyburide	Avoid	Avoid	Hypoglycemia
	Glimepiride	Low dose: 1 mg/day	Avoid	Hypoglycemia
α-Glucosidase inhibitors	Acarbose	SCr >2 mg/dL;Avoid	Avoid	Possible hepatic toxicity
	Miglitol	SCr >2 mg/dL;Avoid	Avoid	
Biguanide	Metformin	Contraindicated: Male: SCr >1.5 mg/dL; Female: SCr >1.4 mg/dL;	Avoid	Lactic acidosis
TZDs	Pioglitazone	No dose adjustment	No dose adjustment	Volume retention
	Rosiglitazone	No dose adjustment	No dose adjustment	Volume retention
Meglitinides	Repaglinide	No dose adjustment	No dose adjustment	
	Nateglinide	Initiate low dose: 60 mg	Avoid	Hypoglycemia
Incretin mimetic	Exenatide	No dose adjustment	No dose adjustment	
Amylin analog	Pramlintide	No dose adjustment GFR <20 mL/min/1.73 m^2: unknown	Unknown	
Dipeptidyl-peptidase IV inhibitor	Sitagliptin	GFR 30-50 mL/min/1.73 m^2; ↓ 25% GFR <30 mL/min/1.73 m^2; ↓ 50%	↓ 50%	Hypoglycemia

Source: National kidney function: KDOQ1 clinical practice guidelines and clinical practice recommentation for Diabetes and CKD. Am J Kidney Dis. 49:51-5180,2007

OTHER ASPECTS OF TREATING DIABETIC KIDNEY DISEASE

Nutritional Considerations in Diabetes and CKD

As GFR decreases, dietary protein nitrogen intake must be reduced. Although debated, a very low-protein diet is a standard dietary therapy for patients to delay kidney pathogenesis. Reduction of dietary protein intake to 0.8 g/kg body weight for CKD stages 1–4 is recommended to try to reduce albuminuria and reduce the rate of loss of kidney function. Thus, for patients with CKD, high-protein diets are not recommended. The food causing hyperkalemia and hyperphosphatemia should be avoided.

HYPERTENSION

Due to increased activation sympathetic system and RAAS system, there is increased incidence of hypertension in CKD especially in type 2 diabetes. Prevalence of hypertension is estimated to range from 30% to 96%, with higher prevalence found to be associated with greater levels of proteinuria. If hypertension is present in DKD, there is rapid progression of microalbuminuria to macroalbuminuria. ACEIs and angiotensin receptor blockers (ARBs) are used in early microalbuminuria patients as it slows the progression.[28] Critical renal-artery stenosis (> 70%) occurs in 17% of hypertensive type 2 diabetic patients and may be associated with hypertension and renal insufficiency (ischemic nephropathy). The use of ACEIs or ANG II type 1 receptor blockers (ARBs) could reduce transcapillary filtration pressure, worsen acute or chronic renal insufficiency, especially if renal artery stenosis affects both kidneys or the sole functioning kidney. A rise in serum creatinine 50% after use of these agents is a clue for the presence of renal-artery stenosis.

However, no randomized clinical trials have shown impact on development of more advanced CKD or mortality in diabetic nephropathy population. In Irbesartan Diabetes Nephropathy Trial and the Reduction of End Points in Non-Insulin-Dependent Diabetes with the ANG II Antagonist Losartan trial. The use of an ARB compared to placebo resulted in a 16–20% risk reduction in the primary composite end point of worsening serum creatinine, development of ESRD, or death from any cause. MICRO-Heart Outcomes Prevention Evaluation (HOPE) study showed that ramipril (10/day) decreased the risk of overt nephropathy by 24% and the risk of cardiovascular death in patients with type 2 diabetes who were greater than 55 years of age with one additional cardiovascular risk factor by 37%. Moreover, ramipril reduced UAE at 1 year and at the end of the study. A few small studies have reported that use of spironolactone, an aldosterone receptor antagonist, may be associated with a reduction of proteinuria and slower progression of kidney disease. But potassium levels should be closely monitored.

HYPERLIPIDEMIA

Dyslipidemia eventually causes worsening of the kidney function. Hence it forms important part of risk factor management. So lipid levels should be measured annually with a target low-density lipoprotein (LDL) cholesterol level less than 100 mg/dL for patients with CKD stages 1–4. The 4D trial was a multicenter, double-blind, placebo-controlled prospective study evaluating 1,255 patients with diabetes who were receiving hemodialysis. This study did not find a significant difference in cardiovascular outcomes between statin therapy and placebo; however, Heart Protection Study, 40 mg simvastatin reduced the rate of major vascular events and GFR decline in patients with diabetes, independent of cholesterol levels at baseline, by 25%. The current recommendation says that no need to start statins early. But patient who are receiving should continue, only started once dyslipidemia ensues, usually no dose adjustments required for atorvastatin, niacin, ezetimibe, but should be considered in using rosuvastatin, simvastatin, fluvastatin.[29]

Other treatment strategy includes evaluation of anemia, correction of anemia to levels of 11–12 g/dL in dialysis patients has been associated with improved quality of life, fewer hospitalizations, and a lower risk of mortality. EPO supplementation and iron supplementation should be given.[30]

Hyperphosphatemia and Secondary Hyperthyroidism

The target serum phosphorus goal is less than 5.5 mg/dL in patients with stage 5 CKD and less than 4.6 mg/dL in stages 3–4 CKD should be promptly treated using calcium salts or sevelamer. In addition, if the intact parathyroid hormone (iPTH) is abnormal, an evaluation for vitamin D deficiency should be sought, with measurement of 25-hydroxyvitamin D and subsequent supplementation.

Newer strategies such as high doses of thiamine and its derivative benfotiamine have been shown to retard the development of microalbuminuria in experimental diabetic nephropathy, probably by decrease of protein kinase C, protein glycation, and oxidative stress. Protein kinase C inhibitor (ruboxistaurin) and sulodexide, a glycosaminoglycan, significantly reduced albuminuria in microalbuminuria or macroalbuminuria. Pimagedine, a second-generation inhibitor of AGEs, reduced urinary protein excretion, are being studied.

REFERENCES

1. Levey AS, Coresh J, Balk E, et al. National Kidney Foundation practice guidelines for chronic kidney disease: evaluation, classification and stratification. Ann Intern Med. 2003;139:137-47.
2. Slee AD. Exploring metabolic dysfunction in chronic kidney disease. Nutr Metab (Lond). 2012;9:36.
3. Zoccali C, Kramer A, Jager KJ. Epidemiology of CKD in Europe: an uncertain scenario. Nephrol Dial Transplant. 2010;25:1731-3.
4. Locatelli F, Pozzoni P, Tentori F, et al. Epidemiology of cardiovascular risk in patients with chronic kidney disease. Nephrol Dial Transplant. 2003;18 Suppl 7:vii2-9.
5. Pelletier S, Chapurlat R. Optimizing bone health in chronic kidney disease. Maturitas. 2010;65: 325-33.
6. Siew ED, Ikizler TA. Insulin resistance and protein energy metabolism in patients with advanced chronic kidney disease. Semin Dial. 2010;23(4):378-82.
7. Coresh J, Astor BC, Greene T, et al. Prevalence of chronic kidney disease and decreased kidney function in the adult US population: Third National Health and Nutrition Examination Survey. Am J Kidney Dis. 2003;41:1-12.
8. Middleton RJ, Foley RN, Hegarty J, et al. The unrecognized prevalence of chronic kidney disease in diabetes. Nephrol Dial Transplant. 2006;21:88-92.
9. Fioretto P, Mauer M. Histopathology of diabetic nephropathy. Semin Nephrol. 2007;27(2):195-207.
10. Bader R, Bader H, Grund KE, et al. Structure and function of the kidney in diabetic glomerulosclerosis. Correlations between morphological and functional parameters. Pathol Res Pract. 1980;167:204-16.
11. Laviano A, Inui A, Marks DL, et al. Neural control of the anorexia-cachexia syndrome. Am J Physiol Endocrinol Metab. 2008;295:E1000-8.
12. Mak RH, Cheung W. Adipokines and gut hormones in end-stage renal disease. Perit Dial Int. 2007;27 Suppl 2:S298-302.
13. Gruys E, Toussaint MJ, Niewold TA, et al. Acute phase reaction and acute phase proteins. J Zheijang Univ Sci B. 2005;6(11):1045-56.
14. Lastra G, Dhuper S, Johnson MS, et al. Salt, aldosterone, and insulin resistance: impact on the cardiovascular system. Nat Rev Cardiol. 2010;7:577-84.

15. Mak RH, Cheung WW, Roberts CT. The growth hormone-insulin-like growth factor-I axis in chronic kidney disease. Growth Horm IGF Res. 2008;18:17-25.
16. Kadowaki T, Yamauchi T, Kubota N, et al. Adiponectin and adiponectin receptors in insulin resistance, diabetes, and the metabolic syndrome. J Clin Invest. 2006;116(7):1784-92.
17. Pelletier S, Chapurlat R. Optimizing bone health in chronic kidney disease. Maturitas. 2010;65: 325-33.
18. Koenig W. Predicting risk and treatment benefit in atherosclerosis: the role of C-reactive protein. Int J Cardiol. 2005;98:199-206.
19. Wang M. The role of glucocorticoid action in the pathophysiology of the metabolic syndrome. Nutr Metab (Lond). 2005;2(1):3.
20. Thomas C, Thomas L. Renal failure—measuring the glomerular filtration rate. Dtsch Arztebl Int. 2009;106(51-52):849-54.
21. Gansevoort RT, Verhave JC, Hillege HL, et al. The validity of screening based on spot morning urine samples to detect subjects with microalbuminuria in the general population. Kidney Int Suppl. 2005;(94):S28-35.
22. Morgan L, Marenah CB, Jeffcoate WJ, et al. Glycated proteins as indices of glycaemic control in diabetic patients with chronic renal failure. Diabet Med. 1999;13:514-9.
23. United Kingdom Prospective Diabetes Study (UKPDS). 13: Relative efficacy of randomly allocated diet, sulphonylurea, insulin, or metformin in patients with newly diagnosed non-insulin dependent diabetes followed for three years. BMJ. 1995;310:83-8.
24. Snyder RW, Berns JS. Use of insulin and oral hypoglycemic medications in patients with diabetes mellitus and advanced kidney disease. Semin Dial. 2004;17:365-70.
25. Krepinsky J, Ingram AJ, Clase CM. Prolonged sulfonylurea-induced hypoglycemia in diabetic patients with end-stage renal disease. Am J Kidney Dis. 2000;35:500-5.
26. Sarafidis PA, Bakris GL. Protection of the kidney by thiazolidinediones: an assessment from bench to bedside. Kidney Int. 2006;70:1223-33.
27. Cavanaugh KL. Diabetes management issues for patients with chronic kidney disease. Clinical Diabetes. 2007;25(3):90-7.
28. Sarafidis PA, Khosla N, Bakris GL. Antihypertensive therapy in the presence of proteinuria. Am J Kidney Dis. 2007;49:12-26.
29. Wanner C, Krane V, Marz W, et al. Atorvastatin in patients with type 2 diabetes mellitus undergoing hemodialysis. N Engl J Med. 2005;353:238-48.
30. KDOQI; National Kidney Foundation. II. Clinical practice guidelines and clinical practice recommendations for anemia in chronic kidney disease in adults. Am J Kidney Dis. 2006;47:S16-85.
31. http//misc.medscape.com/pi/iphone/medscapp/html/A238946-burenes.html.

21

CHAPTER

Metabolic Syndrome: Pathophysiological Lessons for the Diabetes Practitioner

DK Hazra, Padmamalika Khanna-Hazra, Nandita Hazra

INTRODUCTION

The metabolic syndrome was a portmanteau word coined by G Reaven to refer to diabetes and allied disorders notably coronary artery disease, cerebrovascular disease/strokes, hypertension and obesity. Other diseases were soon included such as hyperlipidemia, hyperuricemia/gout, cholecystitis and polycystic ovarian syndrome. Also, diabetes mellitus was realized to be one end of a spectrum of dysglycemic disorders including impaired glucose tolerance and impaired fasting glucose. The common denominator of these diseases was insulin resistance. Thus, the metabolic syndrome was a hydra-headed disorder: we therefore preferred to coin a new term referring to Reaven's syndrome as *the Ravana syndrome!*

Many studies were made on the pathophysiology of these diseases, especially diabetes mellitus and atherosclerosis underlying or accompanying coronary and cerebrovascular disease. Diabetes mellitus is associated with numerous complications which are classified as microangiopathic, macrovascular infective and metabolic. Some of these are aggravated or precipitated by glucotoxicity. Lipotoxicity is also being recognized, and the benefits of very low calorie diets on pancreatic function are partly due to correction of this.

Complications of diabetes usually thought of as microvascular include retinopathy, nephropathy, neuropathy. In addition, microvascular disease contributes to diabetic cardiomyopathy. Microangiopathy exacerbates ischemia of the extremities in the diabetic foot, and can contribute to pancreatic damage.

In prediabetics, it is speculated that these complications may predate clinical diabetes on the diagnostic horizon, and in the Agra Diabetes Preventive Intervention study focusing on bidiabetic couple progeny and multidiabetic families.[1,2] We have observed stigmata of complications even in euglycemic subjects, in the form of cardiac function/carotid intimal medial thickness abnormalities.

To quote from our earlier review:[3]

"Hyperglycemia and hypertension, and possibly lipid abnormalities set the soil for microangiopathy. These trigger multiple pathogenetic sequences, viz. advanced glycation end products (AGEs) formation, protein kinase C (PKC) activation, and increased flux through the polyol (sorbitol) and hexosamine pathways, all of which culminate in oxidative stress resulting in pathological vascular remodeling, altered vascular tone, changes in the basement membrane and permeability. The subsequent changes are peculiar to the target tissue. In nephropathy, the mesangium shows abnormal extracellular matrix accumulation. In the retina, ischemia due to acellular capillaries is coupled with neovascularization triggered by vascular endothelial growth factor (VEGF).

Many of these complications share common pathogenetic mechanisms, although the relative quantum of contribution by each pathogenetic mechanism may differ. The understanding of these mechanisms naturally influences our approach to therapy, and prevention of these complications. Vice versa, epidemiological and/or clinical demonstration of the beneficial effect of various preventive and therapeutic interventions, or the lack of such effect has inevitably colored our concept of pathophysiology".[3]

Rather than detail these pathogenic mechanisms, we propose here to focus on the management of the metabolic syndrome in all its Ravana manifestations.

IMMEDIATE AND LONG-TERM BENEFITS OF TIGHT CONTROL OF HYPERGLYCEMIA

In the 1960s and 1970s, the central question of diabetes management was whether tight diabetes control could ameliorate the devastating consequences of diabetes complications in the target organs such as the kidneys, the retina and the nerves, and there was a continuing debate between the nihilists who felt that complications were inexorable and inevitable, and the optimists who believed that tight control would be beneficial. As a young physician, one deliberately chose to follow the optimists, advocating the skilful use of not only lifestyle modification but also of pharmacological tools including the insulins, the highly purified monocomponent varieties, the human insulins and the designer semisynthetic analogs that were being developed.

The debate seemed to be settled in favor of the advocates of tight control in the 1990s with the publication of the Diabetes Control and Complications Trial (DCCT) and the United Kingdom Prospective Diabetes Study (UKPDS) in type 1 and type 2 diabetes respectively. Between 1983 and 1992, the effect of tight control of hyperglycemia on the prevention and limitation of these microangiopathic complications in type 1 diabetes was conclusively shown in the United States DCCT study. The UKPDS study showed beneficial effects in type 2 diabetes. Today long-term benefits of intensive control have been documented in the Epidemiology of Diabetes Interventions and Complications (EDIC) study of DCCT follow-up and similar follow-up of UKPDS subjects and these observations were summarized in the concept of metabolic memory or legacy effects.

The existence of these continuing benefits has been variously explained, including the long-term effects of AGEs persisting at a higher level in conventional as opposed to intensive therapy. In fact of the at least four distinct pathophysiologic mechanisms that have been incriminated in diabetic microangiopathy viz.: (1) AGEs, (2) activated PKC isoforms, (3) increased sorbitol exposure and (4) increased hexosamine flux, biochemically, the first is most likely responsible for metabolic memory effects and thus the existence of metabolic memory strengthens the case for AGEs as a dominant pathophysiologic mechanism.

All these four mechanisms originate in hyperglycemia. All of them also culminate in increased oxidative stress.[4,5] Increased oxidant generation in the mitochondria may induce damage to the mitochondrial DNA and proteins, which has also been incriminated as a mechanism of metabolic memory.[6] It is postulated that the electron transport chain subunits in the mitochondria get damaged, so that there is superoxide overproduction even in the presence of normal glucose levels.

OXIDATIVE STRESS IN DIABETES

Oxidative stress molecules include reactive species of oxygen, nitrogen and chlorine. Reactive oxygen species (ROS) include free radicals: hydroxyl, superoxide, peroxyl, hydroperoxyl and nonradicals hydrogen peroxide and hypochlorous acid. Reactive nitrogen species include free radicals nitric oxide and nitrogen dioxide and the nonradicals peroxynitrite and alkyl peroxynitrates.

Normally 0.2% of the oxygen used in the mitochondria generates free radicals, and this fraction increases with aging. In diabetics, these increase independent of aging, virtually denoting an accelerated aging process.

The antioxidant defense mechanisms of the body are superoxide dismutase (SOD), manganese based in the mitochondria and copper/zinc based in the cytosol; glutathione peroxidase (GP), catalase (CAT), superoxide reductase (SOR), peroxiredoxin (PRX), glutathione reductase (GR), and thioredoxin reductase (TRX/TRXR). Diabetics show reduced antioxidant defenses.[7] Oxidant stress is believed to have deleterious effects at various levels.

Molecularly, stress signaling pathways are activated, involving gene expression, transcriptional factors and apoptosis. There is damage to DNA, proteins and lipids. Lipid peroxidation adversely affects structure and fluidity of biological membranes. Protein and lipid oxidation degrade enzymes and impair their catalytic function.

Reactive oxygen species arise in the endothelium, and cause low-density lipoprotein (LDL) oxidation and altered smooth muscle function. Because of nitric oxide inactivation, there is impairment in endothelial-dependent vasorelaxation, increased expression of adhesion molecules and recruitment of inflammatory cells into the vessel wall. Smooth muscle phenotype changes from contractile to proliferative.[8,9] ROS also have harmful effects on the kidneys and the nerves.

They activate nuclear factor-kB (NF-kB)-dependent cyclooxygenase-2 expressions in mesangial cells with prostaglandin E2 synthesis. Glomerular hypoxia, inflammatory cell infiltration, impaired endothelium-dependent relaxation and increased basal vascular tone, and hypoxic tubules are implicated.[10] Increased oxidant load in type 1 diabetics with microalbuminuria is evidenced by fluorescent products of lipid peroxidation and malondialdehyde.[11] In the nerves, neurovascular defects associated with hypoxia are observed.[12]

PATHOGENESIS OF DIABETIC RETINOPATHY

As with other diabetic microvascular complications, chronic hyperglycemia is thought to be the primary cause. In the DCCT, intensive insulin therapy reduced the incidence of diabetic retinopathy (DR) by 76%. In the UKPDS, each 1% reduction in HbA_{1c} achieved resulted in 37% reduction of DR. The sheet anchor of primary and secondary prevention of DR is tight control of hyperglycemia and hypertension.

Retinal injury is induced in hyperglycemia by impaired autoregulation of retinal blood flow, sorbitol/AGEs accumulation and PKC activation.

Ordinarily retinal blood flow remains constant until there is at least a 40% rise in arterial blood pressure (BP). But during hyperglycemia, autoregulation fails and increased retinal blood flow leads to shear stresses, stimulating possibly vasoactive substances, vascular leakage, fluid accumulation in the outer retinal layers and macular edema.[13] Sorbitol causes raised intracellular osmolality in the lens cells which swell up and may rupture. Both the high osmolality and the consequent decreased intracellular myo-inositol can impair cell metabolism.[14]

Protein kinase C family comprises eleven isoforms. Hyperglycemia leads to increased glyceraldehydes flux and enhanced synthesis of diacylglycerol (DAG). PKC inhibitors reduce diabetes induced increases in retinal circulation time, apart from reducing PKC effects in the glomeruli.[15,16]

Genetic studies on the aldose reductase gene also support a role of sorbitol in DR.[17] Proliferative changes are related to insulin-like growth factor-1 (IGF-1) and VEGF.[18] Erythropoietin, fibroblast growth factor and hepatocyte growth factor have also been implicated. Pituitary ablation has been used in treating diabetic proliferative retinopathy.[19]

ROLE OF THE RENIN-ANGIOTENSIN-ALDOSTERONE SYSTEM IN DR

Since renin-angiotensin-aldosterone system (RAAS) blockade was demonstrated to be useful in diabetic microangiopathy and in ameliorating harmful left ventricular remodeling, we at Agra, India had been fascinated by the possibilities of using this in DR. In a collaborative study with Prof. SK Satsangi of the Eye Department, SN Medical College, Agra, benefits were observed with the angiotensin-converting enzyme (ACE) inhibitor ramipril in both hypertensive and nonhypertensive diabetics.[20] This was followed by a similar study with the angiotensin receptor blocker losartan.

Impressed by these clinical results, we looked for earlier work to justify our use of ramipril in nonhypertensive diabetics. We discovered that Larsen et al. had reported protective effects of captopril on the blood retinal barrier in normotensive type 1 diabetics.[21] Chase et al. (1993) had reported on a 2-year trial of ACE inhibitor treatment for young normotensive diabetics.[22]

Subsequent to our Agra study, the effects of other agents blocking the RAAS—lisinopril, enalapril, losartan and candesartan have been reported.[23-27] These have been recently reviewed by Sjølie, Dodson and Hobbs in 2011.[28] In the EURODIAB study-EUCLID Controlled trial of lisinopril in insulin-dependent diabetes, Lisinopril use was coupled with a significant reduction in retinopathy progression in normotensive type 1 patients but the reduction in new cases was insignificant. The following DIRECT Diabetic Retinopathy Candesartan trials evaluated 32 mg candesartan versus placebo on new retinopathy and progression of retinopathy involving 1,421 normotensive type 1 patients with no retinopathy (18% reduction in incidence), 1,905 patients with type 1 normotensive with mild to moderate nonproliferative changes (no significant change in DR progress) and 1,905 patients with type 2 cases who had mild to moderate proliferative DR (13% nonsignificant reduction in DR progress, and 34% significant regression in mild retinopathy, even after adjusting for normotension).

In the RASS study, reported in 2009 in the New England Journal of Medicine, 20 mg enalapril, 100 mg losartan angiotensin blocker and placebo were compared. At 5 years, 38% placebo patients had DR progression compared with 25% in the enalapril groups ($p = 0.02$) and 21% patients on losartan ($p = 0.008$) at 5 years.[26]

Laser ablation is a proven treatment to induce regression of retinal neoangiogenesis, but is not 100% effective. It induces some visual field loss, and is less effective for cases in which visual symptoms have already caused severe irreversible retinal damage.

Drug therapy with RAAS blockade offers a valuable medical option in addition to tight glycemic and BP control, especially if one can identify the patients at high risk for DR.

Blood Pressure Control

Data from the ACCORD and ADVANCE study have been analyzed to assess the effects of tight blood glucose control (greater HbA_{1c} reduction than in the UKPDS) and BP control. Intensive glycemia control reduced retinopathy in both the studies but this was significant only in ACCORD.[29,30] In the ACCORD study, intensive BP control (target < 120 mm Hg) was not superior to standard control (< 140 mm) suggesting that beyond a threshold BP lowering does not yield significant benefits in preventing DR.

Lipid Lowering

The ACCORD Eye study reported reduced retinopathy progression when fenofibrate was added to simvastatin therapy (28, loc cit). The Fenofibrate Intervention and Event Lowering in Diabetes (FIELD) study showed that fenofibrate addition reduced the need for laser therapy in DR, but interestingly the benefit was not related to lipid levels suggesting an unknown fenofibrate effect.[30,31]

PRACTICAL MANAGEMENT IMPLICATIONS

1. The late Prof. KN Saxena my teacher in Skin and VD used to remark: "*When you find Gold, be sure to look for Silver!*", alluding to the frequent coexistence of syphilis and gonorrhea. Similarly, my dictum is "*When treating subjects suffering from one form of the metabolic syndrome, look for the other forms*" as well-whether in history, clinical features or pathognomonic laboratory tests.
2. When treating one patient, take a careful family history and institute appropriate diagnostic or preventive measures both in the patient as well as other family members. *You must treat not only the patient, but also the family!*

   This includes controlling or eliminating the use of saturated fats, transfats, sugars, sweets, processed foods, sodas and excessive salt or inappropriately high calories. Making the family aware of what really is a healthy diet also helps reducing in pressure by wives/ mothers/grandmothers that retard the primary patients' efforts at diet reform!

   A healthy lifestyle comprises not only these dietary measures but also promoting calorie expenditure: walking, games and nonexercise calorie expenditure. Activity must be incorporated into the daily routine—walking to colleagues rather than texting across the room!

Yoga, meditation, prayer, relaxation, holidays, humor yield multiple benefits, including destressing which reduces harmful surges in corticosteroids and catecholamines (the spiritual benefits of yoga, meditation and prayer are real but can hardly be discussed here). Such hormonal surges not only cause hypertension and cardiac arrhythmias but also damage hippocampal neurons and accelerate neurocognitive age-related impairment. Similarly avoiding procrastination in meeting deadlines and taking steps toward settling potential litigation issues, or family issues such as the partition of joint family property or businesses can help destressing!

This is important because diabetes, hypertension and the metabolic syndrome are associated with these, and perhaps with Alzheimer's dementia.

3. *Make sure that the patient is not only euglycemic but also normal in weight, blood lipids, BP and uric acid. This we call the "Agra/Boston Medical Center" extended version of the Steno intervention approach.* This may include assessment of thyroid and adrenocortical function. Thyroid-stimulating hormone (TSH) and evening cortisol measurement are simple methods of doing this.

   For treating hypertension, the first choice is ACE inhibitors, followed by angiotensin receptor blockers, and if both are not tolerated, then calcium channel blockers with chlorthalidone type diuretics, with, if indicated, aldosterone/eplerenone.

4. For monitoring euglycemia *estimation of fructosamine or glycated albumin is often more relevant than glycated hemoglobin* for the latter is not only vitiated by hemoglobinopathies and anemias but also does not tell us of recent poor control which is more important for fine tuning management. At the American Diabetes Association (ADA) meeting in Boston (2015), evidence was presented indicating the superior prognostic value of fructosamine/glycated albumin as compared to glycated hemoglobin.

   Control has to be monitored not only in terms of glucose but in terms of outcomes.

   It is no longer universally accepted that obtaining blood sugar and BP reduction suffices irrespective of the agent that achieved these. Measuring the blood sugar or BP during diabetes management is not enough. Further, it is important to look at microangiopathic markers such as microalbuminuria, estimated glomerular filtration rate (e-GFR) and retinal changes, and structural markers such as carotid intimal medial thickness and cardiac function markers for assessing macrovascular disease.

   How we achieve blood sugar control with minimal glycemic variability and hypoglycemias important pathophysiologically. Insulin, exogenous peripheral or endogenous hepatic, or peglispro hepato-preferential, gliptins, glucagon-like peptide-1 (GLP-1) and its analogs, metformin, the glitazones, sodium-glucose cotransporter 2 (SGLT2) inhibitors, newly available glitazaars such as saarglitazaar and the sulfonylureas have distinct effects on weight gain and lipid moieties such as triglycerides, small dense LDL, high-density lipoprotein (HDL) and in all probability on microvascular pathophysiology.

   Even within a class of pharmacological agents such as the sulfonylureas, different members can differ in their microvascular pathophysiological effects. Gliclazide may in contrast to other sulfonylureas have antioxidative properties, reducing oxidized LDL, interfering with monocyte adhesion to the vessel wall, and preventing AGE-induced VEGF expression, interfering with NF-kB and PKC activation, and possibly mitochondrial overproduction of ROS.

5. Because sorbitol has a role in one of the presumed pathophysiological pathways, and sorbitol is linked to fructose metabolism, *use of sorbitol/fructose/high fructose corn syrup/fruit juice should not be encouraged. The only juices permissible are fresh homemade tomato juice or Phalsa juice.* Fructose and sucrose are probably more harmful than glucose.
   The ideal carbohydrate source is of course polysaccharides, preferably from low glycemic index foods such as whole wheat/missi roti/missi parantha. Bread/pizza, biscuits, pasta, bhatura, naan and kulcha derived from maida or refined flour should be discouraged.
   The patient and the entire family should stop buying sugar and sweets. It is difficult to control the patient's intake of sweets if constantly exposed to temptation! Further in view of the family predilection for dysglycemia and the metabolic syndrome, this could be preventive for them as well. Personally we feel that sugar addiction will soon join tobacco addiction as a recognized public health problem at WHO level. Sucralose and Stevia as artificial sweeteners are to be preferred to aspartame and saccharin. Heat labile aspartame converts to toxic methyl alcohol when reheating a cup of aspartame sweetened tea. The long-term effects of sucralose are being debated: perhaps it will be used as a de-escalation/avoidance strategy when abandoning sugars, just as nicotine gums/e-vaps in giving up smoking.
   As regards fats in the diet, the prudential diet advised by my mentor Prof. KS Mathur uses a judicious 1:1:1 mixture of saturated fat (butter), monounsaturated fat (olive oil or mustard oil) and polyunsaturated oil (corn oil/sesame oil/soya oil/linseed oil/flaxseed oil). This option is probably the best, taking care to avoid heating cooking oils beyond their smoking point. Thus, extra virgin olive oil with a low smoking point is preferred for salad dressing, whilst pomace olive oil with a higher smoking point is preferred for cooking. Refined oils have a higher smoking point!
   As regards alcohol, excessive use harms the liver already stressed by the nonalcoholic steatohepatitis (NASH) and fatty liver associated with diabetes. Red wine contains the anti-aging agent resveratrol but this can be derived from other sources, such as red wine vinegar. HDL elevation is another benefit ascribed to moderate alcohol intake. Small doses of alcohol may facilitate destressing. The decision to prescribe alcohol or permit its use in small quantities hinges on a careful analysis of the patient's personality and likelihood of addiction.
   Many "children"—including patients of all ages—rebel against dietary restrictions, and for them one can allow one unrestricted meal out of the 21 meals in the week.
   Imaginative cooking by the meal maker can be inculcated/taught so that the permitted foods are used to construct a tasty, nutritious and wholesome meal e.g. Bhelpuri/salads/falafel to name but a few. Competitions amongst patient families can be organized for inculcating healthy culinary skills.
6. Ban the use of tobacco/congeners as chews/smokes/dental powders. They promote free radical formation and vascular disease. Again the entire family must join in to cut down temptation, and also eliminate passive smoking!
7. Even though the patient has normal renal function avoids allowing the patient becoming habituated to nephrotoxic agents such as nonsteroidal analgesics. This is because the

diabetic or hypertensive needs to conserve renal function, as the kidneys are major target organs.

8. Similar considerations apply to using steroids in subjects of the metabolic syndrome: they contribute to weight gain/hypertension and hyperglycemia. If their use is unavoidable, topical or regional administration is to be chosen, if possible.
9. If possible, extensive intermarriage between strongly diabetic families should be avoided. This is perhaps Utopian advice! It is another matter that diabetes can manifest in the partner after marriage, and here the effects of environmental/lifestyle/dietary stresses may merit consideration.
10. Preventive annual health checkups for members of the family should be instituted, just as in corporate organizations. Group savings/group insurance for the metabolic syndrome family may become available in the future. The metabolic syndrome subject and his family members should be encouraged in financial savings for a rainy day—illnesses, and for extended longevity that medical prevention can confer!
11. There is a deep nexus between the preventive strategies in metabolic disease and the prevention of aging. Free radicals and oxidative stress play a role. Pathophysiologically, the cross-linking of collagen molecules leading to stiffness and reduced physical mobility are features of both. Physical activity can delay both. Mental aerobics—learning new languages/Sudoku/chess/Antakshari/crossword puzzles/scrabble/music and reading (not passive TV viewing) must become a part of the physician's prescription!

CONCLUSION

To conclude, fighting and preventing metabolic disease is a task that needs strategy, dedication and time on the part of both the physician and his health care team, as well as the patient and his family!

It is a labor of love, if the health carer is in love with the profession, and diabetics and the like being so endearing and intelligent, we ourselves have often practically fallen in love with the patient and his/her family.

REFERENCES

1. Hazra D, Gupta A, Jain V, et al. Comparison of MUGA assessment with ANU photo rheography for assessment of early cardiac dysfunction in prediabetics and diabetics. J Nucl Med. 2008;49(Suppl 1):199P.
2. Hazra DK, Gupta AK, Sachan A, et al. The Agra diabetes prevention intervention study in the offspring of biparental diabetics: Cross section analysis initial data. Diabetes Res Clin Pract. 2000;50:139-40.
3. Hazra DK, Viswanathan V. Pathogenesis of diabetic microvascular complications. In: Chandalia HB (Ed). RSSDI Textbook of Diabetes Mallitus. Research Society for the Study of Diabetes: Mumbai; 2014.
4. Mokini Z, Marcovecchio ML, Chiarelli F. Molecular pathology of oxidative stress in diabetic angiopathy: role of mitochondrial and cellular pathways. Diabetes Res Clin Pract. 2010;87:313-21.
5. Brownlee M. Biochemistry and molecular cell biology of diabetic complications. Nature. 2001;414:813-20.

6. Ihnat MA, Thorpe JE, Kamat CD, et al. Reactive oxygen species mediate a cellular 'memory' of high glucose stress signalling. Diabetologia. 2007;50:1523-31.
7. Johansen JS, Harris AK, Rychly DJ, et al. Oxidative stress and the use of antioxidants in diabetes: linking basic science to clinical practice. Cardiovasc Diabetol. 2005;4:5.
8. Taniyama Y, Griendling KK. Reactive oxygen species in the vasculature: molecular and cellular mechanisms. Hypertension. 2003;42:1075-81.
9. Jay D, Hitomi H, Griendling KK. Oxidative stress and diabetic cardiovascular complications. Free Radic Biol Med. 2006;40:183-92.
10. Singh DK, Winocour P, Farrington K. Mechanisms of disease the hypoxic tubular hypothesis of diabetic nephropathy. Nat Clin Pract Nephrol. 2008;4:216-26.
11. Chiarelli F, Cipollone F, Mohn A, et al. Circulating monocyte chemoattractant protein-1 and early development of nephropathy in type 1 diabetes. Diabetes Care. 2002;25:1829-34.
12. Cameron NE, Cotter MA, Archibald V, et al. Antioxidant and pro-oxidant effects on nerve conduction velocity, endoneurial blood flow and oxygen tension in non-diabetic and streptozotocin-diabetic rats. Diabetologia. 1994;37:449-59.
13. Kohner EM, Patel V, Rassam SM. Role of blood flow and impaired autoregulation in the pathogenesis of diabetic retinopathy. Diabetes. 1995;44:603-7.
14. Lee AY, Chung SK, Chung SS. Demonstration that polyol accumulation is responsible for diabetic cataract by the use of transgenic mice expressing the aldose reductase gene in the lens. Proc Natl Acad Sci U S A. 1995;92:2780-4.
15. Ishii H, Jirousek MR, Koya D, et al. Amelioration of vascular dysfunctions in diabetic rats by an oral PKC beta inhibitor. Science. 1996;272:728-31.
16 Koya D, Haneda M, Nakagawa H, et al. Amelioration of accelerated diabetic mesangial expansion by treatment with a PKC-beta inhibitor in diabetic db/db mice, a rodent model for type 2 diabetes. FASEB J. 2000;14:439-47.
17. Ko BC, Lam KS, Wat NM, et al. An (A-C)n dinucleotide repeat polymorphic marker at the 5' end of the aldose reductase gene is associated with early-onset diabetic retinopathy in NIDDM patients. Diabetes. 1995;44:727-32.
18. Ruberte J, Ayuso E, Navarro M, et al. Increased ocular levels of IGF-1 in transgenic mice lead to diabetes-like eye disease. J Clin Invest. 2004;113:1149-57.
19. Watanabe D, Suzuma K, Matsui S, et al. Erythropoietin as a retinal angiogenic factor in proliferative diabetic retinopathy. N Engl J Med. 2005;353:782-92.
20. Satsangi SK, Hazra DK, Mishra V, et al. Evaluation of age inhibitor ramipril in diabetic retinopathy. In: Patney NL (Ed). Clinical Medicine Update. Indian Academy of Clinical Medicine, Kota, India; 1997. pp. 81-7.
21. Larsen M, Hommel E, Parving HH, et al. Protective effect of captopril on the blood-retina barrier in normotensive insulin-dependent diabetic patients with nephropathy and background retinopathy. Graefes Arch Clin Exp Ophthalmol. 1990;228:505-9.
22. Chase HP, Garg SK, Harris S, et al. Angiotensin-converting enzyme inhibitor treatment for young normotensive diabetic subjects: a two-year trial. Ann Ophthalmol. 1993;25:284-9.
23. Chaturvedi N, Sjølie AK, Stephenson JM, et al. Effect of lisinopril on progression of retinopathy in normotensive people with type 1 diabetes. Lancet. 1998:351:28-31.
24. Chaturvedi N, Porta M, Klein R, et al. Effect of candesartan on prevention (DIRECT-Prevent 1) and progression (DIRECT-Protect 1) of retinopathy in type 1 diabetes: randomized, placebo-controlled trials. Lancet. 2008;372:1394-402.
25. Sjølie AK, Klein R, Porta M, et al. Effect of candesartan on progression and regression of retinopathy in type 2 diabetes (DIRECT-Protect 2): a randomized, placebo-controlled trial. Lancet. 2008;372:1385-93.
26. Mauer M, Zinman B, Gardiner R, et al. Renal and retinal effects of enalapril and losartan in type 1 diabetes. N Engl J Med. 2009;361:40-51.

27. Bilous R, Chaturvedi N, Sjølie AK, et al. Effect of candesartan on microalbuminuria and albumin excretion rate in diabetes: three randomized trials. Ann Intern Med. 2009;151:11-20.
28. Sjølie AK, Dodson P, Hobbs FR. Does renin-angiotensin system blockade have a role in preventing diabetic retinopathy? A clinical review. Intern J Clin Pract. 2011;65:148-53.
29. ACCORD study Group; ACCORD Eye Study Group, Chew EY, et al. Effects of medical therapies on retinopathy progression in type 2 diabetes. N Engl J Med. 2010;363:233-44.
30. Beulens JW, Patel A, Vingerling JR, et al. Effects of blood pressure lowering and intensive glucose control on the incidence and progression of retinopathy in patients with type 2 diabetes mellitus: a randomized controlled trial. Diabetologia. 2009;52:2027-36.
31. Keech AC, Mitchell P, Summanen PA, et al. Effect of fenofibrate on the need for laser treatment for diabetic retinopathy (FIELD study): a randomized controlled trial. Lancet. 2007;370:1687-97.

22
CHAPTER

Diabetic Foot and Its Complications

Mumtaz Ahmad Ansari, Vivek Srivastava, Rajgopal Acharya

INTRODUCTION

Diabetes mellitus (DM) refers to a group of common metabolic disorders that share the phenotype of hyperglycemia. This hyperglycemia may be due to any of the following metabolic dysregulations; reduced insulin secretion, decreased glucose utilization and increased glucose production. These metabolic dysregulations lead to secondary pathophysiologic alterations in multiple organ systems that impose a tremendous burden on the diabetic patient as well as health care system. As the incidence of DM is increasing worldwide, there will be a substantial increase in mortality and morbidity due to diabetes and its complications in near future.

Diabetes mellitus is the leading cause of nontraumatic lower extremity amputation in the United States. Foot ulcers and infections are also a major source of morbidity in individuals with DM. Approximately 15% of individuals with DM develop a foot ulcer, the most common sites being great toe or metatarsophalangeal areas. Of these, a significant subset ultimately undergoes amputation.

PATHOPHYSIOLOGY OF DIABETIC FOOT[1]

Diabetic foot is the end result of interaction of several pathogenic factors like neuropathy, abnormal foot biomechanics, peripheral arterial disease (PAD) and poor wound healing. Patients of DM develop peripheral sensory neuropathy which interferes with normal protective mechanisms and make the patient vulnerable to major or repeated minor trauma to the foot, which often goes un-noticed by the patient owing to neuropathy. Likewise, disordered proprioception causes abnormal weight bearing while walking leading to the formation of callus and subsequently, ulceration occurs.

Motor and sensory neuropathy lead to abnormal foot mechanics and to structural changes in the foot (hammer toe, claw toe, prominent metatarsal heads, Charcot joints) (Fig. 1).

Autonomic neuropathy results in anhidrosis and altered superficial blood flow in the foot, which leads to drying of the foot and fissure formation. PAD and poor wound healing together

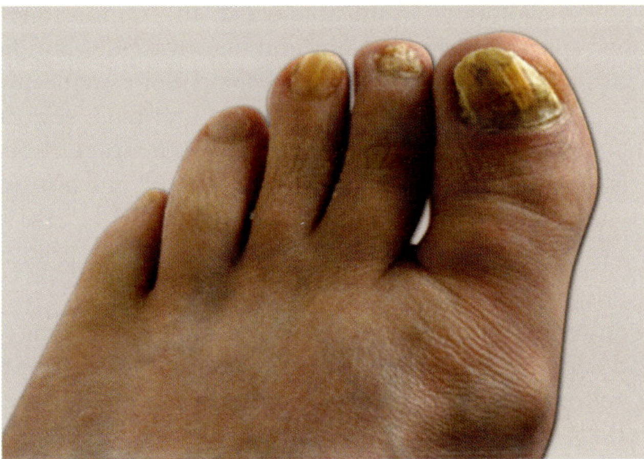

Fig. 1: Structural changes in foot

impede resolution of even minor injuries in the foot, promoting them to enlarge and get infected.

Neuropathy and ischemia, two common complications of DM, are the primary underlying risk factors for the development of foot ulcers and their complications. The presence of symmetric distal polyneuropathy, encompassing motor, sensory and autonomic involvement is one of the most important factors in the development of diabetic foot ulcers. Perhaps one-third of diabetic foot ulcers have a mixed neuropathic and ischemic etiology. Although neuropathy and ischemia are the primary predisposing factors in the formation of diabetic foot ulcers, an initiating factor, such as physical or mechanical stress, is required for an ulcer to develop. Ischemic ulcers develop as a result of low perfusion pressure in a foot with inadequate blood supply, whereas neuropathic ulcers result from higher pressures in a foot with adequate blood supply but loss of protective sensation. In addition to increasing the risk of ulceration, DM also increases the risk of infection by impairing the body's ability to eliminate bacteria.

COMPLICATIONS OF DIABETIC FOOT[2]

- Peripheral neuropathy (20–40% of patients with diabetes)
- Peripheral vascular disease (20–40% of patients with diabetes)
- Foot ulceration (5% of patients with diabetes a year)
- Foot infection and osteomyelitis (22–66% of all foot ulcers)
- Amputation (0.5% of patients with diabetes a year)
- Charcot neuroarthropathy (0.1–0.4% of patients with diabetes a year).

ULCERATION

Despite preventive measures, diabetic foot ulcer is common and a serious concern. The plantar surface of the foot is the most common site of ulceration. Ulcers may be primarily neuropathic (i.e. without accompanying infection) or infected. The pathophysiology of these ulcers is multifactorial, as has been elaborated in the above text. The compartmentalized anatomy of the foot, with its various spaces, tendon sheaths and neurovascular bundles, allows ischemic necrosis to affect tissues within a compartment or spread along anatomic tissue planes. Risk factors for development of ulcers in a patient with DM are: male sex, duration of diabetes greater than 10 years, peripheral neuropathy, abnormal foot structure (bony abnormalities, callus, thickened nails), PAD, smoking, poor glycemic control, and a history of previous foot ulcer or amputation.

Infection

Individuals with DM have a greater frequency and severity of infections (Fig. 2), the reasons being abnormalities in humoral immunity (impaired neutrophil chemotaxis, phagocytosis and intracellular killing), cell-mediated immunity and impaired monocyte-macrophage function, as well as diminished vascularization. These abnormalities correlate with the adequacy of glycemic control. Hyperglycemia aids the growth and colonization of a variety of organisms like *Candida spp* and other fungi. Recurrent infections are common in DM.

Acute infections are usually caused by Gram-positive cocci. *Staphylococcus aureus* is the most important pathogen in diabetic foot infections (DFIs). Diabetic patients have an increased rate of colonization of *S. aureus* in skin folds. It is often present as a monomicrobial infection, but it is also an important pathogen in polymicrobial infections. Chronic wounds, recurrent infections, and infections in hospitalized patients are more likely to harbor complex flora, including aerobes as well as anaerobes. Gas gangrene may develop in the absence of clostridial infection. Among Gram-negative bacteria, family Enterobacteriaceae is common, and *Pseudomonas aeruginosa* may be isolated from wounds that have been treated with hydrotherapy or wet dressings. Enterococci may be isolated from patients previously been treated with cephalosporins. Anaerobic bacteria seldom cause DFIs as a sole pathogen, but may be isolated from deep infections or necrotic tissue. Antibiotic-resistant bacteria, especially methicillin-resistant *S. aureus* (MRSA), may be isolated from patients who have received antibiotics previously or who have been hospitalized for a long time.

Cellulitis without ulceration is also frequent in patients with DM. The cause of persistent cellulitis and nonhealing infection is usually underlying deep infection or *osteomyelitis.*

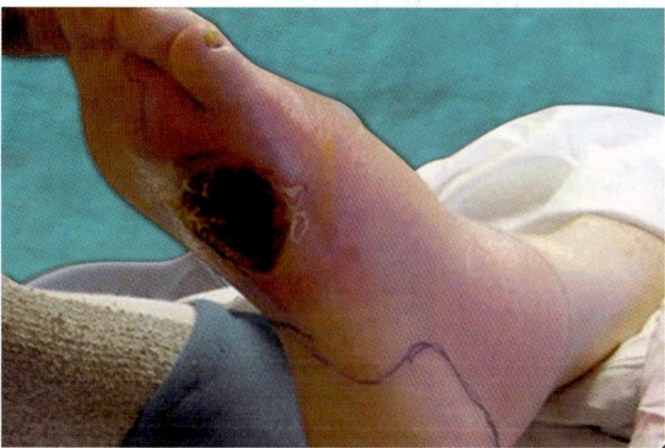

Fig. 2: Foot ulceration

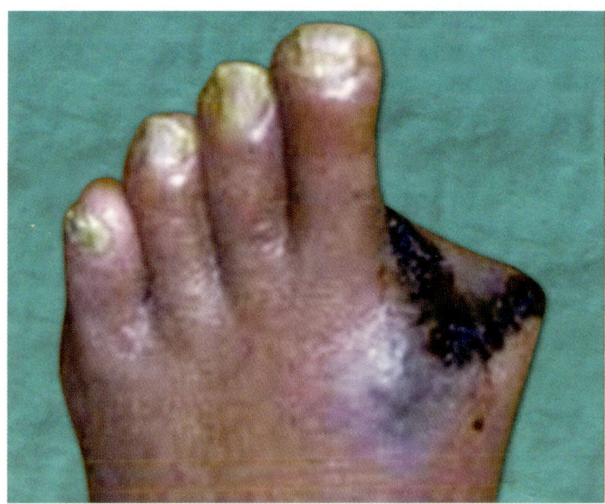

Fig. 3: Recently amputated great toe

Amputation

Despite all preventive measures, around 10–30% of diabetic patients with foot ulceration eventually require amputation (Fig. 3). It is not only associated with functional loss but also emotional stress to the patient and his family that may even culminate in depression.

MANAGEMENT OF DIABETIC FOOT AND ITS COMPLICATIONS

The proper management of a diabetic foot begins with considering the overall complications the diabetic patient has.

History

A complete medical history should be obtained with special emphasis on DM-relevant aspects such as weight, family history of DM, risk factors, lifestyle, etc. In a patient with prior established DM, the initial history should also include special emphasis on prior diabetic care, including the type of therapy, hemoglobin A1c (HbA_{1c}) levels, self-monitoring blood glucose results, assessment of patient's knowledge about DM, exercise and nutrition. Also, history should be taken regarding the presence of DM-related comorbidities such as cardiovascular disease, hypertension, etc.

Physical Examination

A complete physical examination should be done. Careful examination of the lower extremities should be carried out, seeking evidence for peripheral neuropathy, calluses, superficial fungal infections, nail disease, ankle reflexes and foot deformities. Sites of potential skin ulceration should be identified. Moderately advanced diabetic neuropathy can be assessed by detecting ability to sense touch with a monofilament, pinprick sensation and vibratory sense.[1] Vibratory sensation should be assessed using 128-MHz tuning fork at the base of great toe.

After examining the overlying cellulitis, any possible underlying abscess should be examined by palpation for crepitus or detection of drainage of purulent fluid. Cellulitis should not be confused with dependent rubor caused by severe ischemia. The status of arterial circulation should be documented by palpating the lower extremity pulses "bilaterally".

Investigations

The laboratory assessment should first determine whether the patient meets the diagnostic criteria for DM and then assess the degree of glycemic control.

- Plain X-rays with multiple views of the foot can assist in assessing the extent of foot infection. Advanced osteomyelitis can be detected, but plain X-rays fail to show early bone infection. Magnetic resonance imaging (MRI) of the foot is a sensitive imaging modality for detecting soft tissue infection and early osteomyelitis. Indium-labeled white cell studies may be used to determine whether infection involves underlying bone or soft tissue only; however, it is technically demanding and expensive.
- In patients with severe foot edema, the peripheral pulses may be difficult to palpate. In such cases, noninvasive arterial ultrasound can be useful in assessing the extent of arterial disease.
- Routine laboratory investigations should be sent for evaluating presence of sepsis.
- Cultures should be taken from debrided ulcer base or from purulent discharge or aspiration from the wound.

TREATMENT GOALS FOR ADULTS WITH DM[3]

Treatment goals for adults with DM have been shown in Table 1.

Table 1: Treatment goals for adults with diabetes mellitus

• Glycemic control	
– HbA_{1c}	< 7.0
– Preprandial capillary plasma glucose	5.0–7.2 mmol/L (90–130 mg/dL)
– Peak postprandial capillary plasma glucose	< 10 mmol/L (< 180 mg/dL)
• Blood pressure	< 130/80 mm Hg
• Lipids	
– Low-density lipoprotein	< 2.6 mmol/L (< 100 mg/dL)
– High-density lipoprotein	> 1.1 mmol/L (> 40 mg/dL)
– Triglycerides	< 1.7 mmol/L (< 150 mg/dL)

NUTRITIONAL RECOMMENDATIONS FOR ADULTS WITH DM[3]

Fats:

- 20–355% of total caloric intake
- Saturated fat less than 7% of total calories
- Dietary cholesterol less than 200 mg/day
- Two or more servings of fish/week provide omega-3 polyunsaturated fatty acids (PUFAs).

Carbohydrates:
- 45–65% of total caloric intake
- Amount and type of carbohydrate important
- Sucrose-containing foods can be consumed with insulin adjustments.

Proteins:
- 10–35% of total caloric intake.

Others:
- Fiber-containing foods may reduce postprandial glucose excursions
- Non-nutrient sweeteners.

PREVENTION OF DIABETIC FOOT

Prevention is the optimum therapy for diabetic foot ulcers and amputations. This can be accomplished through identification of high-risk patients, education of the patient and institution of measures to prevent ulceration. High-risk patients should be identified during routine foot examination. Patient education should emphasize: careful selection of footwear, daily inspection of feet to detect early signs of ill-fitting footwear or minor trauma, daily foot hygiene to keep skin moist and clean, avoidance of self-treatment of foot abnormalities and high-risk activities (e.g. walking barefoot), and prompt consultation with a health-care provider in case of any abnormality. Measures should be taken aiming at modification of risk factors. These include orthotic shoes and devices (Fig. 4), callus management, nail care and prophylactic measures to reduce increased skin pressure from abnormal bony architecture.

TREATMENT OF DIABETIC FOOT[4]

Due to multifactorial pathogenesis of diabetic foot, its management is multidisciplinary and involves fields such as orthopedics, vascular surgery, endocrinology, podiatry and infectious diseases.

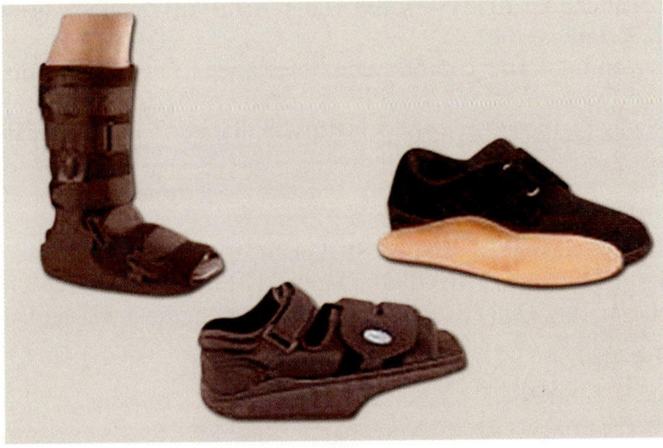

Fig. 4: Offloading devices

A large number of treatments have been proposed for management of diabetic foot;[5] however, efficacy of none has been proved repeatedly in trials. A consensus statement from the American Diabetes Association (ADA)[6] identified six interventions which have demonstrated efficacy in diabetic foot wounds: offloading, debridement, wound dressings, appropriate use of antibiotics, revascularization, and limited amputation. Offloading is the complete avoidance of weight bearing on ulcer, which removes the mechanical trauma that retards wound healing. Bed rest and orthotic devices limit weight bearing on wounds and pressure points. Surgical debridement is of utmost importance in diabetic foot and all necrotic and devitalized tissue should be removed.[7] Dressings such as hydrocolloid dressings promote wound healing by creating a moist environment. Topical antibiotics are of limited use.

Mild or non-limb threatening infections can be treated with oral antibiotics (cephalosporin, clindamycin, co-amoxiclav, fluoroquinolones), wound debridement, local wound care and close surveillance. More severe ulcers may require intravenous (IV) antibiotics and urgent surgical debridement as well as bed rest.[8] IV antibiotics should provide broad-spectrum coverage directed toward *S. aureus*, streptococcus, Gram-negative aerobes and anaerobes. Nonresponding infections should be treated keeping MRSA and *Pseudomonas aeruginosa* as causative agents.

Osteomyelitis is best treated by a combination of prolonged antibiotics and surgical debridement of infected bone.

Newer interventions are being tried for the management of DFIs. These include living skin equivalents and growth factors such as basic fibroblast growth factor and recombinant platelet-derived growth factor.

Referral for physical therapy, orthotic evaluation and rehabilitation should occur once the infection is controlled.

REFERENCES

1. Vinik A, Ullal J, Parson HK, et al. Diabetic neuropathies: clinical manifestations and current treatment options. Nat Clin Pract Endocrinol Metab. 2006;2(5):269-81.
2. Cheer K, Shearman C, Jude EB, et al. Managing complications of the diabetic foot. BMJ. 2009;339:b4905.2007.
3. Townsend CM, Beauchamp RD, Evers BM (Eds). Sabiston Textbook of Surgery, 18th edition. Philadelphia: WB Saunders; 2007.
4. Laing P. The development and complications of diabetic foot ulcers. Am J Surg. 1998;176(2A Suppl):11S-19S.
5. Al-Maskari F, El-Sadig M. Prevalence of risk factors for diabetic foot complications. BMC Fam Pract. 2007;8:59.
6. American Diabetes Association. Clinical practice recommendations 2007. Diabetes Care. 2007;30:S4.
7. Fauci AS, Braunwald E, Kasper DL, Hauser SL, Longo DL, Jameson JL, Loscalzo J (Eds). Harrison's Principles of Internal Medicine, 17th edition. McGraw-Hill: New York; 2008. F, M.
8. Armstrong DG,, Lavery LA. Diabetic foot ulcers: prevention, diagnosis and classification. Am Fam Physician. 1998;57(6):1325-32, 1337-8.

23
CHAPTER

Psychiatric Evaluation in Patient with Insulin Resistance

Vipul Garg, Pankaj Kanaujia, Suchi Dwivedi

INTRODUCTION

Investigation of the relationship between psychiatric disease and insulin resistance among young adults is essential to understand how insulin resistance may be influenced by this. With identification of persons who are at risk of developing insulin resistance in primary care clinics, preventive interventions can be developed to intervene at an early stage. There are many mental disorders which affect insulin resistance in multiple ways, out of which these are most common.

- Depression
- Schizophrenia
- Bipolar disorders.

DEPRESSION

There is abundant evidence that depression in diabetic patients is more frequent, more apt to be severe, recurrent and difficult to treat and strongly correlated with diabetic complications.

The Relationship between Depression and Insulin Resistance

Research has established a positive association between depression and type 2 diabetes that is more commonly found among women than men. A meta-analysis reported that adults with depression (either clinical diagnosed depression or depressive symptoms) had a 37% increased risk of developing type 2 diabetes and the prevalence of depression was twice as high among adults with type 2 diabetes than those without diabetes.

Pathophysiological Link between Depression and Insulin Resistance

Although the underlying mechanism is still unclear, several pathophysiological pathways have been proposed to explain the relationship between depression and insulin resistance, including hypothalamic-pituitary-adrenal (HPA) hyperactivity, increased immunoinflammatory cytokines and lifestyle risk behaviors.

and fat among depressed patients can promote development of obesity and release of various adipokines secreted from adipose tissue. Reduced energy utilization associated with physical inactivity can in turn decrease insulin sensitivity of skeletal muscle.

SCHIZOPHRENIA

Schizophrenia is a neurodevelopmental disorder, which affect 1.4–4.6 per 1,000 of the general population, has an incidence rate of 0.16–0.42 per 1,000 population and is associated with excess mortality.

The association between diabetes and schizophrenia has been recognized for over a century. In 1879, Sir Henry Maudsley in "The Pathology of Mind" commented that, "Diabetes is a disease which often shows itself in families in which insanity prevails". More recent studies have shown that the prevalence of impaired glucose tolerance and diabetes is increased two- to threefold in individuals with schizophrenia. A few recent studies indicate that the prevalence of the metabolic syndrome is increased in people with schizophrenia, and this may provide an explanation for the increased prevalence of diabetes and cardiovascular disease (CVD) in schizophrenia.

The Mechanisms Underlying the Increased Prevalence of Diabetes

The mechanisms that underlie the increased prevalence of diabetes in schizophrenia include hereditary and environmental factors, such as less healthy lifestyles and poorer health care, as well as side effects of antipsychotic medication.

Obesity

Individuals with schizophrenia are more likely to have obese parents. When assessed by CT scanning and anthropometry, drug-naïve and drug-free schizophrenic patients were found to have significantly higher waist-to-hip ratios, and over three times as much visceral fat.

Lipid Profile

The lipid profile in first-episode, drug-naïve patients with schizophrenia was found to be more favorable than in healthy controls, but in contrast high-density lipoprotein cholesterol levels are decreased and triglycerides are increased in chronic schizophrenic patients treated with phenothiazine.

Hereditary Factors

Up to 30% of people with schizophrenia have a family history of type 2 diabetes. Genetic factors appear at least as important in the etiology of schizophrenia as diabetes and hypertension and studies to map diabetes and schizophrenia genes are ongoing. There is strong evidence that gene regions on 6p and 8p contain schizophrenia susceptibility genes, while regions on 6q, 13q and 22q are also being studied. As there is some overlap with the chromosomal regions that have been linked to type 2 diabetes, it is possible that there are areas of linkage disequilibrium that may predispose to both diabetes and schizophrenia.

Lifestyle

Poverty and poor access to good nutrition may also contribute to the increased prevalence of type 2 diabetes. Patients with schizophrenia generally take little exercise. Inactivity and apathy are characteristic of schizophrenia; the physical inactivity may reflect developmental delays as well as social factors, such as high levels of perceived criticism from other family member. Smoking, another risk factor for the metabolic syndrome, is increased in people with schizophrenia.

Antipsychotic Medication

After the introduction of phenothiazine, the prevalence of type 2 diabetes in schizophrenic patients increased.[3] The atypical antipsychotics (AAPs) are associated with weight gain and an increased incidence of metabolic disease including type 2 diabetes mellitus.

BIPOLAR DISORDER

Overweight and obesity are highly prevalent in patients with bipolar disorder. There appears an association between mood disorders and component of metabolic syndromes. Abnormality of hypothalamus pituitary axis is more prevalent in mood disorders, causing insulin resistance. The lifestyle and behavior pattern of individual with bipolar disorder also play important role in the prevalence of metabolic syndrome. Pharmacotherapy used in bipolar disorders such as lithium and valproic acid has been associated with significant weight gain, thus promoting the insulin resistance.

ANTIPSYCHOTIC DRUGS ASSOCIATED WITH INSULIN RESISTANCE

The AAPs are associated with weight gain and an increased incidence of metabolic disease including type 2 diabetes mellitus. Epidemiological, cross-sectional and prospective studies suggest that two of the AAPs, olanzapine and clozapine cause the most dramatic weight gain and metabolic impairments including increased fasting glucose, insulin and triglycerides.[4] Relative to the other AAPs, both olanzapine and clozapine exhibit a particularly high antagonistic affinity for histamine and muscarinic receptors which have been hypothesized as mediators of the reported increase in weight and glucose abnormalities.[5]

Atypical antipsychotics act on multiple receptors subtypes with arrange of affinity for dopamine, serotonin, histamine, muscarinic and adrenergic receptors (Fig. 2).[6] The decreased specificity for dopamine receptors of the AAPs has lessened the motor disorders associated with previous agents such as haloperidol but the lack of specificity may be responsible for the wide spread metabolic side effects associated with the drugs.

Atypical antipsychotics, such as clozapine and olanzapine, induce the most significant weight gain and metabolic disturbances while risperidone and aripiprazole may have modest effects and others, such as ziprasidone, appear to be weight-neutral.[7] These data suggest that subtle differences in receptor binding and affinity may have profound effects on food intake, weight gain and ultimately metabolism (Fig. 3).[8]

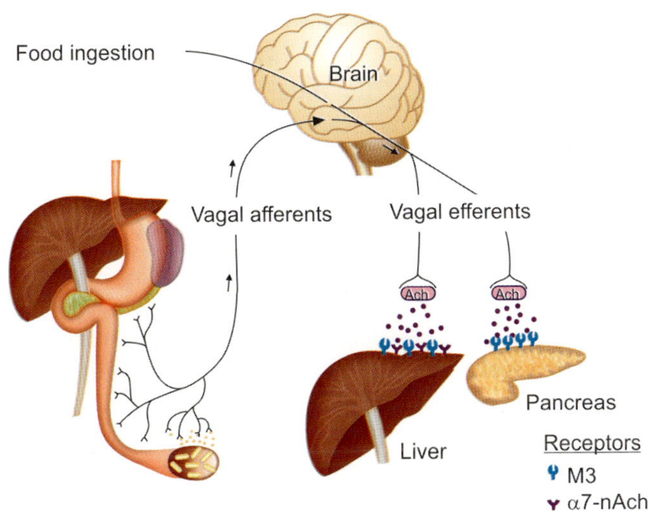

Fig. 2: Role of the vagus nerve in glucose homeostasis. Vagal afferents relay sensory information from peripheral tissues such as the stomach and intestine to the brain which may initiate vagal efferent activation. Food ingestion is required to activate preganglionic vagal efferent fibers terminating on postganglionic intrapancreatic neurons which release acetylcholine. Acetylcholine enhances insulin release to glucose and other nutrients. Physiological studies suggest that the vagal efferent may inhibit hepatic glucose production although the site of hepatic innervation has not been identified. Muscarinic receptors have been shown to mediate vagally mediated insulin secretion. Hepatic responses may be mediated by either nicotinic or muscarinic receptors

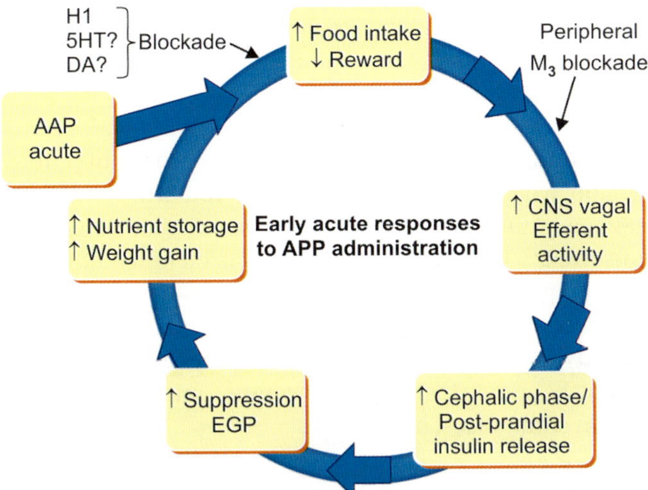

Fig. 3: Acute effects of atypical antipsychotic administration to humans. Initial administration of some atypical antipsychotics increases food intake and decreases the rewarding experience of food ingestion potentially through blockade of histaminergic, dopaminergic and serotonergic receptors in the central nervous system. The increase in food intake results in repetitive stimulation of vagal efferent activity, eliciting cephalic phase insulin release and postprandial hyperinsulinemia which overcomes peripheral muscarinic blockade by the AAPs. The postprandial hyperinsulinemia would then promote nutrient storage and weight gain, exacerbating the effects of increased food intake

Source: Teff KL, Kim SF. Atypical antipsychotics and the neural regulation of food intake and peripheral metabolism. Physiol Behav. 2011;104(4):590-8.

Olanzapine and clozapine exhibit binding affinities for muscarinic receptors of at least two orders of magnitude higher than the other AAPs. Similarly, both these drugs exhibit a high antagonist affinity for H1 receptors. The differential binding affinity of olanzapine and clozapine to muscarinic and histaminergic receptors has led to hypotheses that these receptors play a primary role in the abnormal metabolic and orexigenic properties of these drugs.[9] A number of review articles have reported positive correlations between histamine binding and increased weight gain as well as muscarinic binding and metabolic impairment.

Treating your Diabetes and Depression

Today, depression in diabetes is treated several ways. Treatment includes medication, therapy (also called psychotherapy), or a flexible combination both with relatively good results, comparable to those for patients who have depression but not diabetes.[10]

If you have diabetes and depression, treating your depression is both necessary and beneficial. While some single past studies had shown that depression treatment could improve glycemic control (a recent meta-analysis found that while most antidepressant treatments effectively treated depression, they failed to help improve diabetes-related outcomes, e.g. improved glycemic control). Treatments are needed that effectively improve both depression and diabetes.

Adverse Outcomes Linked to Untreated Depression in Diabetes

- If you have depression and diabetes that remains untreated, you may have difficulty in managing your diabetes.
- Depression and diabetes has been associated with poor medication adherence[11] (Kilbourne et al. 2005), poor glycemic control (McKellar et al. 2004) and with an increased prevalence of complications in type 2 diabetes (Bruce et al. 2005).
- Untreated depression in diabetes can increase your odds of getting diabetes complications, such as heart, kidney and nerve disorders, as well as eye and foot problems.[12]
- Untreated depression will make it less likely that you will be able to care for yourself and properly manage your diabetes. Those with untreated depression are less likely to take care of themselves.[13] This poor self-care which includes nonadherence to diet, less exercise, smoking and not taking medications as directed results in poor overall health and complications (Lin et al. 2004).
- In people diagnosed with type 1 or type 2 diabetes, depression increases the risk for complications such as persistent hyperglycemia, microvascular and macrovascular complications, and in some cases, even death.

Diabetes Disease Process and Treatment Options

- Nutritional management
- Incorporating physical activity into lifestyle
- Using medication(s) safely and for maximum therapeutic effectiveness
- Monitoring blood glucose and other parameters; interpreting and using the results for self-management decision making
- Preventing, detecting and treating acute complications

- Preventing, detecting and treating chronic complications
- Developing personal strategies to address psychosocial issues and concerns, such as stress, anxiety and depression
- Developing personal strategies to promote health and behavior change.

NOVEL DRUGS FOR DIABETES

Hydroxychloroquine

Antimalarial such as hydroxychloroquine, a long-standing safe and inexpensive treatment for autoimmune diseases such as rheumatoid arthritis and systemic lupus erythematous, theoretically may improve glucose tolerance and prevent diabetes mellitus.

In vitro and animal studies indicate that antimalarial improve insulin secretion and peripheral insulin sensitivity. Hypoglycemia is a rare but well recognized adverse effect of treatment with antimalarial, also have been shown to lower glycated hemoglobin levels in patients with type 2 diabetes who have suboptimal glucose control.

Bromocriptine

A formulation of bromocriptine, dopamine receptor agonist has been approved by the US Food and Drug Administration for the treatment of type 2 diabetes. Quick-release bromocriptine (bromocriptine-QR) is highly absorbed quick-release formulation of the dopamine D2 agonist bromocriptine mesylate, an ergot alkaloid derivative. Bromocriptine-QR may act centrally to reset hypothalamic centers regulating postprandial insulin-mediated glucose and lipid metabolism, reducing hyperglycemia and hyperlipidemia. Bromocriptine-QR is administered orally within 2 hours of waking in the morning at 1.6–4.8 mg once daily.

REFERENCES

1. Kim SF, Huang AS, Snowman AM, et al. From the cover: antipsychotic drug-induced weight gain mediated by histamine H1 receptor-linked activation of hypothalamic AMP-kinase. Proc Natl Acad Sci. USA, 2007;104 (9):3456-9.
2. Kinder LS, Kamarck TW, Baum A, et al. Depressive symptomatology and coronary heart disease in Type 1 diabetes mellitus: a study of possible mechanisms. Health Psychol. 2002;21(6):542-52.
3. Starrenburg FC, Bogers JP. How can antipsychotics cause diabetes mellitus? Insights based on receptor-binding profiles, humoral factors and transporter proteins. Eur Psychiatry. 2009; 24(3):164-70.
4. Markowitz JS, Brown CS, Moore TR. Atypical antipsychotics. Part I: pharmacology, pharmacokinetics, and efficacy. Ann Pharmacother. 1999;33(1):73-85.
5. Kroeze WK, Hufeisen SJ, Popadak BA, et al. H1-histamine receptor affinity predicts short-term weight gain for typical and atypical antipsychotic drugs. Neuropsychopharmacology. 2003;28(3):519-26.
6. Bymaster FP, Felder CC, Tzavara E, et al. Muscarinic mechanisms of antipsychotic atypicality. Prog Neuropsychopharmacol Biol Psychiatry. 2003;27(7):1125-43.
7. Nasrallah HA. Atypical antipsychotic-induced metabolic side effects: insights from receptor-binding profiles. Mol Psychiatry. 2008;13(1):27-35.
8. Stahl SM, Mignon L, Meyer JM. Which comes first: atypical antipsychotic treatment or cardiometabolic risk? Acta Psychiatr Scand. 2009;119(3):171-9.

9. Gao Q, Horvath TL. Neurobiology of feeding and energy expenditure. Annu Rev Neurosci. 2007;30:367-98.
10. van Bastelaar KM, Pouwer F, Cuijpers P, et al. Web-based cognitive behavioural therapy (W-CBT) for diabetes patients with co-morbid depression: design of a randomised controlled trial. BMC Psychiatry. 2008;8:9.
11. Kilbourne AM, Reynolds CF, Good CB, et al. How does depression influence diabetes medication adherence in older patients? Am J Geriatr Psychiatry. 2005;13(3):202-10.
12. Kinder LS, Katon WJ, Ludman E, et al. Improving depression care in patients with diabetes and multiple complications. J Gen Intern Med. 2006;21(10):1036-41.
13. Khan A, Khan S, Kolts R, et al. Suicide rates in clinical trials of SSRIs, other antidepressants, and placebo: analysis of FDA reports. Am J Psychiatry. 2003;160(4):790-2.

24

CHAPTER

Diabetes in Pregnancy

V Balaji

INTRODUCTION

Pregnancy induces progressive changes in maternal carbohydrate metabolism. As pregnancy advances insulin resistance and diabetogenic stress due to placental hormones necessitate compensatory increase in insulin secretion. When this compensation is inadequate, gestational diabetes develops. Pregnancy that occurs in a woman who already has diabetes is termed "pre-gestational diabetes mellitus" (pre-GDM). Both these situations are associated with increased maternal and fetal morbidity and rarely mortality. The magnitude of these complications is lesser in woman with GDM than in pre-GDM. Universal screening for GDM is strongly recommended for the population ethnically prone to high prevalence of type 2 diabetes mellitus (T2DM). The screening around 24th to 28th week is usually done, but it is ideal to test for glucose intolerance in the early pregnancy itself. In much of the world, a 75-g glucose tolerance test is performed and GDM is diagnosed if 2-hour plasma glucose (PG) is more than or equal to 140 mg/dL. Pregnant women with gestational diabetes have a significantly increased incidence of cesarean section, pre-eclampsia and macrosomia. It has also been observed that increasing carbohydrate intolerance in women without GDM also do suffer from these perinatal complications. Medical nutrition therapy (MNT) is important in the management of GDM. Women who fail to respond to nutrition therapy are advised insulin and the insulin dose is individualized. Pre-GDM has to be on insulin throughout pregnancy including preconception period.

Gestational Diabetes Mellitus

Gestational diabetes mellitus is defined as carbohydrate intolerance of variable severity with onset or first recognition during the present pregnancy.

The definition applies irrespective of whether or not insulin is used for treatment or the condition persists after pregnancy. It does not exclude the possibility that glucose intolerance may have antedated the present pregnancy. GDM results from sluggish first phase insulin release and in addition to excessive resistance to action of insulin on glucose utilization due to placental hormones (placental lactogen, progestin, prolactin and cortisol). The insulin secretion pattern in both pregnant women with NGT and women with GDM is given in Box 1.

Box 1: Insulin secretion in pregnancy

- Insulin secretion is considerably increased in both pregnant women with NGT and women with GDM.
- Glucose stimulated insulin secretion is increased more in normal pregnant women than in women with GDM.
- Peak plasma insulin during an OGTT occurs later in women with GDM than in women with NGT.
- First phase insulin response to intravenous glucose is more during pregnancy in women with NGT than in women with GDM.
- Increases in second phase insulin responses are of similar magnitude in women with NGT and those with GDM.

Abbreviations: NGT, normal glucose tolerance; GDM, gestational diabetes mellitus

DIAGNOSTIC CRITERIA AND SCREENING OF GESTATIONAL DIABETES MELLITUS

Compared to selective screening recommended by the American Diabetes Association (ADA), universal screening for GDM detects more cases and improves maternal and neonatal prognosis.[1] Hence, universal screening for GDM is essential, as it is generally accepted that women of Asian origin and especially ethnic Indians are at a higher risk of developing GDM and subsequent T2DM.[2]

World Health Organization Procedure

To standardize the diagnosis of GDM, the World Health Organization (WHO) recommends using a 2-hour 75-g oral glucose tolerance test (OGTT) with a threshold PG concentration of greater than 140 mg/dL at 2 hours, similar to that of impaired glucose tolerance (IGT) (>140 mg/dL and <199 mg/dL) outside pregnancy.[3]

American Diabetes Association Procedure

The American Diabetes Association procedure has become obsolete and not being followed anywhere now. ADA has adopted the International Association of the Diabetes and Pregnancy Study Groups (IADPSG) criteria.

The International Association of the Diabetes and Pregnancy Study Groups[4]

Based on the hyperglycemia and adverse pregnancy outcome (HAPO) study, IADPSG suggested the guidelines. In this HAPO study, population from India, China, South Asian countries (except city of Bangkok, Hong Kong), Middle East and Sub-Saharan countries were not included. Thus, essentially HAPO study was performed in Caucasian population.

- The IADPSG recommends that diagnosis of GDM is made when any of the following PG values meet or exceed: fasting: ≥5.1 mmol/L (92 mg/dL); 1-hour: ≥10.0 mmol/L (180 mg/dL); 2-hour: ≥8.5 mmol/L (153 mg/dL) with 75 g OGTT.

- The IADPSG also suggests: fasting plasma glucose (FPG) >7.0 mmol/L (126 mg/dL)/A1c >6.5% in the early weeks of pregnancy is diagnostic of overt diabetes. Fasting >5.1 mmol/L and <7.0 mmol/L is diagnosed as GDM.[4]

Disadvantages of the IADPSG Guidelines

- Most of the time pregnant women do not come in the fasting state because of commutation and belief not to fast for long hours. The dropout rate is very high when a pregnant woman is asked to come again for the glucose tolerance test.[5] Attending the first prenatal visit in the fasting state is impractical in many settings.[4]
- In all GDM, FPG values do not reflect the 2-hour post glucose with 75-g oral glucose (2-hour PG), which is the hallmark of GDM.[6] Ethnically Asian Indians have high insulin resistance and as a consequence, their 2-hour PG is higher compared to Caucasians.[7] The insulin resistance during pregnancy escalates further[8] and hence FPG is not an appropriate option to diagnose GDM in Asian Indian women. In this population by following FPG >5.1 mmol/L as cutoff value, 76% of pregnant women would have missed the diagnosis of GDM made by the WHO criterion.[9]
- Asian and South Asian ethnicity are both independently associated with increased insulin resistance in late pregnancy. A diagnostic FPG was present in only 24% of those with GDM in Bangkok and 26% in Hong Kong.[10]
- Center to center differences occur in GDM frequency and relative diagnostic importance of fasting, 1-hour and 2-hour glucose levels. This may impact strategies used for the diagnosis of GDM.[10]
- The A1c is not possible to perform in the less resource countries, not only because it is expensive but also due to lack of technically qualified staff. The cost and standardization of A1c testing are issues for consideration.[4]

Evidence-based WHO Criterion

Short-term Outcome

Economical test: This procedure requires one blood sample drawn at 2 hours after 75-g oral glucose load for estimating PG. Even if the test is to be repeated in each trimester, the cost in performing the procedure will be 66% less than the cost of performing IADPSG recommended procedure. Thus, WHO procedure is feasible, sustainable, cost-effective and high impact best buy for less resource settings.

Evidence-based

- A study performed by Crowther et al. found that treatment of GDM diagnosed by WHO criterion reduces serious perinatal morbidity and may also improve the women's health-related quality of life.[11]
- Diagnosis of GDM with OGTT 2-hour PG ≥7.8 mmol/L (140 mg/dL) and treatment in a combined diabetes antenatal clinic is worthwhile with a decreased macrosomia rate and fewer emergency cesarean sections. The treatment of GDM women as defined by the WHO criterion was associated with reduced risk of pregnancy outcome.[12]

- Wahi et al. observed in their randomized controlled study, the advantage of adhering to a cutoff level of 2-hour PG ≥7.8 mmol/L in diagnosis and management of GDM for a significantly positive effect on pregnancy outcomes both in relation to mother as well as the child.[13]
- Perucchini et al. also suggest one-step diagnostic procedure (2-hour PG ≥7.8 mmol/L) to diagnose GDM.[14]

Long-term Outcome

A long-term outcome study conducted by Franks et al. documented that when maternal 2-hour PG was ≥7.8 mmol/L, the cumulative risk of offspring developing T2DM was 30% at the age 24 years.[15]

New WHO Criteria

The WHO while endorsing the IADPSG criteria, also recommends "a single-step procedure" to diagnose GDM, which the diabetes in pregnancy study group India (DIPSI) is following.[16]

A Single Test Procedure to Diagnose GDM in the Community (Diabetes in Pregnancy Study Group India)[17]

Note: DIPSI diagnostic criteria of 2-hour PG ≥140 mg/dL is similar to WHO criteria 2-hour PG ≥140 mg/dL to diagnose GDM.

"A single-step procedure" was developed due to the practical difficulty in performing glucose tolerance test in the fasting state, as seldom pregnant women visiting the antenatal clinic for the first time come in the fasting state. If they are asked to come on another day in the fasting state many of them do not return.[18] Hence, it is important to have a test that detects the glucose intolerance without the woman necessarily undergoing a test in the fasting state and it is preferable to perform the diagnostic test at the first visit itself.

Procedure

In the antenatal clinic, a pregnant woman after undergoing preliminary clinical examination has to be given a 75-g oral glucose load, irrespective of whether she is in the fasting or non-fasting state and without regard to the time of the last meal. A venous blood sample is collected at 2 hours for estimating PG by the GOD-POD method. GDM is diagnosed if 2-hour PG is ≥140 mg/dL (7.8 mmol/L). If 75-g glucose packet is not available, remove and discard five level teaspoons (not heaped) of glucose from a 100 g packet which is freely available. In hospitals where glucose is supplied in bulk, a cup or container of 75-g may be used. The glucose marketed is in anhydrous form.

Performing this test procedure in the non-fasting state is rational, as glucose concentrations are affected little by the time since the last meal in a normal glucose tolerant woman, whereas it will, in a woman with gestational diabetes.[19] After a meal, a normal glucose tolerant woman would be able to maintain euglycemia despite glucose challenge due to brisk and adequate insulin response, whereas, a woman with GDM who has impaired insulin secretion,[20] her glycemic level increases with a meal and with glucose challenge, the glycemic excursion exaggerates further.[21] This cascading effect is advantageous as this would not result in false-positive diagnosis of GDM.

Advantages of the DIPSI procedure are:

- Pregnant women need not be fasting.[15]
- Causes least disturbance in a pregnant woman's routine activities.
- Serves as both screening and diagnostic procedure. This single-step procedure has been approved by Ministry of Health, Government of India[22] and also recommended by the WHO.

PHYSIOLOGY OF PREGNANCY AND GLUCOSE METABOLISM AND INSULIN RESISTANCE IN GDM

Maternal and Fetal Adaptations in Pregnancy

A new structure arises de novo during pregnancy, develops and matures till it is expelled at the completion of the gestational period. The metabolic adaptations that occur during pregnancy are to accommodate a rapidly growing tissue transplant, the conceptus. For its own normal growth and development, the conceptus brings about alterations in maternal fuel metabolism and hormones. The placenta facilitates embryogenesis, growth, maturation and survival of the fetus. It has the capacity to synthesize steroid and peptide hormones and to modulate and transport maternal fuel to the fetus.

Fuel Metabolism in Normal Pregnancy

The fuel metabolism during normal (nondiabetic) pregnancy is characterized by:

- Facilitated insulin action during the first half of pregnancy and
- Diabetogenic stress during the second half of pregnancy.

Early Weeks of Gestation

In the early weeks of gestation certain hormonal changes occur:

- Increase in fasting insulin concentration.
- Increase in glucose stimulated insulin release (which reaches a peak at the 18th to 20th week).[23]
- Increase in serum levels of estrogen and progesterone. Progesterone is necessary for the implantation of embryo in the endometrium. Estrogen improves the insulin sensitivity as well as the β cell hyperplasia.

These hormonal changes result in an increased elaboration of insulin (hyperinsulinemia) and heightened sensitivity to insulin. Insulin, being an anabolic and anti-catabolic hormone favors the following:

- Tissue glycogen storage
- Prevents production of glucose from the liver
- Increases peripheral glucose utilization.

The net effect of these anabolic changes is a decrease in fasting blood glucose by 10% compared to non-pregnancy fasting level. The other reason for the decrease in the FPG is due to increase in plasma volume in early gestation and increase in feto placental glucose utilization (Table 1).

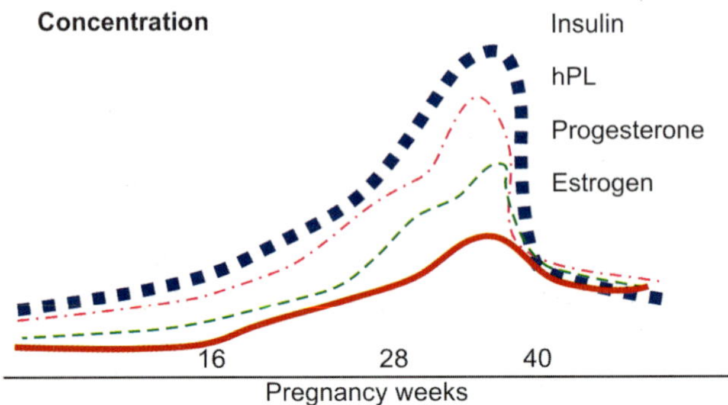

Fig. 1: Hormonal changes during normal pregnancy

Later Weeks of Gestation

During the later half of pregnancy, the facilitated insulin action continues and at the same time, there is an increased elaboration of placental chorionic somatomammotrophin (human placental lactogen, hPL), prolactin and cortisol. These surges in counter hormones result in insulin resistance and stress on the carbohydrate metabolism (diabetogenic stress) and due to this, maternal insulin sensitivity is reduced approximately by 50%.[24] Extra insulin compensates for the 50% reduction in the responsiveness of peripheral tissues to insulin action due to placental hormones (Fig. 1).

Table 1: Carbohydrate metabolism in early pregnancy (to 20 weeks)

Hormonal alteration	*Effect*	*Metabolic change*
↑ Estrogen and ↑ Progesterone ↓ Beta cell hyperplasia and ↑ Insulin secretion	↑ Tissue glycogen storage ↓ Hepatic glucose production ↑ Peripheral glucose utilization	Anabolic ↑ due to sex steroids + Hyperinsulinemia

Source: Adopted from Hollingsworth DR. Maternal metabolism in normal pregnancy and pregnancy complicated by diabetes mellitus. Clin Obstet Gynecol. 1985;28(3):457-72.

In a normal pregnant woman, first and second phase insulin response increases approximately threefold by the third trimester[25] and is associated with maternal B cell hypertrophy and hyperplasia.[26] Overall, the metabolic alterations under the influence of insulin and placental hormones facilitate anabolism during feeding and catabolism during fasting. As the pregnancy advances, the PG during fasting continues to be low, due to constant removal of glucose by the fetus since the fetus is a continually feeding boarder in an intermittently eating host, the mother. The lower level of FPG is also attributed to a fall in circulating amino acids particularly alanine which is needed for gluconeogenesis, a situation of "*substrate deficiency syndrome*". The fetus removes both glucose and amino acids from the maternal circulation, the former by facilitated diffusion and the latter by active transport. Hence during pregnancy, maternal nitrogen is conserved (for the fetal use) by sparing protein and relying as little as possible on proteins and carbohydrates as substrate. The maternal metabolism shifts rapidly to catabolism when exogenous fuel is not available, using fat as the fuel source. Placental hormones help in this metabolic shift by producing ketogenesis and a state of *"accelerated starvation". The metabolic changes which should normally occur after 72 hours of food deprivation in a nonpregnant state occur within 18 hours during pregnancy.*

Glucose and a variety of substrates act in a coordinated manner to regulate insulin and glucagon secretion. Normal alpha cell function serves to protect against hypoglycemia (aminogenic stimulation—gluconeogenesis) and to minimize prandial glucose excursions. During fed state, the levels of insulin and glucose are higher and more prolonged. Following a glucose load, glucagon is more readily suppressed during pregnancy than in the nonpregnant state. The combination of enhanced beta cell response (extra insulin) to glucose and preserved alpha cell response to amino acids leads to "facilitated anabolism" from "mixed meals": the "extra" insulin that is secreted in response to meal blunts the gluconeogenic potential of glucagon during the immediate postprandial hyperglycemia and so "spare" ingested amino acids for maternal or fetal access. Contrariwise, after disposal of the carbohydrate, the responsiveness of the alpha cell to the persistent hyperaminoacidemia could stimulate enough gluconeogenesis to prevent reactive hypoglycemia in the mother[27] (Table 2).

Table 2: Carbohydrate metabolism in late pregnancy (20–40 weeks)

Hormonal change	*Effect*	*Metabolic change*
↑ hCS	"Diabetogenic"	Facilitated anabolism during feeding
↑ Prolactin	↓ Glucose tolerance	Accelerated starvation during fasting
↑ Bound and free cortisol	↑ Insulin resistance	↓
	↓ Hepatic glycogen stores	Ensure glucose and amino acid to fetus
	↑ Hepatic glucose production	

Abbreviation: hCS, human chorionic somatomammotropin

In short, facilitated anabolism in the fed state and accelerated starvation in the fasted state characterize the maternal fuel adaptations during pregnancy. These hormonal and metabolic changes are geared toward facilitated anabolism under the actions of insulin throughout pregnancy. However, in the second half of the pregnancy, insulin resistance and diabetogenic stress due to placental hormones necessitate compensatory increased insulin secretion. Hence, the clinical expression of gestational diabetes occurs, where this compensation is inadequate, usually during the second half of pregnancy. Changes in maternal metabolism are given in the Box 2.

Box 2: Changes in maternal metabolism during normal pregnancy

- Decreased fasting plasma glucose level
- Increased postprandial plasma glucose level
- Increased fasting and postprandial plasma insulin levels
- Cell hypertrophy and hyperplasia
- Decreased insulin sensitivity (↑ Insulin resistance due to placental hormones)
- Enhanced lipolysis.

PATHOGENESIS OF GLUCOSE INTOLERANCE DEVELOPING DURING PREGNANCY

Genetic Factors

The relative importance of genetic factors has not yet been established. Increasing maternal age and obesity are significant contributing and compounding factors.

Gestational Factors

Islet Secretion

In gestational diabetes, during OGTT, the early insulin release is sluggish (Fig. 2). They have significantly lower insulin response at 30 and 60 minutes after oral glucose, compared with glucose tolerant controls. Due to this, as the pregnancy progresses the time to reach the maximum glucose concentration increases.

The mean time to reach the peak PG level is 55 minutes at 38 weeks of gestation compared to 34 minutes in the nonpregnant state.[23] There is no diminution in the biologic activity of circulating insulin and the alpha cell function in gestational diabetes.

Insulin Resistance and Hormones of Gestation

- In about 20% of gestational diabetics, the sluggish early insulin secretion cannot be demonstrated. It may be that in these individuals, there is an increased elaboration and/or

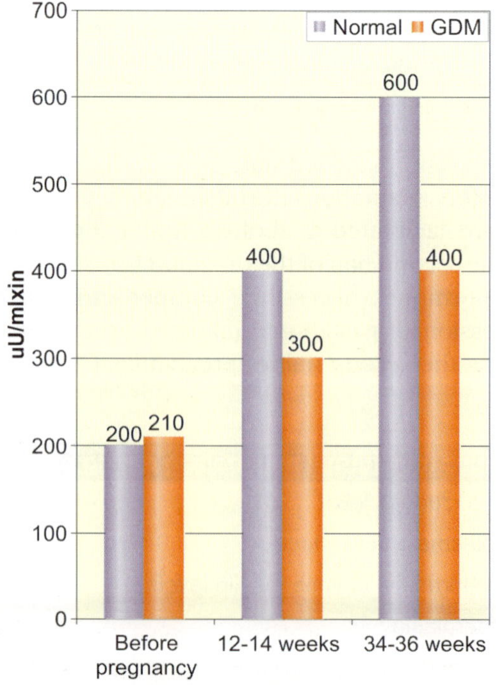

Fig. 2: First phase insulin response

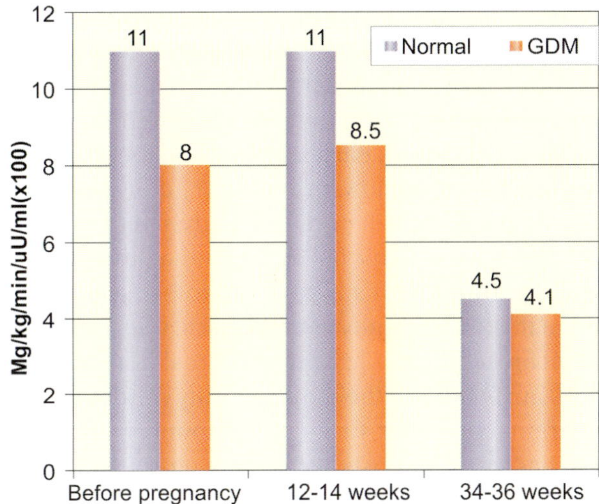

Fig 3: Insulin sensitivity

heightened sensitivity to one or more of the gestational counter hormones like hPL leading to decreased insulin sensitivity (Fig. 3).

- The postreceptor defects in the insulin signaling cascade appears to be a cause for the decreased insulin sensitivity in both pregnant women with normal glucose tolerance and gestational diabetes[28] compared to weight matched nonpregnant controls.
- Insulin receptor substrate (IRS-1) expression is decreased in all pregnant women compared to nonpregnant controls. The downregulation of IRS-1 protein parallels the decreased ability of insulin in inducing further steps in insulin signaling cascade. The factors affecting IRS-1 function in the signaling cascade is due to cytokine tumor necrosis factor-α.[29]
- In other words the pathophysiology of gestational diabetes has been related to excessive insulin antagonism by the pregnancy contra-insulin factors. When maternal insulinogenic compensation is inadequate to offset these factors, gestational diabetes will supervene.
- Further when gestational diabetics who had reverted to normal glucose tolerance following delivery and women with normal glucose tolerance during pregnancy were given prednisolone or hPL in the postpartum period and challenged with oral glucose load (OGTT), the former failed to increase plasma insulin levels above those in the latter, despite greater hyperglycemia. Thus the decreased beta cell function that occurs in GDM women may be the indication for the future susceptibility to diabetes.[30,31]

GDM AND ITS PREVENTION

Medical Nutrition Therapy

All women with GDM should receive nutritional counseling. The meal pattern should provide adequate calories and nutrients to meet the needs of pregnancy. The expected weight gain during pregnancy is 300–400 g/week and total weight gain is 10–12 kg by term. Hence the meal plan aims to provide sufficient calories to sustain adequate nutrition for the mother and fetus and to avoid excess weight gain and postprandial hyperglycemia. Calorie requirement depends on age, activity, prepregnancy weight and stage of pregnancy. Approximately 30–40 kcal/kg ideal body weight or an increment of 300 kcal/day above the basal requirement is needed (Table 3). Pregnancy is not the ideal time for obesity correction. Underweight subjects or those not gaining weight as expected, particularly in the third trimester, require admission to ensure adequate nutrition to prevent low birth weight infants.

As a part of the MNT, pregnant diabetic woman are advised to wisely distribute their calorie consumption especially the breakfast. This implies splitting the usual breakfast into two equal halves and consuming the portions with a 2-hour gap in between. By this the undue peak in PG levels after ingestion of the total quantity of breakfast at one time is avoided. For example, if four *idlis/chapthi*/slices of bread (applies to all type of breakfast menu) is taken for breakfast at 8 am and 2 hours PG at 10 am is 140 mg: the same quantity divided into two equal portions, i.e. one portion at 8 am and remaining after 10 am, the 2 hours postprandial PG at 10.00 am falls by 20–30 mg. This advice has scientific basis as the peaking of PG is high with breakfast (due to dawn phenomenon) than with lunch and dinner. Further in a normal person, insulin secretion is also high with breakfast than with lunch or dinner.[32] GDM mothers have deficiency in first phase insulin secretion and to match this insulin deficiency the challenge of quantity of food at one time should also be less.

Table 3: Dietary allowances for women 25–50 years of age

Constituent	*Nonpregnant*	*Pregnant*	*Increase*
Protein (g)	50	60	10
Average (kcal)*	2,200	2,500	300
Vitamin C (mg)	60	70	10
Vitamin B6 (mg)	1.6	2.2	0.6
Folate (µg)	180	400	220
Calcium (mg)	800	1,200	400
Magnesium (mg)	280	320	40
Iron (mg)	15	30	15
Zinc (mg)	12	15	3

* Additional calories are needed during the second and third trimesters only

Source: Adapted from American Diabetes Association: Nutritional management during pregnancy in preexisting diabetes. In: Jovanovic-Peterson L (Ed). Medical Management of Pregnancy Complicated by Diabetes. Alexandria, VA: American Diabetes Association; 1993. pp 47-56.

Insulin Treatment

Insulin is essential if MNT fails to achieve euglycemia. In normal (nondiabetic) pregnancy, the FPG concentration ranges between 55 and 70 mg/dl, the 1-hour postprandial glucose level is <120 mg/dL.[33]

Various criteria have been proposed for the initiation of insulin therapy (Table 4). To interpret these values, one must take into account the following:

- The relationship between plasma and whole blood glucose concentrations,

Table 4: Criteria recommended for the initiation of insulin therapy in women with gestational diabetes

*Fasting**	*Postprandial**	*Reference*
105†	None	Metzger
>95	2-hour >120	Langer et al.
>100	1-hour >130	Ramus and Kitzmiller
>90	1-hour >120	Jovanovic-Peterson

* Glucose concentrations (mg/dL) measured in finger-stick whole blood samples unless designated otherwise.

† Venous plasma sample.

- The site of sampling
- Whether the value is a fasting or a postprandial one.

It is enough to realize that a plasma value is approximately 12% higher than a whole blood value. A finger-stick yields arterialized blood, which does not influence the fasting glucose concentration because in the fasting state there is little glucose uptake by muscle tissue. After eating, however, muscle glucose utilization becomes a factor. Measurement of glucose concentrations in blood samples obtained by a finger-stick yields higher values than if a venous sample had been obtained. This is because the arterialized blood has not yet traversed muscle and hence glucose removal by this tissue has not occurred.

If the FPG concentration on the OGTT is ≥120 mg/dL, then the patient is started on insulin immediately along with meal plan. Other GDM women are seen within 3 days and are also taught self-monitoring of blood glucose (SMBG). SMBG is to be performed before breakfast and 2 hours after each meal. GDM women usually have high post-breakfast PG level compared to post-lunch and post-dinner. A few GDM women do have post-dinner PG also high. Insulin is started within 1–2 weeks, if the majority (i.e. at least 4 of 7 per week) of fasting values exceeds 90 mg/dL. Similarly, if the majority of postprandial values after a particular meal exceed 120 mg/dL, insulin is started. Pen injectors are very useful and the patient's acceptance is excellent.

The initial dose of NPH insulin could be as low as 4 units and the dose of insulin can be adjusted on follow up (Flow chart 1). A few GDM patients may require combination of short-acting insulin and intermediate-acting insulin in the morning and evening.

- If a patient has elevated prelunch blood sugar, regular insulin is usually necessary in the morning to handle the post-breakfast hyperglycemia, as there is a lag period before the intermediate-acting insulin begins to work. The above regimen of regular- and intermediate-acting insulin in the morning controls hyperglycemia in most cases.
- If the post-dinner blood sugar is high, a small dose of regular insulin is necessary before dinner in addition to the regular- and intermediate-acting insulin given in the morning.
- Combination of regular and intermediate-acting insulin before dinner may be necessary if fasting blood sugar is high. This combination of short- and intermediate-acting insulin in the morning and as well as in the evening is known as mixed and split dose of insulin regimen. In this regimen two-thirds of the total daily dose of insulin is given in the morning and one-third in the evening. For each combination, one-third dose should be regular insulin and two-third intermediate-acting insulin. With this regimen if the patient continues to have fasting hyperglycemia, the intermediate-acting insulin has to be given at bedtime instead of before dinner. Insulin dose is individualized.

Flow chart 1: Algorithm for insulin initiation

1. Preferable to start with Premix insulin 30/70 of any brand*
Starting dose: 4 units before breakfast

↓

Every 4th day increase 2 units till 10 units

↓

If FPG remains > 90 mg/dL advise → 6 units before breakfast and 4 units before dinner

↓

Review with blood sugar test → Adjust dose further

↓

Total insulin dose per day can be divided as two-third in the morning and one-third in the evening

↓

2. If GDM is diagnosed in the third trimester; MNT is advised for a week. Insulin is initiated if MNT fails

↓

3. If 2-hour PG > 200 mg/dL at diagnosis, a starting dose of 8 units of premixed insulin could be administered straightaway before breakfast and the dose has to be titrated on follow-up. Along with insulin therapy, MNT is also advised.

***Abbreviations*:** GDM, gestational diabetes mellitus; MNT, medical nutrition therapy
*Initially if post-breakfast plasma glucose is high → Start Premix 50/50

Ultrasound Fetal Measurement

GDM management based on fetal growth combined with glycemic criteria provides outcomes equivalent to management based on strict glycemic criteria alone. Inclusion of fetal growth might provide the opportunity to reduce glucose testing in low-risk pregnancies.[34]

Target Blood Glucose Levels

Maintenance of mean blood glucose level around 105 mg% is ideal for good fetal outcome.[35] A study by Karlson and Kjellman from Sweden showed that perinatal mortality is proportional to maternal blood glucose level during the last weeks of pregnancy[36] (Table 5).

Table 5: Target of blood glucose level

Mean glucose level	*Perinatal mortality*
>150 mg%	24%
100–150 mg%	15%
<100 mg%	4%

Hesitancy to start insulin treatment may be due to misconception that insulin administration may produce hypoglycemia in the newborn. Contrary to this belief, the maintenance of mean PG around 105 mg% would protect the newborn from hypoglycemia (fasting 85 ± 5 mg% and 2-hour post-meal 115 ± 5 mg%) (Table 6). When this is not achieved, excess glucose crosses the placenta and stresses the fetal beta cells which respond by increased elaboration of insulin. As long as fetus is in the uterine compartment, it has enough fuel to maintain its blood glucose level. When the fetus is expelled at the termination of pregnancy, the super charged beta cells of the neonate continue to secrete insulin but there is no fuel supply from the maternal compartment and the newborn develops hypoglycemia. On the contrary, if PG of the mother had been maintained at the acceptable level with diet and insulin, an excess flow of glucose from maternal to fetal compartment cannot occur and thereby the fetal beta cells are not stimulated and the newborn of this mother would not develop hypoglycemia. The fact that maternal hypoglycemia does not jeopardize fetal outcome, is very well brought out by a study done in Düsseldorf, Germany. Out of seventy-seven pregnant women with type 1 diabetes mellitus (T1DM), 32 had 94 episodes of severe hypoglycemia with loss of consciousness requiring hospital admission in some. There was no difference in fetal outcome between those mothers who had severe hypoglycemia and those who did not. *Nevertheless all efforts should be taken to avoid hypoglycemia in the pregnant mother.*

To summarize, neonatal hypoglycemia is due to poor control of diabetes in the mother, rather than the amount of insulin taken by the mother.

Insulin

Human insulin is being extensively used during pregnancy, but due to the pharmacokinetic action of this insulin a considerable segment of pregnant women with diabetes fails to achieve optimum glycemic control, mostly the postprandial PG. In them the best option is to administer ultra-short acting analogs, insulin lispro (Humalog) or insulin Aspart (Novo rapid). These analogs improve the postprandial glucose in pregnant women with both T1DM and T2DM and are safe and effective.[37,38] Insulin Aspart has received further approval in the EU for the use in pregnancy. This approval follows results of the largest ever randomized controlled trial of modern insulin in pregnant women with diabetes. Novo rapid significantly improves first and third trimester postprandial glycemic control compared to human insulin for the both mother and the child in terms of (a) fewer preterm deliveries, (b) reduced risk of neonatal hypoglycemia requiring treatment, (c) consistently lower rates of major hypoglycemia (24 hr, nocturnal and daytime), (d) reduced risks to the fetus, with outcomes at least comparable to human insulin.[39]

Oral Antidiabetic Drugs

Sometimes a hitherto undiagnosed type 2 diabetic woman may progress through the early weeks of gestation at the risk of malformation in her offspring or a known type 2 diabetic woman who is already on oral hypoglycemic agent may present to antenatal clinic after conception and at times in second or third trimester of pregnancy. The best course at this juncture is to withdraw oral hypoglycemic agents and introduce insulin. Though oral antidiabetic drugs are not recommended, the outcome in diabetic women who have conceived and continued to be on oral antidiabetic drugs is not gloomy, since many workers have used these drugs successfully in pregnant diabetics.[40] Recently reports have shown good fetal outcome in GDM women who were on glyburide (micronized form of glibenclamide). A randomized unblinded clinical trial compared the use of insulin and glyburide in women with GDM who were not able to meet glycemic goals on meal plan. Treatment with either agent resulted in similar perinatal outcomes. All these patients were beyond the first trimester of pregnancy at the initiation of therapy.[41]

A few more studies are required before routinely recommending glyburide during pregnancy especially during the first trimester itself. Metformin has been found to be useful in women with polycystic ovarian disease who failed to conceive. Continuing this drug after conception is still a controversy. But there are a few studies favoring continuation of metformin throughout pregnancy.[42]

Table 6: Target plasma glucose levels

Fasting plasma glucose	*Postprandial plasma glucose*	*Mean plasma glucose level*
80 mg% ↕ 90 mg%	110 mg% ↕ 120 mg%	95 mg% ↕ 105 mg%

Monitoring Glycemic Control

The success of the treatment during GDM depends on the glycemic control maintained with meal plan or pharmacological intervention. To know the effectiveness of treatment, monitoring of glycemic control is essential.

The glycemic control maintained with meal plan or pharmacological intervention. Studies suggest 1-, 1.5- and 2-hour post-meal for monitoring glycemic control.[43] 2-hour post-meal monitoring is preferred as the diagnosis of GDM is also based on 2-hour PG. It is easier to remember this timing, as the time for diagnosis and also for monitoring is the same, i.e. 2 hours. However, whichever time is targeted for monitoring glycemic control and adjusting insulin dose, blood tests must be performed at the same time at each visit. They should be advised to perform SMBG on a daily basis, failing which, at least weekly monitoring should be encouraged. If self-monitoring is not possible, laboratory venous PG has to be estimated for adjusting the dose of insulin.

For women with T1DM and T2DM who are already on treatment, intensive monitoring is required from the day 1 of conception. They will have to do SMBG or get the levels checked at a laboratory at least once a week to adjust the dosage of insulin.

- Once target blood glucose is achieved, woman with GDM till the 28th week of gestation require monitoring of both fasting and 2 hours post-breakfast once a month and at other time of the day as the clinician decides.
- After the 28th week of gestation, the monitoring should be more frequent at least once in 2 weeks, if need be more frequently.
- After 32 weeks of gestation, monitoring should be done once a week till delivery.
- In high-risk pregnancies, frequency of monitoring may be intensified with SMBG.
- Continuous glucose monitoring devices are available but these equipment need special training and further are expensive. These devices may be useful in high-risk pregnancies to know the glycemic fluctuations and to plan proper insulin dosage.

Measuring Other Parameters

It is rewarding if blood pressure is monitored during every visit along with examination of the fundus and estimation of microalbuminuria, every trimester.

A1c Levels

If the glucose intolerance is detected in the early pregnancy, A1c level will be helpful to differentiate between a pre-GDM and GDM. If the A1c level is more than 6%, she is likely to be a pre-GDM. A1c is useful in monitoring the glucose control during pregnancy, but not for the day-to-day management. A1c level may serve as a prognostic value.

MANAGEMENT OF DIABETES IN PREGNANCY

Pre-gestational Type 1 and Type 2 Diabetic Women

The congenital malformation remains the leading cause of mortality and serious morbidity in infants of mother with T1DM or T2DM, in spite of advancement in understanding pregnancy metabolism and treatment. Studies have established association between elevated maternal glucose during embryogenesis and high rates of spontaneous abortions and major malformations in newborn. Clinical trials also have established preconception care to achieve tight glycemic control during first trimester have resulted in striking reductions in malformations. Unfortunately unplanned pregnancy occurs in a considerable number of women with diabetes resulting in fetal mortality and morbidity.

The perinatal morbidity attributable to conditions such as macrosomia and metabolic disorders remain relatively high in women who develop glucose intolerance of any degree with onset or first recognized during pregnancy (gestational diabetes mellitus). Yet another observation was that in pregnant women with one elevated blood glucose during formal glucose tolerance test has abnormal glucose values under continuous ambulatory glucose monitoring.[44] These elevated ambulatory glucose values were significantly correlated with fetal macrosomia. Thus the fetus of pre-gestational diabetic women, gestational diabetic women or women with any degree of abnormal glucose tolerance during pregnancy is at risk of developing either congenital malformation or morbidity in the form of macrosomia.

To minimize the occurrence of lethal malformations, pre-gestational counseling is essential. The pregnant women with diabetes need standard care throughout pregnancy. The goal for glycemic management in the preconception period and during the first trimester should be to obtain the lowest A1c test level possible without undue risk of hypoglycemia in the would be mother.

Practical self-management skills are essential for attaining good glycemic control in preparation for pregnancy and during pregnancy.

- Use of appropriate meal plan
- Self-monitoring of blood glucose
- Self-administration of insulin and adjustment of insulin doses
- Treatment of hypoglycemia (patient and family members)
- Incorporate safe physical activity
- Development of techniques to reduce stress and cope with the denial.

All these measures are applicable in women with gestational diabetes also.

Insulin Requirement in Pre-GDM

If appropriate prepregnancy counseling has occurred and near euglycemia had been achieved before conception and if the prepregnancy insulin regimen incorporates two or more insulin injections a day, it may be suitable to achieve the near euglycemia necessary for a successful outcome of the pregnancy.

- NPH insulin given before dinner has the likelihood of producing overnight hypoglycemia if the dose is increased to control the next morning's fasting value (even though the patient eats a bedtime snack). This happens because the peak action of the intermediate-acting insulin occurs during the middle of the night.
- Moving the pre-dinner NPH insulin to bedtime shifts the time of peak action toward early morning and minimizes the possibility of overnight hypoglycemia.
- Injecting NPH insulin in the morning, however, limits a patient's flexibility in regard to eating and exercise patterns. Unanticipated changes are more difficult to deal with because once the intermediate-acting insulin is given, it exerts its preordained effect for many hours.
- In a few pregnant women, a split/mixed regimen (NPH and regular or insulin analogs) given in the morning and evening may achieve good glycemic control.
- Using three injections of regular human insulin or rapid-acting insulin analogs (Humalog/ Novorapid) with each meal gives a patient more flexibility with regard to eating and exercise.
- Preprandial regular- or rapid-acting insulin analogs can be particularly helpful during the first trimester, when nausea and anorexia (morning sickness) are common.
- Controlling the FPG concentration requires pre-dinner or bedtime NPH insulin.

Regular insulin is usually given half hour before a meal because it does not start to work until approximately 30 minutes after injection. On the other hand, the new rapid-acting insulin analogs administered with meal, starts to act within 10-15 minutes, hence they are much more effective in controlling the postprandial peaks.

Adjusting insulin doses is simpler with SMBG four times a day because each component of the insulin regimen affects only one SMBG value. Monitoring before meal and 2 hours after a meal is recommended as the postprandial peak in diabetic pregnancies occurs at approximately 90 minutes after meals.[45] Most high-risk and precious pregnancies may require frequent SMBG to find out the fluctuations in levels and adjust the dose of insulin accordingly. Continuous glucose monitoring system and the GlucoWatch are useful in this regard.

In a pre-gestational type 1 diabetic woman, the requirement of insulin may fall during the early part of first trimester due to increased insulin sensitivity. Insulin requirement increases during later half of pregnancy because of the increased concentration of circulating contra-insulin placental hormones. Constant insulin adjustment is necessary to keep up with the increasing insulin requirement of pregnancy (Fig. 4).

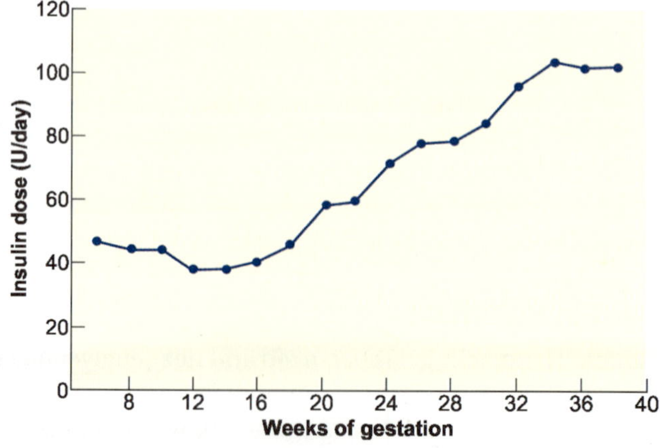

Fig. 4: Usual changes in insulin requirements in a patient with T1DM

The insulin dose is increased from 0.7 U/kg/day in the first trimester to 0.8 U/kg/day at week 18, 0.9 U/kg/day at week 26 and 1.0 U/kg/day at week 36 in women who maintained within 15% of ideal body weight. The insulin doses vary from person to person though the weight is almost the same. In a study of 11 patients who were markedly obese at the start of pregnancy, 6 required 1.2 U/kg/day at term, 3 required 2 U/kg/day at term and 2 required 3 U/kg/day at term.

Further *T2DM patients* require significantly higher dose of insulin during each trimester compared to T1DM. During first trimester no difference was found between T1DM and T2DM subjects. During the second trimester, a significant increase in insulin requirement was observed. (10% increase for patients with T1DM compared with 33% for those with T2DM). In the third trimester a 40% increase was found for women with T2DM (Fig. 5). This has been attributed to increased body mass and heightened insulin resistance in type 2 diabetic women during pregnancy.[46]

Rarely pre-gestational type 2 diabetic women may require a very high dose of insulin even up to 200 units/day given in divided doses. It is appropriate to use the dose needed to achieve near normoglycemic level without giving undue concern about giving too much insulin to the patient. *The main concern should be blood glucose results rather than the dose of insulin.*[47] Failure to require increased insulin dose as pregnancy advances reflects poor placental growth, intrauterine growth retardation and impending intrauterine death. This situation requires close coordination with obstetrician. A few pregnant women may require less insulin in the last week of pregnancy attributed to fetal handling of maternal glucose due to hypertrophic fetal beta cells. At approximately 36 weeks, placental growth ceases and contra-insulin hormone production plateaus. Thus insulin requirement may decline.

OBSTETRIC CONSIDERATIONS

Sudden intrauterine fetal demise in the third trimester of diabetic pregnancy is not uncommon. To avoid this risk, preterm delivery is recommended. But with this, respiratory distress syndrome is likely to occur. Administering steroids for lung maturity or β-adrenoreceptor agonist to inhibit premature uterine contractions are likely to induce adverse metabolic effects due to their glycolytic, glycogenolytic and lipolytic effects. In this situation, extra insulin may

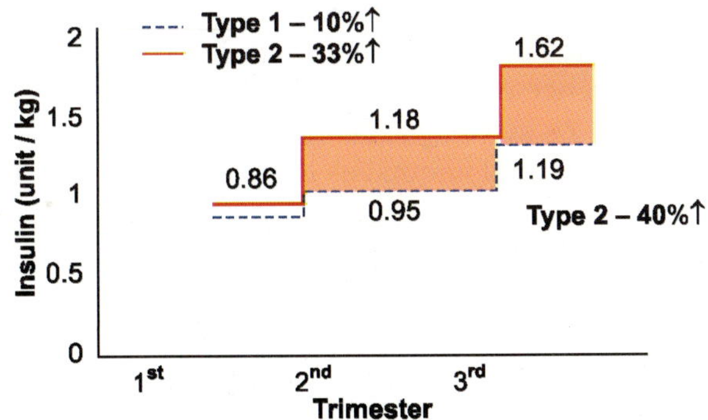

Fig. 5: Insulin requirement in T1DM and T2DM women during pregnancy

be required to maintain euglycemia. Fetal demise can also occur due to preeclampsia, which can produce fetal hypoxia via decreased uteroplacental perfusion. The recent advances in techniques for detecting fetal wellbeing are given in the Table 7. Some centers allow women with uncomplicated diabetes to go into spontaneous labor irrespective of the gestational age, *but most still advocate delivery at 38 weeks* as perinatal mortality and morbidity appear to increase after this time. Induction at 38 weeks gestation may be slow or unsuccessful due to unfavorable conditions of the cervix but this has to be balanced against the poorly defined and predictable risk of late intrauterine death if pregnancy is allowed to continue more than 38 weeks. Fetal health may deteriorate suddenly, hence obstetric management should not be rigid and each case needs individual care and attention. Having a neonatologist support at the time of delivery is advisable.

Table 7: Obstetrical management procedures

Procedure	***Risk based on glycemic control, vascular disease***	
	Low risk	***High risk***
Dating ultrasound	8–12 weeks	8–12 weeks
Prenatal genetic diagnosis	As needed	As needed
Targeted perinatal ultrasound: fetal echocardiography	18–22 weeks	18–22 weeks
Fetal kick counts	28 weeks	28 weeks
Ultrasound for fetal growth	28 and 37 weeks	Monthly
Antepartum FHR monitoring, backup c biophysical profile	36 weeks, weekly	27 weeks, 1–3/week
Amniocentesis for lung maturity	—	35–38 weeks
Induction of labor	41 weeks[1]	35–38 weeks

[1]Earlier for obstetrical reasons or for impending fetal macrosomia

Abbreviation: FHR, fetal heart rate

FETAL EVALUATION

An ultrasound scan has to be performed around 18–20 weeks of gestation focusing on structures namely the spine, skull, kidney and heart. Fetal echocardiography has to be done around 20–24 weeks which allows to view all the four chambers of the heart. From 26th week onwards, fetal growth and liquor volume has to be monitored every 2–3 weeks.

Fetal abdominal circumference provides baseline for further serial measurements which gives growth acceleration or restriction. Fetal movements are monitored from 20 weeks onwards. Screening for chromosomal anomalies is necessary in pre-GDM. Screening should be done for Down syndrome, alpha-fetoprotein for neural defects and human chorionic gonadotropin to identify any chromosomal abnormalities.

Mid-pregnancy (16–20 Weeks) to Detect Fetal Anomalies

- Maternal serum alpha-fetoprotein
- Screening for chromosomal anomalies

- Ultrasonography
- Fetal echocardiography.

Late Pregnancy (28 week to delivery) to Assess Fetal Wellbeing

- Maternal assessment of fetal activity (<4/hr indicate fetal jeopardy)
- Non-stress test
- Contraction stress test
- Fetal biophysical profile
- Ultrasonography
- Lecithin-to-sphingomyelin (L/S) ratio (>3.0), lung profile.

INTRAPARTUM DIABETIC MANAGEMENT

Metabolic studies of nondiabetic pregnant women during labor revealed that glucose turnover increased fourfold with little change in insulin levels.[42] This strongly suggests that muscle contractions (probably both uterine and skeletal) independent of insulin are the predominant determinant of glucose utilization during labor. During active labor, the insulin requirement was zero while glucose requirements were relatively constant at 2.6 mg/kg/min or approximately 10 g/h in a 60 kg woman.[48] The following approach is suggested for treating an *insulin requiring woman with pre-gestational diabetes* as she progresses through labor and delivery.

- If labor is to be induced, induction should start in the morning.
- The usual dose of evening NPH insulin is taken, but no subcutaneous morning insulin is given.
- The goal is to maintain the PG between 90 mg/dL and 100 mg/dL (95 ± 5 mg/dL). Most labor and delivery units have the ability to measure finger-stick glucose concentrations, and this should be done every hour.
- If labor is to be induced, intravenous saline is used as the medium until active labor begins.
- If the initial PG is <70 mg/dL, 5% dextrose is infused at 100 mL/h until the glucose level is in the appropriate range. The IV fluids and insulin dose to be given on monitoring the blood glucose level is given in the Table 8.
- When active labor begins, the same insulin infusion rate described earlier is used, depending on the glucose concentration at this time as well.
- Most often in known diabetics, the dose of insulin required is highly individualized and has to be adjusted by monitoring blood glucose.

In contrast, a *woman with GDM* does not require insulin once labor begins.

- If labor is to be induced in GDM, the usual evening NPH insulin should be taken the night before, but no subcutaneous insulin is given the following morning when induction begins and to follow the guidelines given in the Table 8.
- In a gestational diabetic, the requirement of insulin is likely to fall precipitously and no insulin may be required immediately after expulsion of placenta.

Table 8: Plasma glucose and insulin IV fluid

Plasma glucose	*Insulin/IV fluids*
<70 mg/dL	5% GNS 100 mL/hr
90–120 mg/dL	NS 100 mL/hr
120–140 mg/dL	NS 100 mL/hr plus 4 units of regular insulin added with IV fluid
140–180 mg/dL	NS 100 mL/hr plus 6 units of regular insulin added with IV fluid
>180 mg/dL	NS 100 mL/hr plus 8 units of regular insulin added with IV fluid

Abbreviation: NS, normal saline

PREEXISTING METABOLIC DISORDERS AND DIABETES IN PLANNING OF PREGNANCY AND ITS MANAGEMENT

Consequences of Diabetes on the Fetus

Consequences of the changes in fuel metabolism during pregnancy on the fetal development revolve around "maternal hyperglycemia and fetal hyperinsulinemia" (Fig. 6).

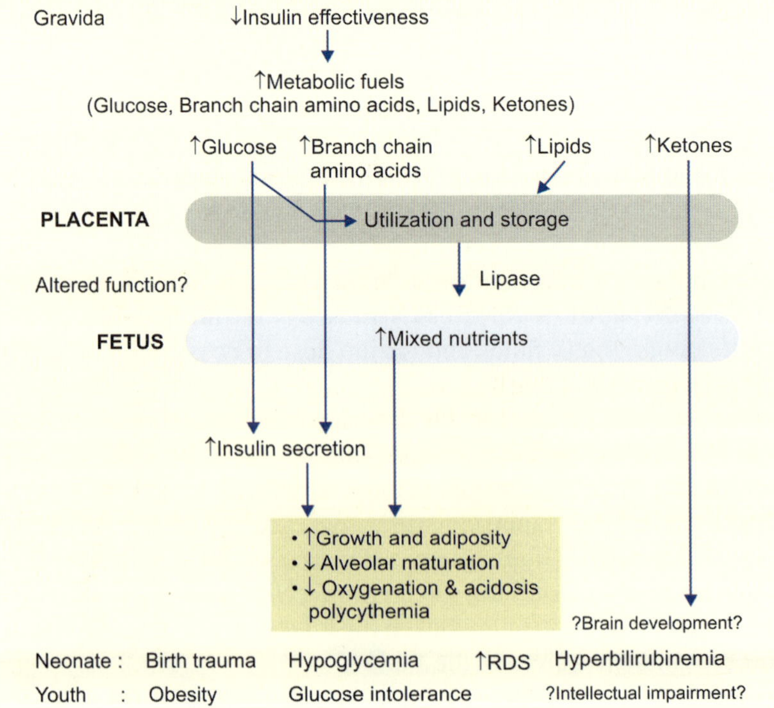

Fig. 6: Model of maternal gestational diabetes, fetal hyperinsulinemia and infant outcome (Modified Pedersen Hypothesis)

Pregnancy is considered as a tissue culture experiment[49] implicating that placenta and fetus develop in an incubation medium that is totally derived from maternal fuels[50] consisting of glucose, amino acids and lipids. The glucose traverses the placenta by facilitated diffusion and amino acids by active transport and enters the fetal circulation (Fig. 7). The recent concept is that the placental glucose transport is dependent on the glucose transporter (GLUT) family and GLUT-1 is the principal transporter which is located in the syncytiotrophoblast.[51] GLUT-1 is present both on the microvillus and basal membranes. With the advancing gestation, there is a twofold to threefold increase in the expression of syncytiotrophoblast glucose transportation.[52] The role of GLUT-3 and GLUT-4 remains speculative. Amino acids are actively transported across the concentration gradient from the mother to fetus and placenta via energy requiring amino acid transporters. These processes are regulated by insulin and hence any disturbance in the secretion and action of insulin will influence the whole nutrient composition to which fetus is exposed and may lead to fetal hyperinsulinemia. The abnormal mixture of maternal nutrients gain access to the developing fetus and modify phenotype gene expression in newly forming cells and thereby causing permanent short- and long-term effects in the offsprings. Accordingly the fetal and neonatal complications occur when the fetus is exposed to the abnormal fuel mixture during different periods of gestation (Table 9).

First Trimester

In the first trimester, the exposure to abnormal mixed nutrients during organogenesis (first 6–8 weeks of gestation) may cause spontaneous miscarriage, intrauterine growth retardation and malformations (Table 10).

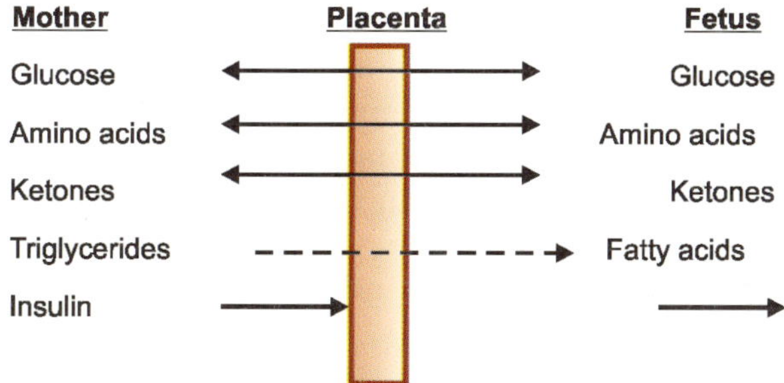

Fig. 7: Schematic representation of maternal–fetal nutrient transport in humans

Table 9: Fetal problems associated with maternal hyperglycemia by trimester

First trimester	*Second trimester*	*Third trimester*
Malformations	Hypertrophic cardiomyopathy	Hypoglycemia
Growth retardation	Polyhydramnios	Hypocalcemia
Fetal wastage	Erythemia	Hyperbilirubinemia
	Placental insufficiency	Respiratory distress syndrome
	Preeclampsia	Macrosomia
	Fetal loss	Hypomagnesemia
	Low IQ	Intrauterine death

Table 10: Types and timing of malformations in infants of diabetic mothers

Type of anomaly		*Timing of lesion (Weeks postconception)*
Skeletal	Caudal regression	3
	Spina bifida	6
Neural	Hydrocephalus	4
	Anencephaly	4
	Myelocele	5
Cardiovascular	Dextrocardia	4
	Conus arteriosus defects	5
	Ventricular septal defects	6
Renal	Renal agenesis/hypoplasia	6

Studies have shown that the maternal metabolic abnormalities are the most important cause for the increased risk of malformations in diabetic pregnancies. The mechanisms suggested for the teratogenic effect in the early postimplantation stage of the embryo are:

- Disruption of normal functioning of the yolk sac which regulates nutrient transport from maternal plasma to embryo during early neural tube development
- Diffusion of intracellular myoinositol with resultant disruption of arachidonic acid and prostaglandin metabolism
- Oxidative metabolism and generation of free oxygen radicals that may be toxic to the embryos, and
- Glucose induced mutations in embryonic DNA.

If this fuel mediated teratogenesis is to be avoided, then excellent control of maternal metabolism must commence before conception and must be maintained during the first 8 weeks, a critical period when many women may not be aware that they are pregnant. Preventive medicine necessarily starts before conception reflecting the importance of prepregnancy counseling. Supplementation with folic acid dose (0.4 mg), myoinositol and antioxidants may play a role in the prevention of malformations and lower the ratio from 7.5% to 0.8%.[53]

Second Trimester

- The formation and the development of brain cells take place in the second trimester. Hyperglycemia during this trimester alters the behavioral, intellectual and psychological pattern in childhood.[54,55]
- Insulin is detectable in the fetal pancreas as early as 9th week after conception. Beta cell growth and replication are regulated by nutritional insulin secretagogues such as glucose, mannose and essential amino acids.[56]
  - Human studies have shown an increase in pancreatic fetal cell mass and insulin secretion in fetuses of poorly controlled diabetic women of 16th week of gestation and both these abnormalities increase throughout second trimester until 26th week of gestation.[57]
  - This priming of beta cell in mid-gestation may account for the persistence of fetal hyperinsulinemia throughout the pregnancy and the risk of accelerated fetal growth even when mother achieves a good metabolic control in later pregnancy.[58]

Third Trimester

- Maternal hyperglycemia in the third trimester causes proliferation of fetal adipocytes, muscle cells and pancreatic beta cells and neuroendocrine systems and they form the base for macrosomia and for the development of obesity, IGT and T2DM in later life.[59]
- Stillbirth in diabetic pregnancies is still unexplained, although both maternal hyperglycemia and fetal macrosomia are associated.[36]
- *Mechanisms implicated are fetal hypoxia, acidosis, hypokalemia leading to dysrhythmias and placental dysfunction and competition for essential nutrients.*[60]
- In an unexplained stillbirth, the possibility of undiagnosed GDM must be considered and at autopsy the fetus may have islet cell hyperplasia (in the absence of rhesus problem) and increased interstitial tissue in the testis or luteinization of the theca interna of the ovary.

NEONATAL COMPLICATIONS

Hypoglycemia

Due to the endogenous hyperinsulinemia and suppression of endogenous glucose production, the infant of the diabetic mother is at increased risk of hypoglycemia at 1–3 hours after birth. About 50% of the hypoglycemic babies may remain asymptomatic. Twitching of the limbs, hypotonia, tachypnea and rarely seizures in severe hypoglycemia are the clinical presentations. Hypoglycemia is defined as blood sugar level less than 44 mg/dL in any infant regardless of gestational age. Once hypoglycemia is confirmed, IV glucose as an initial bolus of 200 mg/kg must be given and is followed by a continuous glucose infusion at 8 mg/kg/mt. The factor mainly protective against fetal hypoglycemia is the optimal control of maternal hyperglycemia especially during the third trimester and during labor. It has been shown that a mean maternal PG >105 mg/dL during the last 4 hours of labor in a diabetic mother leads to a higher incidence of neonatal hypoglycemia.[61]

Hypocalcemia

About 25% of the infant of the diabetic mothers may present with serum calcium of <7 mg/dL and this may remain mostly asymptomatic and is usually detectable during the 2nd or 3rd day of the birth. Asphyxia and prematurity, operating through elevated cortisol, induces vitamin D antagonism at the intestinal level. Respiratory distress and fetal metabolic acidosis may result in calcium being shifted from intracellular to extracellular pools and reversal of this shift during correction of the acidotic event may produce hypocalcemia. Hypomagnesemia may coexist and may require correction.

Respiratory Distress Syndrome

Respiratory distress syndrome is observed in about 5% of infants of diabetic mothers. In vitro studies indicate that insulin antagonizes the stimulatory effects of cortisol on fibroblasts to induce the synthesis of fibroblast-pneumocyte factor, which in turn inhibits type II cells and phosphatidyl choline production.

Measurement of phosphatidyl glycerol alone or in combination with the lecithin phosphatidyl choline may be a more reliable indicator of lung maturity in diabetic pregnancies than the L/S ratio alone.

- Prophylactic steroids to accelerate the lung maturity may be indicated if the L/S ratio is less than 2:1.
- Such obstetric situations, requiring steroids or beta sympathomimetics drugs (e.g. salbutamol) may worsen the diabetic control and calls for frequent monitoring of blood sugar and correction with soluble insulin.

Polycythemia

It is relatively common in infants of diabetic mothers. This is mostly due to the hypoxic stimulus by the placental insufficiency and elevated glycohemoglobin. Over transfusion from the large placenta of diabetic pregnancy may also contribute. The resultant hyperviscosity may induce congestive heart failure and vascular thrombosis accounting for the increased risk of renal vein thrombosis in these infants.

Hyperbilirubinemia

This common abnormality is due to increased bilirubin production and decreased lifespan of the RBCs with glycosylated cell membranes. Hepatic conjugation of bilirubin may be impaired due to an immature liver.

Macrosomia

Neonates weighing more than 4 kg are considered to be macrosomic. *The Indian consensus is that newborn baby's weight ≥3.5 kg should be considered as macrosomia*[62] Macrosomic babies have considerable greater shoulder/head and chest/head differences and are prone to shoulder dystocia.

Fetal hyperinsulinemia per se is accompanied by excessive transfer of nutrients to the fetus and external somatic growth. This phenomenon usually manifest around 28th week gestation. The fetal insulin has a central role in fetal growth and development around the last 10 weeks of gestation. Meticulous control of maternal metabolism (substrate concentration) tends to normalize the fetal growth to a certain extent.

Two types of macrosomic infants can be identified:

1. *Constitutional macrosomia*, which represents the genetic drive to growth, this infant is large for gestational age (≥90th percentile) already in the second trimester and will continue to grow on its own growth curve during pregnancy.
2. *Metabolic macrosomia*, which represents diabetic fetopathy as a result of abnormal glucose metabolism, this infant is characterized by increased liver and spleen size (greater abdominal circumference) and normal head size (head circumference). In addition, this infant suffers from an enlarged heart and increased subcutaneous fat.[63]

CONSEQUENCES OF DIABETES ON THE PREGNANT MOTHER

Complications of diabetes in pregnancy occur almost exclusively in pre-gestational diabetic women.

Hypoglycemia: Hypoglycemia may occur in the first trimester of the pregnancy. This is due to combination of physiological adaptation, attempt for strict control and the nausea of early pregnancy.

Diabetic ketoacidosis: As pregnancy has some features of starvation state, ketoacidosis is a real hazard. Diabetic ketoacidosis has deleterious effect on the fetus.

Retinopathy: Background diabetic retinopathy (BDR) can develop or worsen during pregnancy. It is not a risk for vision and usually regresses postpartum. If BDR is already present, may progress to proliferative diabetic retinopathy (PDR). Therefore, it is essential to perform periodic ophthalmic examination and in a few photocoagulations may be necessary. The pregnant women with poor glycemic control and with hypertension are at an increased risk of developing PDR. These risks can be minimized by instituting preconception control of diabetes and hypertension.

Nephropathy: The risk of worsening diabetic nephropathy depends on baseline renal function and the degree of hypertension. Diabetic women with microalbuminuria may develop albuminuria during pregnancy with regression postpartum. Some among them are likely to develop preeclamptic symptoms. If the initial renal function is impaired in pregnancy, almost 50% of them are likely to show further decline in renal function.

Hypertension: The safe and effective antihypertensive drug during pregnancy is methyldopa. The other alternate drugs are diltiazem, clonidine and prazosin. Beta-blockers are to be avoided due to possible association with fetal growth retardation. Angiotensin inhibitors should never be used due to potential damage to the fetal kidneys.

Diabetic gastropathy: This condition severely exacerbates nausea and vomiting. The drug such as cisapride or mosapride may give relief.

Polyhydramnios: This occurs in poorly controlled diabetic mothers and is attributed to increased glucose content in the amniotic fluid, creating an osmotic pressure that equilibrates in the presence of an increased volume of amniotic fluid.

SUMMARY

The fuel metabolism during normal (nondiabetic) pregnancy is characterized by facilitated insulin action during the first half of pregnancy and diabetogenic stress during the second half of pregnancy.

- In the early weeks of gestation, fasting insulin concentrations rise as does glucose stimulated insulin release reaching a peak at the 18th to 20th week.
- During the later half of pregnancy, the facilitated insulin action continues and at the same time, there is increased elaboration of placental chorionic somatomammotrophin (hPL), prolactin and cortisol.

Facilitated anabolism in the fed state and accelerated starvation in the fasted state characterize the maternal fuel adaptations during pregnancy. Insulin secretion is considerably increased in both pregnant women with normal glucose tolerance and women with GDM. Peak plasma insulin during an OGTT occurs later in women with GDM than in women with normal glucose tolerance. However, in the second half of the pregnancy, insulin resistance and diabetogenic stress due to placental hormones necessitate compensatory increased insulin secretion. The clinical expression of gestational diabetes occurs, where this compensation is inadequate.

Consequences of the changes in fuel metabolism during pregnancy on the fetal development revolve around "maternal hyperglycemia and fetal hyperinsulinemia". Pregnancy is considered as tissue culture experiment implicating that placenta and fetus develop in an incubation medium that is totally derived from maternal fuels consisting of glucose, amino acids and lipids. The fuels traverse the placenta by facilitated diffusion and active transport and enter the fetal circulation.

In the *first trimester*, the exposure to abnormal mixed nutrients during organogenesis (first 6–8 weeks of gestation) may cause spontaneous miscarriage, intrauterine growth retardation and malformations.

Hyperglycemia, during the *second trimester* when the formation and the development of brain cells takes place, alters the behavioral, intellectual and psychological pattern in childhood.

Maternal hyperglycemia in the *third trimester* causes proliferation of fetal adipocytes, muscle cells and pancreatic beta cells and neuroendocrine systems which form the base for macrosomia and for the development of obesity, IGT and T2DM in later life.

Practically all pregnant women should undergo screening for glucose intolerance and it is imperative for the high-risk group. Universal screening is recommended in population ethnically more prone to develop glucose intolerance during pregnancy.

The important predictor of fetal outcome either in pre-gestational or gestational diabetes is the glycemic control attained immediately before and during pregnancy. The PG level of normal pregnant women is less than 90 mg% and 120 mg% respectively during fasting and non-fasting states.

The congenital malformation remains the leading cause of mortality and serious morbidity in infants of mother with diabetes. To minimize the occurrence of lethal malformations, pre-gestational counseling is essential.

If appropriate prepregnancy counseling has occurred and near euglycemia had been achieved before conception and if the prepregnancy insulin regimen incorporates two or more insulin injections a day, it may be suitable to achieve the near euglycemia necessary for a successful outcome of the pregnancy.

All women with GDM should receive nutritional counseling. The meal pattern should provide adequate calories and nutrients to meet the needs of pregnancy. Insulin is essential if MNT fails to achieve euglycemia. Maintenance of mean blood glucose level around 105 mg% is ideal for good fetal outcome.

Oral glucose lowering agents have generally not been recommended during pregnancy. However, one randomized unblinded clinical trial compared the use of insulin and glyburide in women with GDM (not in pre-GDM) who were not able to meet glycemic goals on meal plan. Treatment with either agent resulted in similar perinatal outcomes. All these patients were beyond the first trimester of pregnancy at the initiation of therapy. Metformin has been used in women with polycystic ovarian syndrome with successful fetal outcome.

Unless maternal or fetal complications arise, the goal for timing of delivery should be 39–40 weeks. An ultrasound scan has to be performed around 18–20 weeks of gestation focusing on structures namely the spine, skull, kidney and heart. Fetal echocardiography has to be done around 20–24 weeks which allows to view all the four chambers of the heart.

During intrapartum management of diabetes, the goal is to maintain the glucose concentration between 90 mg/dL and 100 mg/dL (95 ± 5 mg/dL). A woman with GDM does not require insulin once labor begins. In a gestational diabetic, the requirement of insulin is likely to fall precipitously and no insulin may be required immediately after expulsion of placenta. In a known diabetic, the dose of insulin has to be adjusted by monitoring blood glucose.

The future risk of developing diabetes for a gestational diabetic is twofold, if she becomes overweight; but maintaining ideal weight approximately halves the risk. The maternal health and fetal outcome depends upon the care by the committed team of diabetologists, obstetricians and neonatologists.

A short-term intensive care gives a long-term pay off in the primary prevention of obesity, IGT and diabetes in the offspring, as the preventive medicine starts before birth.

REFERENCES

1. Cosson E. Screening and insulin sensitivity in gestational diabetes. Abstract volume of the 40th Annual Meeting of the EASD, September 2004; A 350.
2. Dornhorst A, Paterson CM, Nicholls JS, et al. High prevalence of gestational diabetes in women from ethnic minority groups. Diabet Med. 1992;9(9):820-5.
3. Alberti KG, Zimmet PZ. Definition, diagnosis and classification of diabetes mellitus and its complications. Part 1: diagnosis and classification of diabetes mellitus provisional report of a WHO consultation. Diabet Med. 1998;15(7):539-53.
4. Metzger BE, Gabbe SG, Persson B, et al. International association of diabetes and pregnancy study groups recommendations on the diagnosis and classification of hyperglycemia in pregnancy. Diabetes Care. 2010;33(3):676-82.
5. Magee MS, Walden CE, Benedetti TJ, et al. Influence of diagnostic criteria on the incidence of gestational diabetes and perinatal morbidity. JAMA. 1993;269(5):609-15.
6. Weiss PA, Haeusler M, Tamussino K, et al. Can glucose tolerance test predict fetal hyperinsulinism? BJOG. 2000;107(12):1480-5.
7. Mohan V, Sandeep S, Deepa R, et al. Epidemiology of type 2 diabetes: Indian scenario. Indian J Med Res. 2007;125:217-30.
8. Das S, Behera MK, Misra S, et al. B-cell function and insulin resistance in pregnancy and their relation to fetal development. Metab Syndr Relat Disord. 2010;8(1):25-32.
9. Balaji V, Balaji M, Anjalakshi C, et al. Inadequacy of fasting plasma glucose to diagnose gestational diabetes mellitus in Asian Indian Women. Diabetes Res Clin Pract. 2011;94(1):e21-3.
10. Sacks DA, Hadden DR, Maresh M, et al. Frequency of gestational diabetes mellitus at collaborating centers based on IADPSG consensus panel-recommended criteria: the hyperglycemia and adverse pregnancy outcome (HAPO) study. Diabetes Care. 2012;35(3):526-8.
11. Crowther CA, Hiller JE, Moss JR, et al. Effect of treatment of gestational diabetes mellitus on pregnancy outcomes. N Engl J Med. 2005;352(24):2477-86.

12. Gayle C, Germain S, Marsh MS, et al. Comparing pregnancy outcomes for intensive versus routine antenatal treatment of GDM based on a 75 gm OGTT 2- h blood glucose (>140 mg/dL). Diabetologia. 2010;53:S435.
13. Wahi P, Dogra V, Jandial K, et al. Prevalence of gestational diabetes mellitus (GDM) and its outcomes in Jammu region. J Assoc Physicians India. 2011;59:227-30.
14. Perucchini D, Fischer U, Spinas GA, et al. Using fasting plasma glucose concentrations to screen for gestational diabetes mellitus: prospective population based study. BMJ. 1999;319(7213):812-5.
15. Franks PW, Looker HC, Kobes S, et al. Gestational glucose tolerance and risk of type 2 diabetes in young Pima Indian offspring. Diabetes. 2006;55(2):460-5.
16. Diagnostic criteria and classification of hyperglycemia in pregnancy. WHO/NMH/MND/13.2
17. Anjalakshi C, Balaji V, Balaji MS, et al. A single test procedure to diagnose gestational diabetes mellitus. Acta Diabetol. 2009;46(1):51-4.
18. O'Sullivan JB, Mahan CM. Criteria for the oral glucose tolerance test in pregnancy. Diabetes. 1964;13:278-85.
19. Gough WW, Shack MJ, Bennett PH, et al. Evaluation of glucose in the Pima Indians by longitudinal studies (abstract). Diabetes. 1970;19(Suppl. 1):388.
20. Kühl C. Insulin secretion and insulin resistance in pregnancy and GDM. Implications for diagnosis and management. Diabetes. 1991;40(Suppl 2):18-24.
21. Catalano PM, Tyzbir ED, Wolfe RR, et al. Carbohydrate metabolism during pregnancy in control subjects & women with gestational diabetes. Am J Physiol. 1993;264(1 Pt 1):E60-7.
22. Government of India, Ministry of Health and Family Welfare, Nirman Bhavan, New Delhi (DO No. M-12015/93/2011-MCH/2011).
23. Lind T, Billewicz WZ, Brown G. A serial study of changes occurring in the oral glucose tolerance test during pregnancy. J Obstet Gynaecol Br Commonw. 1973;80:1033-9.
24. Buchanan TA, Metzger BE, Frienkel N, et al. Insulin sensitivity and β-cell responsiveness to glucose during late pregnancy in lean and moderately obese women with normal glucose tolerance or mild gestational diabetes. Am J Obstet Gynecol. 1990;162:1008-114.
25. Catalano PM, Huston L, Amini SB, et al. Longitudinal changes in glucose metabolism during pregnancy in obese women with normal glucose tolerance and gestational diabetes mellitus. Am J Obstet Gynecol. 1999;180:903-16.
26. Van Assche FA, Aerts L, De Prins F. A Morphological study of the endocrine pancreas in human pregnancy. Br J Obstet Gynaecol. 1978;85:818-20.
27. Metzger BE, Unger RG, Frienkel N. Carbohydrate metabolism in pregnancy. XIV. Relationships between circulating glucagons, insulin, glucose, and amino acids in response to 'mixed meal' in late pregnancy. Metabolism 1977;26:151-6.
28. Friedman JE, Ishizuka T, Shao J, et al. Impaired glucose transport and insulin receptor tyrosine phosphorylation in skeletal muscle from obese women with gestational diabetes. Diabetes. 1999;48:1807-14.
29. Catalano P, Highway T, Huston L, et al. Relationship between reproductive hormones/TNF α and longitudinal changes in insulin sensitivity during gestation. Diabetes. 1996;45:175A.
30. Buchanan TA, Xiang A, Kjos SL, et al. Gestational diabetes: antepartum characteristics that predict postpartum glucose intolerance and type 2 diabetes in Latino women. Diabetes 1998; 47:1302-10.
31. Buchanan TA, Xiang AH, Peters RK, et al. Response of pancreatic cells to improved insulin sensitivity in women at high risk for type 2 diabetes. Diabetes. 2000;49:782-8.
32. Polonsky KS, Given BD, Van Cauter E. Twenty four hour profiles and pulsatile patterns of insulin secretion in normal and obese subjects. J Clin Invest. 1988;81:442-8.
33. Seshiah V, Cynthia A, Balaji V, et al. Detection and care of women with gestational diabetes mellitus from early weeks of pregnancy results in birth weight of newborn babies appropriate for gestational age. Diabetes Res Clin Pract. 2008;80(2):199-202.

34. Schaefer-Graf UM, Kjos SL, Fauzan OH, et al. A randomized trial evaluating a predominately fetal growth–based strategy to guide management of gestational diabetes in Caucasian women. Diabetes Care. 2004;27(2):297-302.
35. Langer O, Levy J, Brustman L, et al. Glycemic control in gestational diabetes mellitus: how tight is tight enough: small for gestational age versus large for gestational age? Am J Obstet Gynecol. 1989;161:646-53.
36. Karlsson K, Kjellmer I. The outcome of diabetic pregnancies in relationship to the mother's blood sugar level. Am J obstet Gynaecol. 1972;112:213-20.
37. Hermansen K, Colombo M, Stogaard H, et al. Improved postprandial glycemic control with biphasic human insulin in patients with type 2 diabetes. Diabetes Care. 2002;25:883-8.
38. Jovanovic L, Ilic S, Pettitt DJ, et al. Metabolic and immunologic effects of insulin lispro in gestational diabetes. Diabetes Care. 1999;22:1422-7.
39. Hod M, visser G, Damm P, et al. Safety and perinatal outcome in pregnancy: a randomized trial comparing insulin aspart with human insulin in 322 subjects with type 1 diabetes. ADA. Poster 1805-p. Diabetes. 2006, June Supplement.
40. Coetzee EJ, Jackson WPU. The management of non-insulin dependent diabetes during pregnancy. Diabetes Res Clin Pract. 1986;1:281.
41. Langer L, Conway DL, Berkus MD, et al. A comparison of glyburide and insulin in women with gestational diabetes mellitus. N Engl J Med. 2000;343:1134-8.
42. Jakubowicz DJ, Iuorno MJ, Jakubowicz S, et al._Effects of metformin on early pregnancy loss in the polycystic ovary syndrome. J Clin Endocrinol Metab. 2002;87(2):524-9.
43. Buhling KJ, Winkel T, Wolf C, et al. Optimal timing for post-prandial glucose measurement in pregnant women with diabetes and a non-diabetic pregnant population evaluated by the continuous glucose monitoring system (CGMS). J Perinat Med. 2005;33(2):125-31.
44. Oded Langer. Scientific rational for management of diabetes in pregnancy. Recent Approaches with innovative computer based technology. Diabetes Care. 1988;11(Suppl. 1):67-72.
45. Ben-Haroush A, Yogev Y, Chen R, et al. The post prandial glucose profile in the diabetic pregnancy. Am J Obstet Gynecol. 2004;191(2):576-81.
46. Langer O, Anyaegbunam A, Brustman L, et al. Pregestational diabetes: insulin requirements throughout pregnancy. Am J Obstet Gynaecol. 1988;159:616.
47. Oded Langer. Maternal glycemic criteria for insulin therapy in gestational diabetes mellitus. Diabetes Care. 1998;21(Suppl 2):B91-8.
48. Maheux PC, Bonin B, Dizazo A, et al. Glucose homeostasis during spontaneous labor in normal human pregnancy. J Clin Endocrinol Metab. 1996;81:209.
49. Frienkel N. Of pregnancy and progeny. Diabetes. 1980;29:1023-35.
50. Pederson J. Foetal mortality in the pregnant diabetic and her newborn. Baltimore: Williams & Wilkins; 1967. pp 108-27.
51. Barros LF, Yudilevich DL, Jarvis SM, et al. Quantitation and immunolocalization of glucose transporters in the human placenta. Placenta. 1995;16:623-33.
52. Jansson T, Wennergren M, Illsley NP. Glucose transporter expression and distribution in the human placenta throughout gestation and in intrauterine growth retardation. J Clin Endocrinol Metab. 1993;77:1554-62.
53. Hod M. Clinical and experimental advances in diabetic embryopathy. Diabetes Reviews International. 1997;6:10-4.
54. Philips AF, Porte PJ, Stabinsky S, et al. Effects of chronic fetal hyperglycemia upon oxygen consumption in the bovine uterus and conceptus. J Clin Invest. 1984;74:279-86.
55. Rizzo T, Metzger BE, Burns WJ, et al. Correlation between antipartum maternal metabolism and intelligence of offspring. N Engl J Med. 1991;325:911-6.
56. Swenne I. Pancreatic beta - cell growth and diabetes mellitus. Diabetologia. 1992;35:193-201.

57. Reiher H, Fuhramann K, Noack S, et al. Age dependent insulin secretion of the endocrine pancreas in vitro from fetuses of diabetic and non diabetic patients. Diabetes Care. 1983;6:446-51.
58. Carpenter MW, Canick JA, Hogan JW, et al. Amniotic fluid insulin at 14 - 20 weeks gestation: associated with later maternal glucose intolerance and birth macrosomia. Diabetes Care. 2001;24:1259-63.
59. Silverman BL, Metzger BE, Cho NM, et al. Impaired glucose tolerance in adolescent offspring of diabetic mothers - relationship to foetal hyperinsulinism. Diabetes Care. 1995;18:611.
60. Salafia CM. The foetal, placental & neonatal pathology associated with maternal diabetes. In: Reece EA, Coustan BR (Eds). Diabetes Mellitus in Pregnancy: Principles & Practice. New York: Churchill Livingstone; 1988. pp 143-81.
61. Curet LB, Izquierdo LA, Gilson GJ, et al. Relative effects of antepartum and intrapartum maternal blood glucose levels on incidence of neonatal hypoglycemia. J Perinatol. 1997;17:113-5.
62. Vinod K Paul, Ashok K Deorari, Meharban Singh. Management of Low Birth Weight Babies. In: Parthasarathy A (Ed). IAP Textbook of Pediatrics, 2nd edition, New Delhi: Jaypee publications; 2002. p 60.
63. Langer O, Kagan-Hallet K. Diabetic vs. Non-diabetic infants: a quantitative morphological study. Proceedings of the 38th Annual Meeting of the Society for Gynaecologic Investigation, San Antonio, Texas, 1992.

25
CHAPTER

Continuous Glucose Monitoring and Its Role in Management of Diabetes

Sunil M Jain

INTRODUCTION

Various methodologies have been used for assessment of glycemic control. In current era of technology, we are now moving toward continuous monitoring of glucose.[1,2] Once upon a time, laboratory glucose measurement and urine glucose testing was the only method to know the glucose level and physician has to take treatment decisions based on this limited information. Advent of home glucose testing technology in the 1970s started a new era and subsequently made urinary glucose testing obsolete. Simultaneously HbA1c measurement became possible which gave us overall glycemic assessment of last 3 months. In spite of so many ways to assess glucose control of a patient, need of a technology to know a continuous change in glucose trend was felt because the biggest challenge in diabetes management is to achieve normoglycemia with minimizing hypoglycemia. So far used traditional methods to assess glucose control limit our ability to meet glycemic goals. A need of a better technology was always felt. This need has been fulfilled by CGMS or continuous glucose monitoring system. Urine glucose was giving indirect and incorrect information, laboratory testing was giving very limited information, self-monitoring of plasma glucose (SMPG) provides "snapshot" information thus missing many peaks and troughs, HbA1c giving an average only that may be a mix of extreme highs and extreme lows while CGMS can provide all information and variations in glucose values, what we now label as glycemic variability. In addition, A1C-derived average glucose (ADAG) study has shown the wide range of average glucose for the same HbA1c.

Thus, the current understanding of glycemia based on HbA1c seems to be incomplete and thus, the era of "actual control" measurement by CGMS is going to begin soon. Physicians and diabetologists should understand this new technology of glycemic control assessment. Many patients have started using CGMS as a monitoring tool and no wonder if SMPG is replaced by CHGM or continuous home glucose monitoring. This chapter will be covering CGMS in following subsections:

- What is CGMS?
- How CGMS is performed?
- Where to insert sensor?

- Which glucose is measured by CGMS?
- How CGMS sensor works?
- Types of CGMS
- Available options in India
- Need of SMPG during CGMS: concept of calibration
- Clinically useful information from CGMS
- Role of CGMS in diabetes therapeutic decision making
- CGMS as education tool
- CGMS during emergencies and hospitalized patients
- CGMS technology in India vs. developed countries
- Future of CGMS.

WHAT IS CGMS?

CGMS (Continuous Glucose Monitoring System)

This is a technology which measures glucose levels continuously and hence the only technology which provides information about glycemic variability in an individual. In glucose meter, a strip used and a drop of blood is placed on this strip.

This strip contains enzymes which generate H_2O_2 and followed by the generation of a signal which is measured by reader in glucose meter and converted to glucose number which is then displayed on glucose meter screen as glucose values. Higher is glucose, more H_2O_2 generation and thus higher glucose value and vice versa. Same technology is used in CGMS where a similar enzyme coated platinum sensor is placed in subcutaneous tissue; glucose present in subcutaneous tissue comes in contact with sensor. Enzyme present in sensor generates H_2O_2, and this quantity of generated H_2O_2 depends on glucose levels in subcutaneous tissue. H_2O_2 is measured by sensor every 10 seconds and an average value during a period of 5 minutes is transferred to a system which then converts this to glucose value as done by glucose meter.

HOW CGMS IS PERFORMED?

In CGMS technology,[3] a glucose sensor, which looks like a needle (Fig. 1) is placed into the subcutaneous tissue.

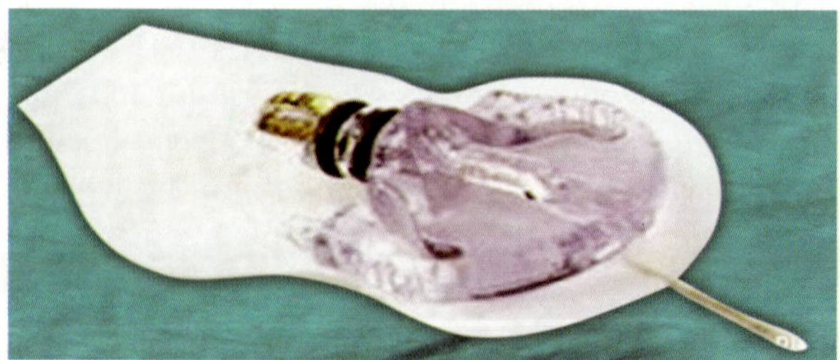

Fig. 1: Glucose sensor

This sensor is then attached to a recorder or a transmitter (Fig. 2). If sensor is attached to a recorder, it will save all data. Sensor will measure glucose and these values will be saved in recorder. Once CGMS is completed, sensor will be removed and this recorder will be connected to computer and all data will be extracted and a report will be generated. This is also known as retrospective CGMS. Here, during CGMS glucose values are stored in recorder, patient is not aware of these values. These values will become visible at the end of CGMS process when sensor will be removed and data from recorder are transferred to a computer (Fig. 3).

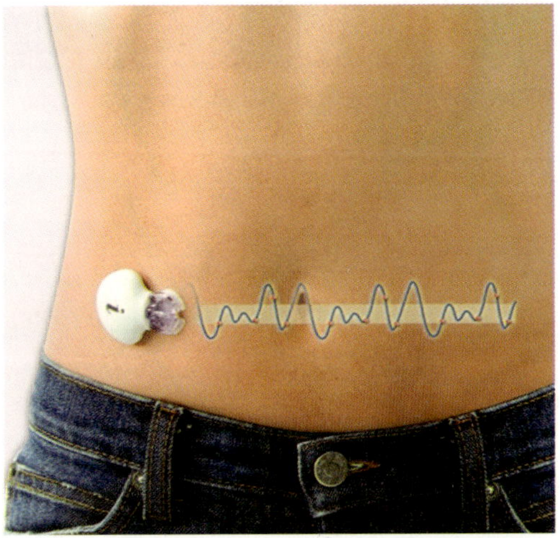

Fig. 2: Sensor attached to a recorder

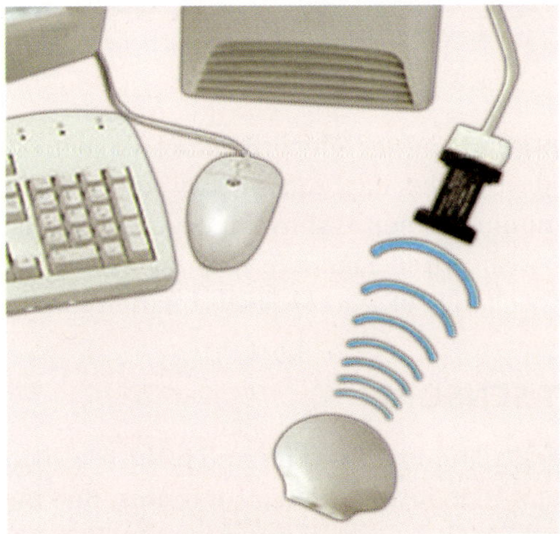

Fig. 3: Data from the recorder transferred to the computer

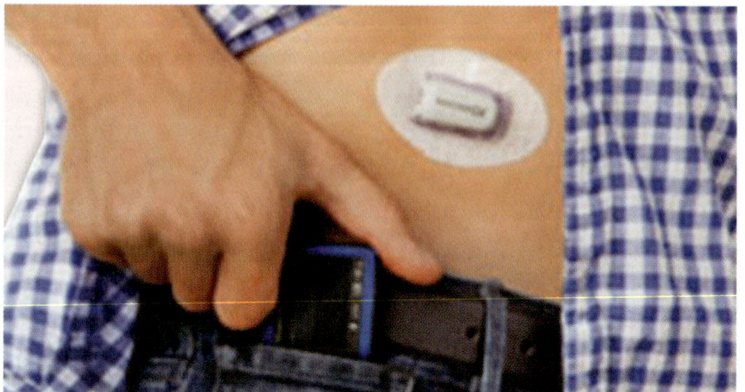

Fig. 4: CGMS with glucose values continuous display

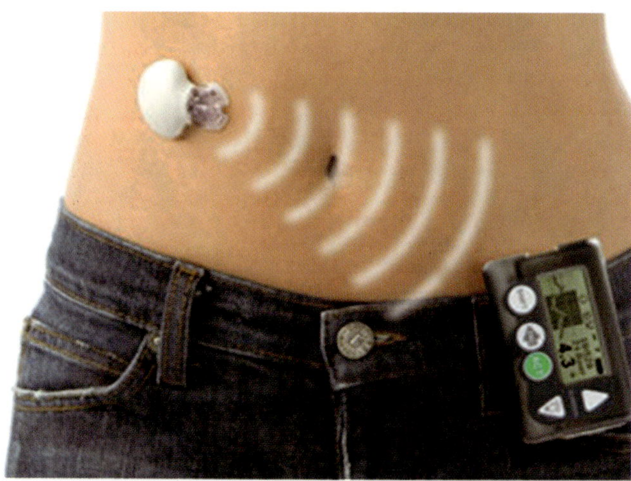

Fig. 5: CGMS with glucose value and trend display

If sensor is attached to a transmitter, glucose values measured by sensor will be sent to transmitter which then will send this data to a display screen and thus glucose value will be continuously visible on a monitor screen as shown in Figure 4. This is also known as prospective CGMS. One more CGMS is shown in Figure 5. In prospective CGMS, patient can see their glucose levels as well rate of change of glucose levels on their monitor.

WHERE TO INSERT SENSOR?

For sensor insertion, generally abdomen is preferred place (Fig. 6), though it can be placed at arms also (Fig. 7). If a patient is on insulin therapy, it is must that insulin should be injected in subcutaneous tissue at least 3 inches away from sensor site. This needle like sensor is inserted with the help of a device which makes sensor insertion virtually painless.

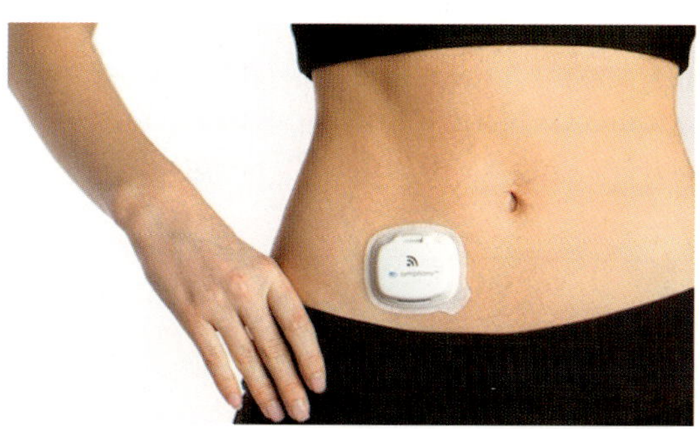

Fig. 6: Placement of sensor on the abdomen

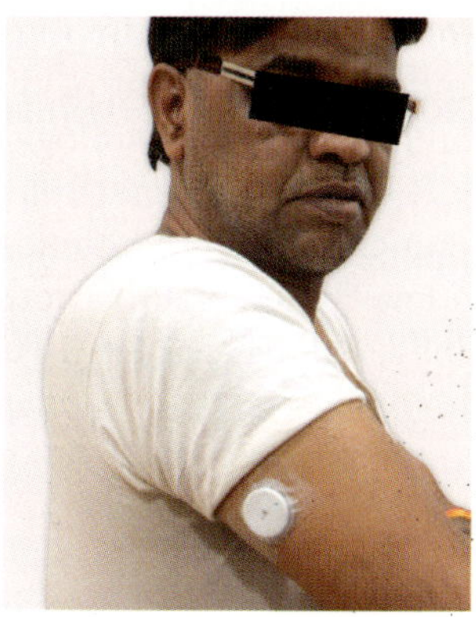

Fig. 7: Placement of sensor on the arms

WHICH GLUCOSE IS MEASURED BY CGMS?

Glucose measurements in laboratory are done in venous plasma, while glucose meter are measuring estimated capillary plasma glucose (Fig. 8).

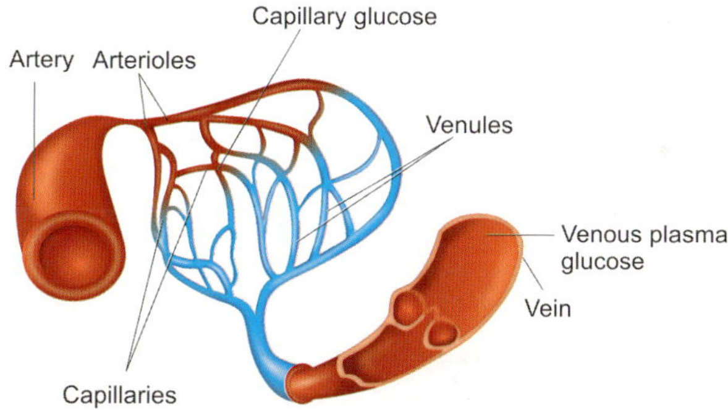

Fig. 8: Blood glucose level measurement—venous plasma (laboratory) or capillary plasma (glucose meter)

While in CGMS, glucose level in another compartment, i.e. interstitial fluid (IF), is measured[4] (Fig. 9).

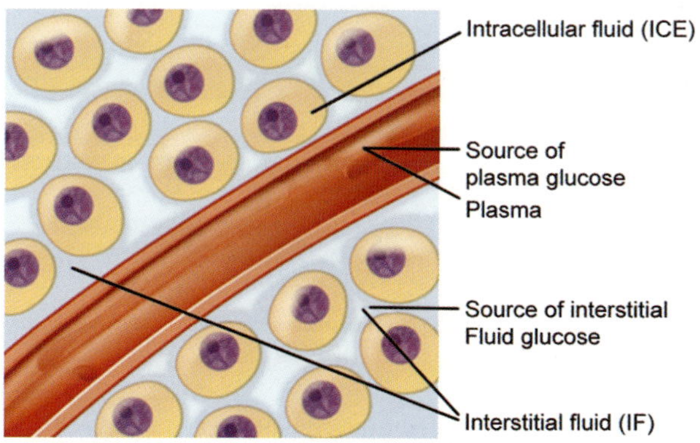

Fig. 9: CGMS measures interstitial fluid glucose level

For the understanding and interpretation of glucose measured by CGMS, there is need to understand concept of IF glucose. Interstitial fluid glucose and capillary glucose have a difference due to physiology of glucose movement from capillaries to IF. Thus to understand how IF glucose differs from capillary or venous plasma glucose, we need to understand difference of glucose kinetics between IF and blood vessels including capillaries. Glucose in blood will reach first to arterioles and capillaries, from here it will diffuse to IF space, and will be delivered to cells (Fig. 10).

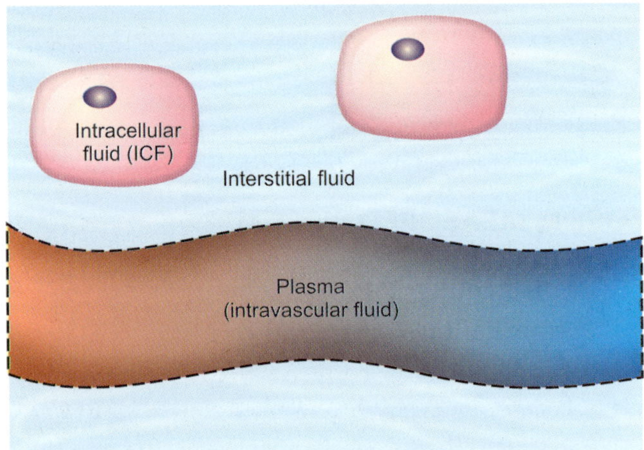

Fig. 10: Concept of interstitial fluid glucose

Continuous glucose monitor (CGM) sensor is placed in subcutaneous tissue, and thus it measures glucose in the IF, while glucose meters measure glucose from mixed capillaries. Glucose takes time to move from capillaries to interstitial space. If glucose levels are stable, such as in the fasting or pre-meal state, both compartments are in equilibrium. In this scenario, glucose levels in both IF and capillaries will be nearly identical. If there is rapid change in glucose level, this will happen first at capillary level, and after few minutes, it will be in equilibrium with IF compartment (Fig. 11).

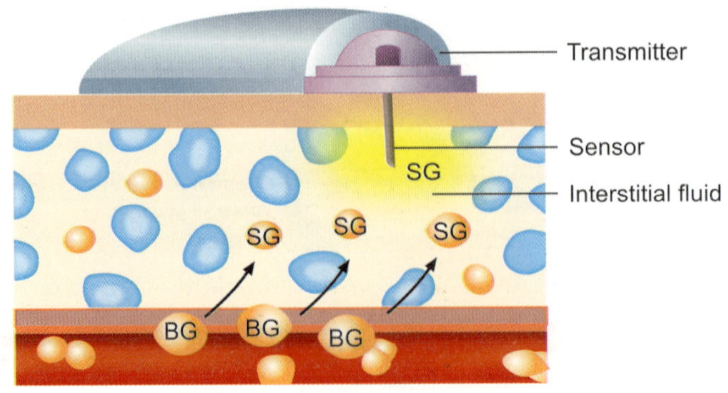

Fig. 11: Capillary glucose reaches to interstitial fluid and measured by sensor

Abbreviations: BG, blood glucose; SG, sensor glucose

Thus, when glucose levels are rapidly changing, such as after a meal, glucose will rise first in blood vessels and capillaries and then will move to interstitial space and if a measurement is done at this time, capillary glucose and thus glucose meter value will be higher than IF glucose or CGM sensor measured value (Fig. 12).

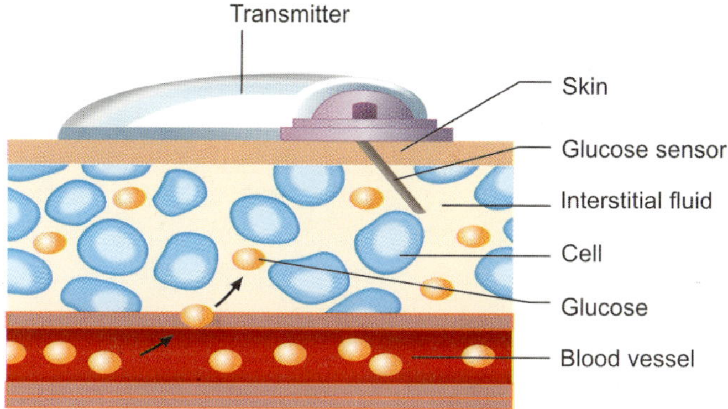

Fig. 12: Rapid rise in glucose, interstitial fluid values relatively low

Similarly, if glucose is falling rapidly as happen in hypoglycemia, changes in glucose level will happen first in capillary glucose and thus glucose meter value will be lower than CGM sensor value (Fig. 13).

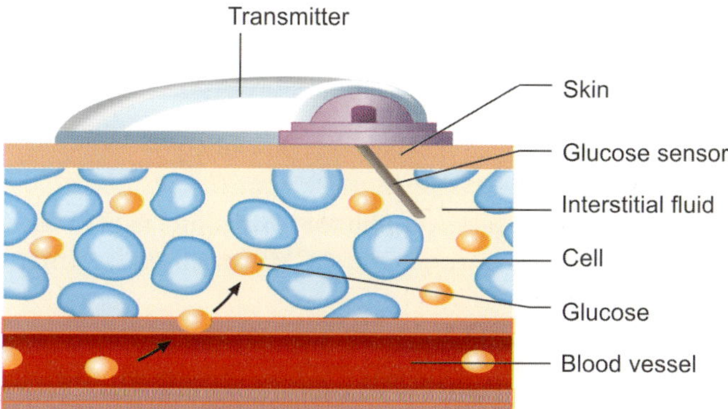

Fig. 13: Rapid fall in glucose, interstitial fluid values relatively high

Thus as a concept, during steady state capillary glucose values are similar to IF glucose while during rapid change in glucose level, CGM sensor value or IF glucose lag behind capillary/metered glucose. This delay is physiological and called lag time. Any interpretation and understanding of CGMS values has to be done in the light of lag time concept.

HOW CGMS SENSOR WORKS?

This sensor consists of two semipermeable membranes containing glucose oxidase enzyme (Fig. 14). Once inserted in subcutaneous tissue, glucose present in interstitial space passes through the semipermeable membrane of sensor to react with the glucose oxidase enzyme in the presence of oxygen. This generates hydrogen peroxide which leads to electron release and produce an electronic signal.[20] The "signal" is then recorded and converted into glucose value. If glucose levels in IF are higher than signal strength will be higher while when glucose levels are lower, signal strength will be lower. Sensor keeps on measuring glucose continuously in this manner.

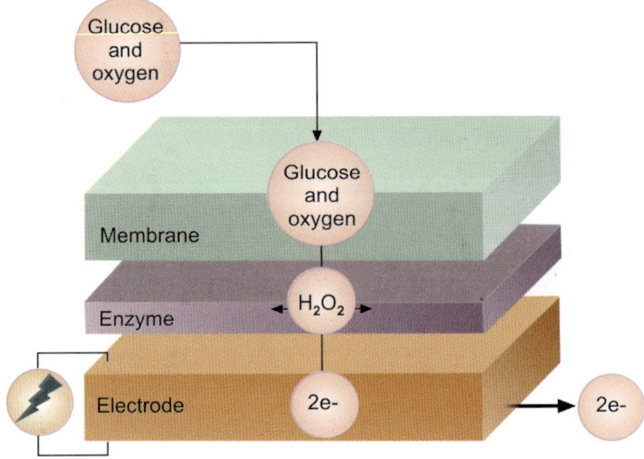

Fig. 14: Glucose measurement by CGMS sensor

Current sensor measures glucose every 10 seconds, an average of such multiple values is converted every 5 minutes to one figure and thus current most CGMS software store and provide glucose value every 5 minutes and 288 glucose values in 24 hours.

TYPES OF CGMS

Continuous glucose monitoring systems can be for physicians use. In these systems, glucose data are blinded to patient, analysis is done after CGMS and then treatment is planned.

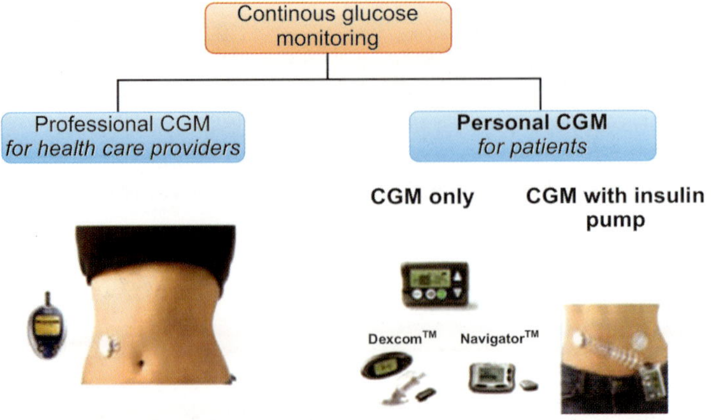

Fig. 15: Various types of CGMS

These are also called as retrospective CGMS. Similarly, CGMS primarily made for patient use are called personal or prospective CGMS. These systems may be a part of sensor augmented insulin pumps or may be CGMS only system (Fig. 15).

Professional CGMS

This consists of a glucose sensor and a recorder to store data. The glucose sensor is inserted under the skin to check glucose levels in subcutaneous tissue fluid. The glucose sensor has an adhesive patch to hold it on skin. The glucose sensor is inserted with help of a device. iPro 2 is one such CGMS. The most common site for iPro 2 sensor is abdomen. Sensor lasts for 5 days. Recently FreeStyle Libre Pro Flash sensor is launched in India. This sensor works for 14 days. Site for insertion of this sensor is arm. Once CGMS duration is over, sensor is removed and data stored in recorder are converted to report by software. This report provides every 5 minutes glucose value, daily graphs, glucose value in relation to meals, medication and physical activity, parameters of glycemic variability, etc. In this CGMS, glucose values are not visible to patient. Physician has to modify treatment based on this retrospective information.

Personal CGMS[6]

This consist of the same sensor as used for professional CGMS, a transmitter to transmit glucose data and a small external monitor (which may be built-in to an insulin pump or a stand-alone device) to view glucose levels, trends, graphs, etc.

Glucose sensor will measure glucose, this glucose value will be gathered by the transmitter attached to sensor; this information is sent wirelessly to the glucose monitor unit. This glucose monitor unit may be mobile phone like device (Fig. 16) or in case of sensor augmented pumps, insulin pump screen will be a monitor.

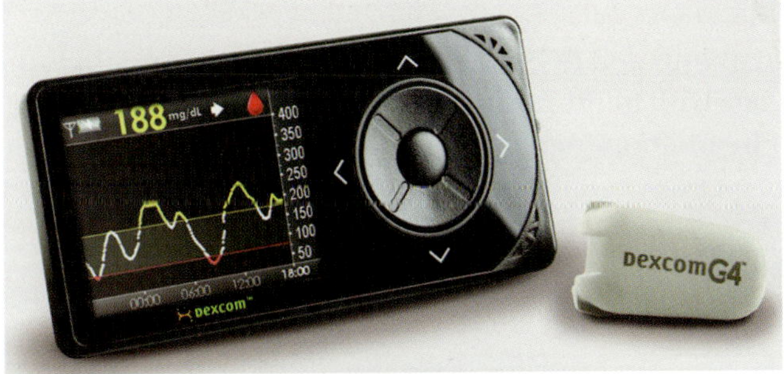

Fig. 16: Personal CGMS (Dexcom G4)

Thus, patient can see glucose value being displayed on monitor screen every 5 minutes. In addition, glucose trend that is glucose is stable, rising or falling is also visible on the monitor screen. This kind of information can warn patient about hypoglycemia in advance. Thus, this CGMS provides a prospective information on which patient can react and act so as to keep in normoglycemic range.

AVAILABLE OPTIONS IN INDIA

Currently available options: In India following CGMS options are available.
Professional CGMS
- iPro 2
- FreeStyle Libre Pro Flash

Personal CGMS
- Guardian RT
- Dexcom G4

NEED OF SMPG DURING CGMS: CONCEPT OF CALIBRATION[7,8]

With most available CGMS devices, patient has to measure glucose level by glucose meter and enter the data into system. This is called as calibration. The concept of calibration is based on the fact that currently, CGM systems are to be cross checked with glucose meter reading. If sensor IF glucose and SMPG value correlate well, only then CGMS will provide glucose readings. This is must at beginning as well at nearly 12 hours interval.[9] This process of cross check of SMPG value with sensor value is called calibration. SMPG is the reference for glucose levels, so the CGM sensor needs to be calibrated using a meter blood glucose value as the reference. In simple words, CGMS sensor measures and generates a raw glucose value, it needs a confirmation from glucose meter reading and if both values are similar or nearly equal, only then CGMS sensor will provide continuous data. As a rule calibration has to be done during steady state, at a time when IF and capillary glucose are expected to be same. The new FreeStyle Libre Pro Flash CGMS will not require such calibration.

CLINICALLY USEFUL INFORMATION FROM CGMS

This will depend on type of CGMS used.

Personal CGMS

In sensor augmented pumps and CGMS like Guardian RT, Dexcom G4 systems, FreeStyle Libre Pro Flash real-time data with trend are available. Here glucose value at every 5 minutes interval is visible on screen. In addition, real-time information about rate of change and direction of change is also visible on screen. Rate and direction of change is represented by arrows coming with glucose value. For example, if screen shows a glucose value of 108 mg, and there is one arrow with downward (Fig. 17) direction also shown, this indicates glucose is currently falling at 1 mg/minute.

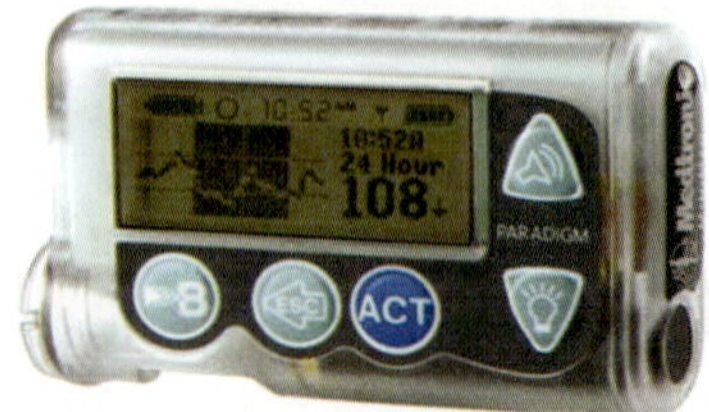

Fig. 17: CGMS showing change and direction of change of glucose value

If there are two arrows and a down arrow, this is an indication that glucose is falling at a rate of 2 mg/minute or more. The opposite is also true that is one up arrow indicates glucose rising by 1 mg/minute and two arrows indicate glucose rising by 2 mg/minutes. If there is no arrow, this is an indication that glucose value is stable. This real-time trend is very helpful to detect hypoglycemia very early, and thus prevent a hypoglycemic episode.[10] If a patient see glucose as 78 mg, and there is no arrow, that mean no need to worry while glucose 78 mg with two arrows down is an indication of hypoglycemia in next few minutes and by needful action, patient can prevent this episode to happen.

Personal CGMS also provides continuous trends in a graph diagram as well as information about parameters of glycemic variability. Data of this CGMS can be downloaded and a report can be prepared for treatment planning by physician.

Professional CGMS

Here CGMS is done, data will not be visible to patient. When patient comes to clinic, data from CGMS will be downloaded and then all glucose values will become visible. In India, as of now, there are two CGMS systems in use for professional—iPro 2 and FreeStyle Libre Pro Flash.

In iPro 2, sensor is fixed, mostly on abdomen and data are downloaded after sensor removal. We get 5 days data with following information (Fig. 18).

Daily graphs and one summary showing all graphs together.[11] Through this summary, we can see pattern of glucose control in a patient. These graphs start from 12 o'clock midnight to next day 12 o'clock midnight. First look at overnight glucose trend and then look at pre- and post-meal glucose trends. Table below the graphs in Figure 18 gives information about highest, lowest and average glucose of the day as well as standard deviation. Numbers of excursions are shown in a table (Fig. 18) in the same report and duration of time spent in hypo-, hyper- and normoglycemia is depicted by pie diagrams (Fig. 18).[5] In addition, a data table with time and every 5 minutes glucose value is also available.

In FreeStyle Libre Pro Flash, sensor is fixed on arm, it works for 14 days, and data can be downloaded with help of a reader during these 14 days (Fig. 19).

Multiple downloads are possible during these 14 days. The software of this CGMS provides data in a format called accelerated graphics port (AGP) (Fig. 20). The graph in AGP shows 1 SD variability from mean.

These data can help in a precise and accurate decision making for choosing therapies for diabetes, particularly selecting regimen and adjusting dose for insulin based treatment.

ROLE OF CGMS IN DIABETES THERAPEUTIC DECISION MAKING[12,13]

Certain patients like type 1 diabetes mellitus (T1DM),[14,15] pregnancy[16,17] and diabetes, unpredictable hypoglycemia, fluctuating type 2 diabetes[10] where physician finds difficulty in adjusting treatment, CGMS provides a detailed information. CGMS is a very useful patient education tool. Apart from such patients, CGMS can be helpful in measuring and reducing glycemic variability for most of patients.

Sensor Data (mg/dL)

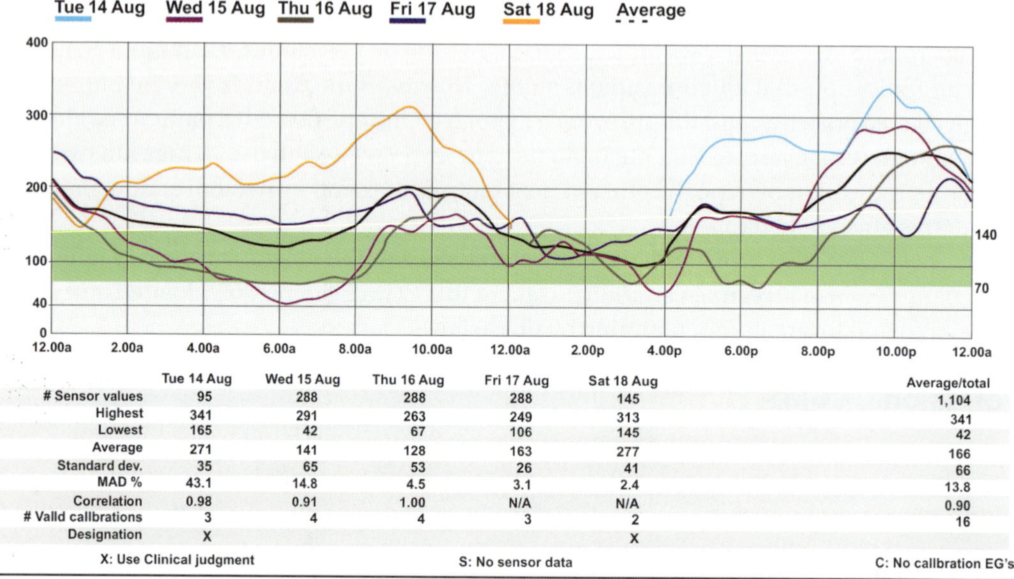

	Tue 14 Aug	Wed 15 Aug	Thu 16 Aug	Fri 17 Aug	Sat 18 Aug	Average/total
# Sensor values	95	288	288	288	145	1,104
Highest	341	291	263	249	313	341
Lowest	165	42	67	106	145	42
Average	271	141	128	163	277	166
Standard dev.	35	65	53	26	41	66
MAD %	43.1	14.8	4.5	3.1	2.4	13.8
Correlation	0.98	0.91	1.00	N/A	N/A	0.90
# Valid calibrations	3	4	4	3	2	16
Designation	X				X	

X: Use Clinical judgment S: No sensor data C: No calibration EG's

Excursion summary (mg/dL/day)

	Tue 14 Aug	Wed 15 Aug	Thu 16 Aug	Fri 17 Aug	Sat 18 Aug	Average/Total
# excursions	1	4	4	2	0	11
# High excursions	1	2	3	2	0	8
# Low excursions	0	2	1	0	0	3
AUC above limit	131.1	26.2	16.7	25.2	86.9	40.4
AUC below limit	0.0	2.1	0.0	0.0	0.0	0.5

Duration Distribution (hh:mm)

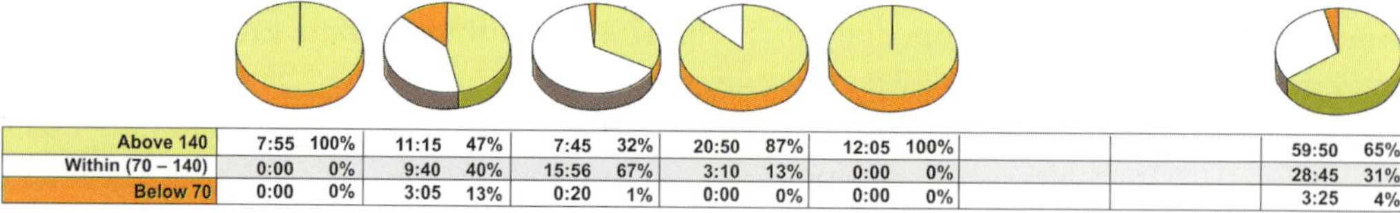

	Tue 14 Aug		Wed 15 Aug		Thu 16 Aug		Fri 17 Aug		Sat 18 Aug				Average/Total	
Above 140	7:55	100%	11:15	47%	7:45	32%	20:50	87%	12:05	100%			59:50	65%
Within (70 – 140)	0:00	0%	9:40	40%	15:56	67%	3:10	13%	0:00	0%			28:45	31%
Below 70	0:00	0%	3:05	13%	0:20	1%	0:00	0%	0:00	0%			3:25	4%

Fig. 18: Information from iPro 2 CGMS

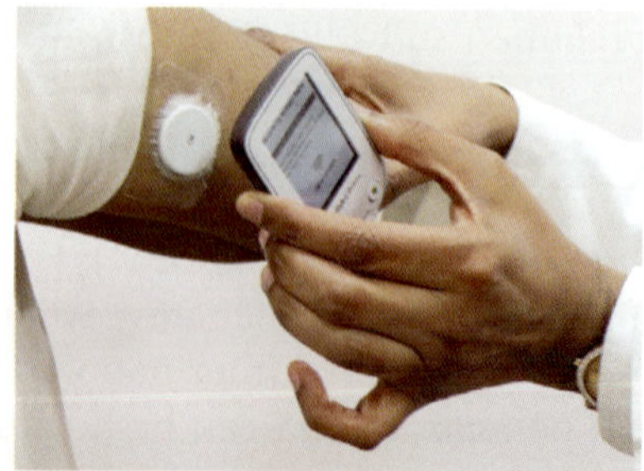

Fig. 19: Data downloading from the FreeStyle Libre Pro Flash Sensor

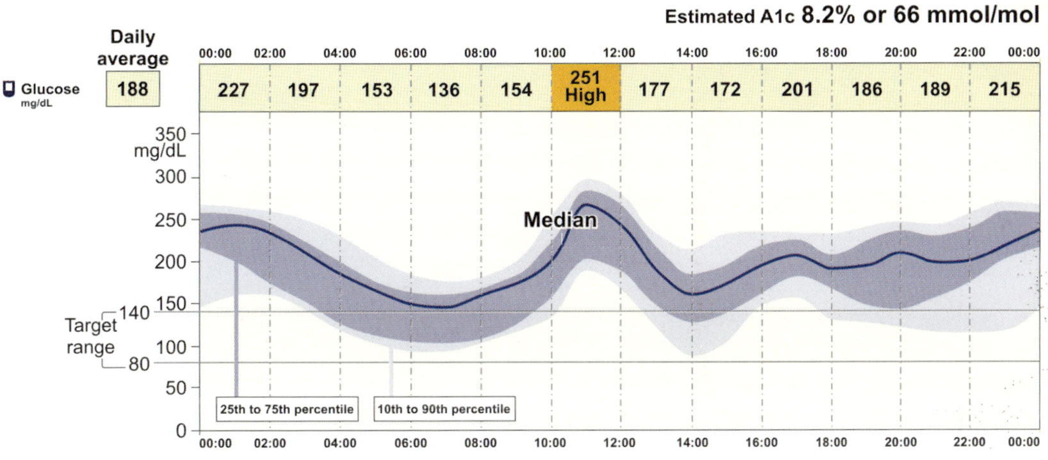

Fig. 20: Data of CGMS in the AGP format

CGMS AS EDUCATION TOOL

Diet compliance is a major practical issue in patients with diabetes. In spite of all knowledge and information, patients do not follow basic rules which lead to unstable glycemic control. CGMS provides glucose value at every 5–15 minutes interval and also provides glucose graphs which makes patient easily understand their role in worsening of hyperglycemia primarily due to food factor. Many patients find this as a great learning. I have seen this effect in few of my patients and just a CGMS changed their HbA1c as well as glycemic variability. Figure 21 shows CGMS of one such patient. This patient had many fluctuations in glucose values. Patient was receiving insulin therapy along with metformin.

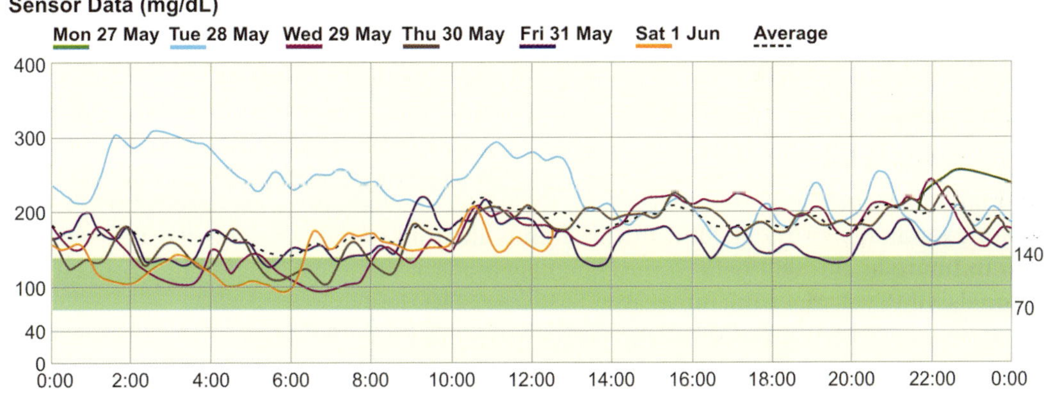

Fig. 21: CGMS data of patient on insulin + metformin

CGMS DURING EMERGENCIES AND HOSPITALIZED PATIENTS[19]

Few studies are performed in critically ill hospitalized patients. These studies have shown that CGMS is reliable in critically ill patients but since CGMS measures IF glucose which may

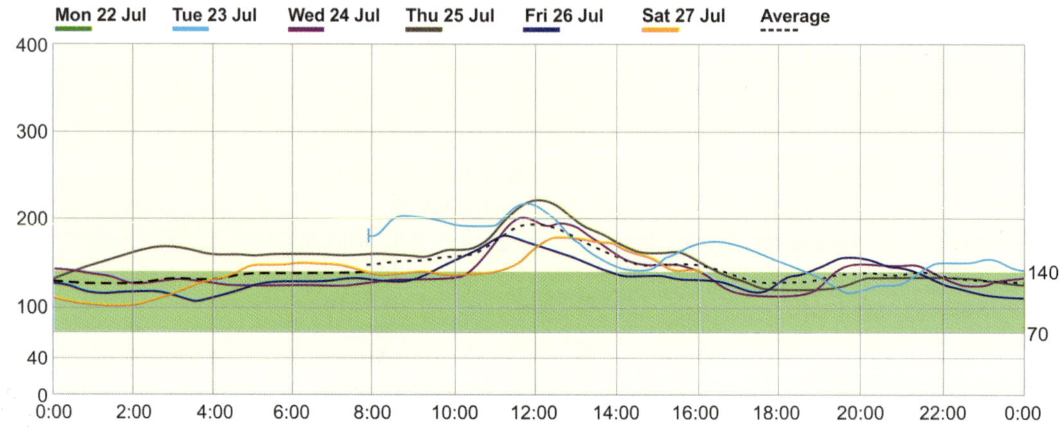

Fig. 22: Repeat CGMS recording of the same patient

be affected with hypotension in sick patients and many drugs may also interfere in sensor function, CGMS is not approved for use in critically ill patients. It may be used in non-critically ill hospitalized patients. More studies are needed in this area and may be in future CGMS may be cleared for critically ill patients as well.[18]

CGMS TECHNOLOGY IN INDIA VERSUS DEVELOPED COUNTRIES

In developed countries, personal CGMS devices and sensor augmented insulin pumps are very often used. Use of this technology has made it possible to bring HbA1c goal to near normal even in T1DM. In India, as of now CGMS use is less. The reason for under usage of CGMS includes cost, lack of training to interpret the report, need of calibration, need of trained manpower, etc. Soon all these obstacles will be taken care by easier and lower priced technologies.

Future of CGMS

Since last few years, avoiding hypoglycemia and improving quality of life have become important goals for diabetes management. CGMS technology provides opportunity to study glycemic variability, to understand glucose trends and thus CGMS is expected to be used more often in future as this will help in micromanagement of diabetes. In addition, popularity of personal CGMS will make the move from SMPG to CHGM.

REFERENCES

1 Bolinger J, Hagestrom-Toft E, Ungerstedt U, Arner P. Selft-monitoring of blood glucose in type 1 diabetic patients: Comparison with continuous microdialysis measurements of glucose in subcutaneous adipose tissue during ordinary life conditions. Diabetes Care. 1997;20:64-70.
2. Klonoff D. Continuous glucose monitoring roadmap for the 21st century diabetes therapy. Diabetes Care. 2005;28:1231-39.

3. Hirsh I, Abelseth J, Bode B, et al. Sensor-augmented insulin pump therapy: results of the first treat-to target study. Diabetes Technol Ther. 2008;10:413-4.
4. Boland E, Monsod T, Dulucia M, Brandt CA, Fernando S, Tamborlane WV. Limitations of conventional methods of self-monitoring of blood glucose: lessons learnt from 3 days of continuous glucose sensing in pediatric patients with type 1 diabetes. Diabetes Care. 2001;24:1858-62.
5. Garg SK, Zisser H, Schwartz S, Bailey T, Kaplan R, Ellis S, Jovanovic L. Improvement in glycemic excursions with a transcutaneous, real-time continuous glucose sensor. Diabetes Care 2006;29: 44-50.
6. The Diabetes Research in Children Network (DirectNet) Study Group: Accuracy of the modified continuous glucose monitoring system (CGMS) sensor in an outpatient setting: result from a diabetes research in children network (DirectNet) study. Diabetes Technol Ther. 2005;7:109-14.
7. Djakoure-Planatoff C, Redermercker R, Reach G, Shama G, Selam JI. Accuracy of the continuous glucose monitoring system in inpatient and outpatient conditions. Diabetes Metab. 2003;29:159-62.
8. International Organization for Standardization. Requirements for in vitro blood glucose monitoring systems for self-testing in managing diabetes mellitus. ISO/TC 212/WG3. Draft International Standard ISO/DIS 15197. Geneva, International Organization for Standardization, 2001.
9. Metzger M, Leibowitz G, Waenstein J, Glaser B, Raz I. Reproducibility of glucose measurements using the glucose sensor. Diabetes Care. 2002;25:1185-91.
10. Conrad SC, Mastrototataro JJ, Gitelman SE. The use of a continuous glucose monitoring system in hypoglycemic disorders. J. Pediatr Endocrinol Metab. 2004;17:281-8.
11. Rodbard D. Interpretation of continuous glucose monitoring data: Glycemic variability and quality of glycemic control. Diabetes Technol Ther. 2009;11(Suppl 1);555-67.
12. Maran A, Crepaldi C, Tiengo A, Grassi G, Vitali E, Pagano G, et. el. Continuous subcutaneous glucose monitoring in diabetic patients: A multicenter analysis. Diabetes Care. 2002;25:347-52.
13. Weinzimer SA, Tamborlane WV, Chase HP, Garg SK. Continuous glucose monitoring in type 1 diabetes. Curr Diab Rep. 2004;4:95-100.
14. Deiss D, Bollinder J, Riveline JP, et al. Improved glycemic control in poorly controlled patients with type 1 diabetes using real-time continuous glucose monitoring. Diabetes Care. 2006;29:2730-2.
15. O' Connell MA, Donath S, O' Neal DN, et al. Glycemic impact of patient-let use of sensor-guided pump therapy in type 1 diabetes: A randomised control trial. Diabetologia. 2009;52:1250-7.
16. Byrne EZ, Zisser HC, Jovanovic L. Continuous glucose monitoring: is it helpful in pregnancy? Curr Diabetes Rev. 2008;4:223-6.
17. Seigmund T, Rad NT, Ritterath C, Seibert G, Henrich W, Buhling KJ. Longitudinal changes in the continuous glucose profile measured by the CGMS in healthy pregnant women and determination of cut-off values. Eur J Obstet Gynecol Reprod Biol. 2008;139:46-52.
18. Tanenberg R, Bode B, Lane W, Laretan C, Mestman J, Harmel AP, et al. Use of continuous glucose monitoring system to guide therapy in patients with insulin-treated diabetes: a randomised control trial, Mayo Clin Proc. 2004;79:1521-6.
19. Godberg PA, Seigel MD, Russell RR, Sherwin RS, Halickman JI, Cooper DA, et al. Experience with the continuous glucose monitoring system in a medical intensive care unit. Diabetes technol Ther 2004;6:339-47.
20. Potts RO, Tamada JA, Tierney MJ. Glucose monitoring by reverse ionophoresis. Diabetes Metab Res Rev. 2002;18 (Suppl. 1):s49-s53.

26

CHAPTER

Management of Diabetes in Geriatric Population

Murlidhar S Rao

INTRODUCTION

With increasing aging of the population and changes in the lifestyle, the prevalence of diabetes is likely to increase among the older individuals aged more than or equal to 65 years. The most recent estimates of International Diabetes Federation (IDF) indicate that globally 8.3% of adult people (i.e. 382 million) have diabetes. This figure may go beyond 592 million cases in the coming 25 years.[1] At least 20% of the patients more than or equal to 65 years have diabetes and this number is expected to grow rapidly in the coming decades. Around 10% of people aged 65–74 years and 20% over 80 years of age are affected by diabetes.[2] An additional 25% of the older people have impaired glucose tolerance (IGT) and impaired fasting glucose (IFG), IGT is known to increase the propensity of the individual for cardiovascular disease (CVD) (macrovascular and atherosclerotic) similar to diabetes [National Health and Nutriton Examination Survey (NHANES)].[3] Nearly half of the elderly diabetics are undiagnosed. Older diabetics have higher rates of premature death, functional disability and coexisting illnesses such as hypertension (HTN), coronary heart disease (CHD), and stroke than those without diabetes.

The care of the older diabetics is complicated by their clinical and functional heterogeneity. Some older individuals develop diabetes years earlier and have significant complications. Others newly diagnosed and may have years of undiagnosed diabetes with resultant complications, and still other older diabetics with truly recent onset disease have few or no complications. In another study conducted in India,[4] elderly people contribute about 9% of the general population.

In this, IFG was seen in 10.6% and diabetes in 21.9%. About 10–15% of the people over the age 70 years have type 1 diabetes (T1DM) or latent autoimmune diabetes of adults.[4] Diabetes also tends to be more among women with advancing age. One study[5] has shown that increasing age, BMI, waist-to-hip ratio and urbanization are the best predictors of type 2 diabetes (T2DM). IGT and T2DM increase with age more in urban than rural population. Glucose intolerance is primarily manifested as postprandial hyperglycemia almost at the rate of 15 mg/decade from the age of 30 years. Eventually by the age of 75 years, 40% of all individuals would have some form of "dysglycemia".

EPIDEMIOLOGY

Elderly population (≥65 years) contributed to 7% of the total population in India in 2001; it will rise to 9% in 2016. By 2010, 100 million people will be in this age group and by 2020, it will rise to 177 million. According to an estimate, they will contribute 1/3 of the population by the year 2050. Prevalence of diabetes in such elderly population is estimated to be 20% or more. Majority of the elderly have T2DM manifesting in two forms:[6]

1. Preexisting diabetes since its onset in young or middle age. These diabetics have increased insulin resistance (IR), increased hepatic output of glucose and have abnormal plasma insulin response to glucose load.
2. New onset diabetes in geriatric age; these diabetics are lean and secrete markedly less insulin, have less IR and secrete less insulin in response to glucose load. These patients have marked postprandial hyperglycemia and near normal fasting blood glucose levels.

The epidemic of T2DM is clearly linked to increasing rates of overweight and obesity and aging of the population not only in Western population and also in Indian population especially the urban.[4,7]

The International Diabetes Federation (2013) estimates the global prevalence of diabetes among people between 60 years and 79 years of age to be 18.6%, i.e. more than 134.6 million people accounting for over 35% of all cases of diabetes in adults. By 2035 this number is projected to increase beyond 252.8 million. Older people with diabetes have increased rate of diabetes-related complications and also comorbid conditions like physical disability, cognitive dysfunction, falls and fractures, defective vision and hearing, depression, pressure ulcers, etc. A personalized approach to diabetes management is therefore essential. Yet there is a paucity of clinical trials involving older people and hence lack of evidence-based diabetes care guidelines.[1]

Prevalence of diabetes in older people continues to increase with age. However, there is leveling off and in some cases a downward trend as mortality increases after the age of 80 years. A tailored approach to care for the older people with diabetes is imperative in order to minimize potentially severe adverse effects, besides, comorbidities, complications, person's functional ability and level of frailty have to be identified and managed.

ETIOPATHOGENESIS OF DIABETES IN OLDER ADULTS

Both normal insulin secretion by beta cells of the pancreas and normal glucose utilization by peripheral tissues are essential for normal glucose homeostasis. In old age overweight as well as reduced physical activity predisposes the older people to develop IR, IGT and diabetes. Apoptosis of beta cells resulting in defective insulin secretion predominates over IR in lean older diabetics and the reverse happens in the overweight and obese older diabetics. Besides, there is also the diminution of incretin hormones in patients with T2DM. Etiological factors predisposing the elderly to diabetes are as follows.[7,8]

- Age-related decrease in insulin secretion due to apoptosis of beta cells.
- Age-related increase in IR and decreased muscle mass, i.e. sarcopenia.
- Overweight and adiposity.
- Reduced physical activity.

- Polypharmacy (drugs like thiazides, steroids and psychiatric drugs).
- Genetic factors.
- Coexisting illness.
- Noninsulin mediated glucose uptake (70% in central nervous system).
- Reduced secretion of incretin hormones in T2DM.
- Inhibition of glucagon secretion.

Further, there is a slow progressive decline of glomerular filtration rate (GFR) with aging and also development of HTN along with diabetes in most elderly patients. There is a change in pharmacokinetics and pharmacodynamics of the drugs besides dietary constraints of the older people with diabetes. Older adults with diabetes are at risk of developing a similar spectrum of macro- and microvascular complications as their younger counterparts with diabetes. However, their absolute risk of CVD is much higher than younger adults. Skeletal muscle which is the main site of age-related IR is due to decline of insulin sensitivity with advancing age. Visceral adiposity and associated adipokines, oxidative stress, mitochondrial dysfunction and possibly intrinsic decline in insulin sensitivity in muscle fibers are the main cellular and molecular pathophysiological mechanisms which are involved in etiopathogenesis of T2DM. Convergence of various pathways underlying diabetes and CVD on inflammation, oxidative stress and endothelial dysfunction suggests that these age-related diseases might arise from a common foundation (common soil).[9]

Preventive strategies in diabetes that can be efficiently implemented in clinical settings and in the community have been developed and evaluated but as yet there has been little focus on older adults in the translational studies.

In summary etiological factors include:

- Decreased insulin secretion by beta cells due to aging (apoptosis).
- Increased IR due to decreased skeletal mass as age advances and increased adiposity along with decreased physical activity.
- Decreased secretion of incretin hormones in older patients with diabetes; decreased oral glucose-dependent insulin release.
- Decreased glucagon secretion.

CLINICAL PRESENTATION OF ELDERLY PATIENTS WITH DIABETES

Since symptoms are nonspecific and often attributed to aging, diabetes may go undiagnosed in the older people for months together unless routine periodical checkups including blood glucose [oral glucose tolerance test (OGTT)] are done when diabetes may be revealed. Around 50% of older people with diabetes can be asymptomatic.

Fatigues, lethargy, "not being well" are common manifestations of diabetes in old age. Besides, there could be in course of time weight loss, cachexia (neuropathic), periarthritis of the shoulder, extreme muscle weakness (amyotrophy), erectile dysfunction and chronic unexplained pain in the body. Over the months and years, these elderly diabetics are prone to get various chronic complications like macrovascular [atherosclerotic CVD and myocardial infarction (MI)] and microvascular (nephropathy. neuropathy and retinopathy), occlusive peripheral arterial disease (PAD) resulting in limb ischemia, gangrene of the foot and occasionally amputation (Box 1).

Box 1: Symptomatology of diabetes in elderly

- Fatigues, lethargy, "not being well" weight loss, cachexia (neuropathic), periarthritis of the shoulder, extreme muscle weakness (amyotrophy), erectile dysfunction and chronic unexplained pain in the body old age.
- Chronic complications like macrovascular (atherosclerotic CVD and myocardial infarction) and microvascular (nephropathy. neuropathy and retinopathy), occlusive peripheral arterial disease hyperosmolar non-ketotic coma

Of particular importance is to recognize the hyperosmolar non-ketotic coma in the elderly diabetics which could be the presenting symptom.

Common geriatric syndromes in old age are cognitive impairment and hypoglycemia unawareness, falls and fractures, depression, polypharmacy have to be looked for. Besides, urinary incontinence and recurrent urinary tract infections, vaginal infections, neurogenic bladder and polyuria are frequently observed.

DIAGNOSIS OF DIABETES IN THE ELDERLY

The diagnostic criteria for diabetes and prediabetes are same as in general population as per the American Diabetes Association (ADA) criteria.

- Diabetes: (1) Fasting plasma glucose level (PGL) more than or equal to 126 mg/dL. (2) 2 hours post 75-g oral glucose load, PGL more than or equal to 200 mg/dL. (3) Random PGL more than or equal to 200 mg or more/dL with symptoms.
- Prediabetes: (1) IGT: 2 hours post 75-g oral glucose load PGL less than or equal to 140 mg/dL to more than 200 mg/dL. (2) IFG: fasting PGL more than 100 mg/dL to less than 126 mg/dL.
- Type 1 diabetes: Living up to older age: serum C-peptide: Cutoff value off 0.68 mmol after 100 g of oral glucose.

One-third of the elderly have prediabetes and another one-third have diabetes. In the elderly, 2 hour OGTT may be more useful and sensitive than fasting PGL alone. HbA1C has high specificity but less sensitivity (48%) than fasting PGL as a diagnostic tool for diabetes in the elderly. Serum fructosamine may be a useful tool in monitoring of diabetes in the elderly although this has not been fully validated in this set up.

HbA1C can be used as a diagnostic test with a cutoff level of more than or equal to 6.5% diagnosing diabetes. It has the advantage of convenience of patients, less day-to day variability, specificity for diabetes and it is standardized internationally. However, because of low sensitivity, it can miss more than half of subjects with diabetes. Hence HbA1C should be interpreted cautiously in the elderly keeping in view the comorbidities in the changing body physiology. For instance, in a rapid cell turnover states like hemolytic anemia HbA1C could be falsely low. During treatment with iron, vitamin B12 or erythropoietin [in chronic kidney disease, (CKD)], there may be rapid cell turnover and could be falsely low. In contrast, in low cell turnover states especially iron, B12 or folate deficiency or in the very elderly when marrow turnover is low, HbA1C may be high.

SCREENING FOR DIABETES

All the elderly people should be screened for diabetes every 3 years by fasting plasma glucose level (PGL) estimation in the high-risk elderly population with a family history of diabetes, obesity, ethnicity, HTN and IGT. OGTT should also be done to detect cases of IGT which is quite common in the elderly.

COMORBIDITY BURDEN

Chronic complications of diabetes are common among older people with diabetes. Patients have at least one comorbid chronic disease in addition to diabetes and nearly 40% patients have at least three conditions. The comorbidity burden is even higher in the diabetic elderly patients living in the "home for the aged" or "in old age homes". The CVD, visual problems, pressure sores, limb amputations and end-stage renal disease (ESRD) occur more commonly among the diabetic elderly than among nondiabetic patients. Both macrovascular disease (atherosclerotic CVD, PAD and stroke) and microvascular disease (nephropathy, neuropathy and retinopathy) develop faster in the elderly diabetics especially with poor glycemic control. HTN another important comorbidity appears to develop in most T2DM patients even from the onset of diabetes. HTN accelerates both atherosclerotic CVD and microvascular disease. Diabetes, HTN, dyslipidemia, smoking and lack of exercise are risk factors for CHD and these should be well controlled and treated thoroughly in the elderly diabetics. BP threshold for treating T2DM elderly patients with HTN is 150/90 mm Hg and acceptable BP target in this group of patients is below 150/90 mm Hg. Stroke in the elderly has high morbidity and mortality. PAD is two- to fourfold more prevalent in the elderly diabetics, and increased rate of limb amputation is common in elderly diabetics than nondiabetics. The increased comorbidities in the older diabetic people could be related to improved survival and their longevity.

TREATMENT OF DIABETES IN OLDER ADULTS AND THE COMORBIDITIES

Increasing age is a significant risk factor for T2DM, but the diagnosis is often missed or delayed because the clinical presentation is different from that in younger people. Diabetes is a leading cause of death in older adults due to CVD and other related medical comorbidities.

The long-term studies in older adults demonstrating the benefits of intensive glycemic, BP and lipid control are very few and currently there is no evidence to suggest that tight glycemic control will have a positive impact on the outcomes relevant to older people with diabetes. Important factors to consider for diabetes management in older adults are:

- Patient's remaining life expectancy.
- Availability of support services (from the family, government or private agencies).
- Economic issues.
- Coexisting health problems, viz. cognitive disturbances/depression, diabetic complications, polypharmacy and any other medical problems.

ADA (2015) guidelines are as follows:[2]

Category 1: Those older diabetic adults who are functional with long enough life expectancy, no other medical problems and no long-term complications can be treated using the therapeutic interventions and goals similar to those of younger adults with diabetes.

Category 2: Glycemic goals for older adults not meeting the above criteria may be relaxed using individualized criteria avoiding acute hyper- or hypoglycemic complications.

Category 3: Other cardiovascular (CV) risk factors should be treated in the older adults with diabetes keeping in mind the consideration of the time-frame of the benefits and the individual patient. Treatment of HTN is indicated in virtually in all older adults with diabetes. Lipid control and aspirin therapy may benefit those with life expectancy at least equal to time-frame of primary or secondary prevention trials.

Category 4: For patients with advanced diabetic complications and/or substantial cognitive or functional impairment, it is reasonable to set less intensive glycemic targets/goals. ADA treatment goals for glycemia, BP and dyslipidemia in older diabetics are as per the Table 1.

Table 1: Treatment goals for glycemia, BP and dyslipidemia

Category of patients	*HbA1C (%)*	*FPG/PPG (mg/dL)*	*BP (mm Hg)*	*Lipids*
1	<7.5	90–130	<140/90	Statin
2	<8	90–150	<140/90	Moderate dose statin
3 and 4	<8.5	100–180	<150/90	Statin (moderate–high)

Abbreviations: FPG, fasting plasma glucose; PPG, postprandial plasma glucose

Most guidelines are based mainly on expert consensus and clinical expertise and there is not much evidence from clinical trials to support the recommendation meant for older diabetic patients. Main theme of management will be to individualize the treatment considering the functional capacity.

In summary, guidelines generally recommend strict glucose control in healthier, older patients and lax approach in frail patients with multiple comorbidities and high risk of hypoglycemia. In older patients who are overweight/obese, healthy lifestyle modification, weight reduction, exercise and smoking cessation are beneficial as in younger people.

MANAGEMENT

Lifestyle Modification

Since hyperglycemia tends to be mild in most cases, diet therapy can be enough to achieve euglycemia. Individual's food habits, mental status, lack of appetite and taste and depression-all have to be taken in to the account. Smoking cessation and restriction of alcohol use should be strictly advised. Avoidance of hypoglycemia is the key while optimizing the glycemic control. In general, protein content of the diet should be increased, fat content reduced and increase the minerals and vitamins. Exercise therapy has to be individualized in older diabetics.

Oral Antidiabetic Drugs (Oral Hypoglycemic Agents)

Oral antidiabetic drugs [oral hypoglycemic agents (OHAs)] is given in the Table 2.

Table 2: Oral antidiabetic drugs

Biguanides [Metformin (MF)]	• If serum creatinine is >1.5% mg/dL in men and >1.4% mg/dL in women or if the GFR drops to <30 mL/minute • Cardiac failure, dehydration or acute illness due to the increased risk of lactic acidosis
Sulfonylureas (SUs)	• High risk of hypoglycemia • Short-acting SUs such as gliclazide or glipizide are more suitable • Active liver disease • Show significantly higher CV events (IHD, MI, TIA, PAD)
Meglitinides	• Less hypoglycemia
Glitazones [Thiazolidinediones (TZDs)];	• Atherogenic lipid profile and increased risk of cardiovascular events including MI and death especially rosiglitazone • Pioglitazone is useful in obese patient • Pioglitazone is contraindicated in CCF class III or IV and acute MI • Pioglitazone cause fractures
Alpha-glucosidase inhibitors	• Flatulence and diarrhea are common with these drugs
Dipeptidyl peptidase-4 inhibitors (Gliptins)	• No risk of hypoglycemia • Weight-neutral • Low risk of drug-to-drug interaction • Patients with renal insufficiency require dose adjustments of sita, vilda and saxagliptins but not of linagliptin • Hepatic insufficiency is a contraindication for vildagliptin but not for other gliptins • Gliptins are considered cardio safe and hence have been used even in acute coronary syndrome I
GLP-1 Therapies	*Shown evidence* of pancreatitis Renal derangement
Sodium-Glucose transporters-2 (SGLT-2) inhibitors	Increased incidence of UTI and fungal infections

Biguanides (Metformin)

Biguanides; metformin (MF) is a good first-line therapy in older people due to low risk of hypoglycemia and potential weight loss in obese patients. MF is contraindicated if serum creatinine is more than 1.5% mg/dL in men and more than 1.4% mg/dL in women or if the GFR drops to less than 30 mL/minute. Patients with cardiac failure, dehydration or acute illness should not receive MF due to the increased risk of lactic acidosis. MF acts by increasing hepatic glucose output and increasing muscle glucose uptake.

The most common side effects of MF therapy are gastrointestinal (nausea, diarrhea and abdominal pain). Patients receiving MF should be monitored for vitamin B12 and folic acid deficiency by estimating blood levels. Major advantage of MF is its proven cardioprotective effects as shown in the landmark trial UKPDS-34.[10] MF should be stopped temporarily during iodinated contrast radiographic studies.

Sulfonylureas

They are insulin secretagogues. Glibenclamide and Glimepiride are associated with fairly high risk of hypoglycemia and hence are not suited for older diabetic patients. Short-acting sulfonylureas (SUs) such as gliclazide or glipizide are more suitable for these older diabetics. All SUs are metabolized through liver and hence should not be used in patients with active liver disease. SU-treated T2DM patients aged 75 years on an average, show significantly higher CV events (IHD, MI, TIA, PAD) compared to those treated with MF alone. Occasionally glimepiride or repaglinide may be required to achieve better control.

Meglitinides (Repaglinide)

Meglitinides (repaglinide) is a short-acting non-SU insulin secretagogue and is preferred in the elderly diabetics. Repaglinide stimulates insulin secretion through a different site compared to SUs. It is primarily metabolized by the liver and has a short half-life of 1 hr. Hypoglycemia is less likely and postparindal regulation is better. It can be freely used in type 2 diabetic patients with CKD. Repaglinide is more effective than nateglinide and is safer.

Glitazones (Thiazolidinediones)

Rosiglitazone and Pioglitazone reduce the IR and improve the insulin sensitivity. They may also increase insulin secretion in response to glucose at least in patients with IGT. Only pioglitazone is used to treat some older patients with T2DM and is preferred over rosiglitazone which results in atherogenic lipid profile and increased risk of CV events including MI and death.[11] Rosiglitazone is banned in Europe and USA and removed from Indian market. Pioglitazone is beneficially used in obese T2DM as insulin sensitizer along with MF.[12]

Pioglitazone however causes mild slow water retention and hence is contraindicated in CCF class III or IV and acute MI. Glitazones in general may result occasionally in fractures among old patients with diabetes. New concerns regarding the increased risk of bladder cancer with long-term use of moderate to high dosage of pioglitazone (30–45 mg/day) have been raised.[13] However, this concern is to be taken with caution as shown in some of the later studies. Pioglitazone can be used in patients who have impaired renal function. Pioglitazone in a recent study (ACTNOW)[14] reduced the carotid intima-media thickness (IMT), a subclinical measure of atherosclerosis and is independent of various risk factors in patients with T2DM and IGT. Pioglitazone has been shown to reduce carotid IMT much more compared to glimepiride in a study.[15]

Alpha-Glucosidase Inhibitors

Alpha-glucosidase inhibitors (acarbose, voglibose and miglitol) inhibit the GI alpha-glucosidase that converts dietary starch and other complex carbohydrates to monosaccharaides, thereby slowing the absorption of glucose. Therefore, the postprandial plasma concentration of glucose rises slowly. They may be used alone or with any other OHAs or insulin. Flatulence and diarrhea are common with these drugs. Since they are weak, hypoglycemic agents are suitable as add-on therapy in older people with diabetes. They may increase insulin sensitivity but not insulin release.

Dipeptidyl Peptidase-4 Inhibitors (Gliptins)

Of the various drugs belonging to this class, sitagliptin, vildagliptin, saxagliptin, linagliptin and alogliptin are available for use. DPP-4 is a unique enzyme that deactivates a variety of bioactive peptides including glucagon-like-peptide-1 (GLP-1) and glucose-dependent insulinotropic polypeptide. Gliptins have been shown to be more effective in the elderly perhaps because the levels of DPP-4 increase with advancing age. DPP-4 inhibitors suppress DPP-4 enzyme and ultimately increase GLP-1 and also suppress glucagon and as a result glucose-mediated insulin secretion is augmented.

Gliptins are oral drugs and can be given along with OHAs. However, they are weak antidiabetic drugs, have no risk of hypoglycemia, are weight-neutral and have low risk of drug-to-drug interaction. Patients with renal insufficiency require dose adjustments of sita, vilda and saxagliptins but not of linagliptin. Hepatic insufficiency is a contraindication for vildagliptin but not for other gliptins. Gliptins are considered cardio safe and hence have been used even in acute coronary syndrome (ACS) settings as well. A recent clinical trial assessing saxagliptin on vascular outcomes in patients with diabetes[16] evaluated saxagliptin and the results showed those on saxagliptin were more likely to be hospitalized for heart failure (HF) than were those who were given placebo (3.5% vs 2.8%).[17] In general gliptins are safe to be used in T2DM more so in older diabetics where the benefits also may be more.

GLP-1 Therapies

Liraglutide and exenatide are administered parenterally—exenatide subcutaneous (SC) twice daily and also weekly (depo preparation) and liraglutide once daily SC. They reduce the weight and can be given to obese diabetic patients and not for frail diabetic subjects.

Oral glucose has greater stimulatory effect on insulin secretion than IV glucose. This is called in cretin effect which is mediated by several GI peptides particularly GLP-1. Exenatide, liraglutide and albiglutide are GLP-1 agonists which can be used as mono therapy or in combination with other OHAs. Some post-marketing reports have shown acute pancreatitis and deterioration of renal function in diabetics taking GLP-1 agonists. However, there are insufficient data to know about their causal relationship.

Bromocriptine: Timed release bromocriptine is approved for use in T2DM. It acts by resetting the hyper-dopaminergic tone of the hypothalamus which is disturbed in diabetes. Its action occurs through the dopaminergic receptors. It is cardio safe but it has limited efficacy in general.

Pramlintide

It is administered as meal time SC injections with insulin. It can be used for both T1DM and T2DM. It requires multiple SC injections and hence its use in older diabetics is limited. It is an amylin analog.

Sodium-Glucose Transporters-2 Inhibitors

This new class of oral agents acts by inhibiting the reabsorption of glucose in the proximal convoluted tubules of the kidneys leading to increased excretion of glucose in urine thereby decreasing the PGLs. This is a sort of insulin independent mechanism to lower blood glucose.

Dapagliflozin of this class is widely studied and in doses of 5, 25 and 100 mg given orally improves the glycemic control and also reduces the weight. It can be given singly or with MF. It is recently approved in the USA and Europe.

Insulin

Insulin is often underutilized in older patients of diabetes because of the fear by the clinician, patients or family. However insulin should be used in elderly patients when OHAs are not tolerated or insufficient to achieve satisfactory glycemic control. The new long-acting insulin analogs are suitable for older people due to the ease of use and lower risk of hyperglycemia. Aged patients and their caretakers should be adequately familiar with use of insulin pen and patient cognitively capable of drawing up and giving the appropriate dosage of insulin either through pen or vials and syringe, monitoring blood glucose levels and recognizing and treating hypoglycemia. Insulin remains the most cost-effective treatment of diabetes in both old and the young patients. With modern insulin analogs, viz., rapid acting as part, lispro and glulisine, premixed as part and lispro as well as basal detemir, glargine and degludec, the safety and the convenience of insulin therapy has improved. Insulin is a first-line therapy for diabetes with severe symptomatic hyperglycemia. Insulin has no upper dosage limit and it has no contraindications to its use. Insulin titration in the elderly with cognitive dysfunction and depression, cardiac or renal failure is a real challenge. Technical superiority of a product (analogs vs conventional) or an injection device (pen vs syringe) should play a role in planning insulin therapy in the elderly to make it more comfortable.

Glycemic targets: For healthier, fit, older people with recently diagnosed T2DM, tight glycemic control with HbA1C of 7% is reasonable. For frail older people and/or with CV risk, a safer target of HbA1C 7.5–8% is appropriate. For very frail older people with limited life expectancy, a target of HbA1C 8–9% is appropriate. Very tight glycemic control in this population may be harmful by inducing hypoglycemia and even death.

Methods of Insulin Administration

- *Premixed*: (a) Human insulin short acting + long acting. (b) Insulin analogs. Rapid (aspart, lispro or glulisine) + long acting.
- *Basal insulin*: NPH insulin and analogs detemir, glargine or degludec.
- *Basal-bolus insulin*: A combination of long-acting insulin and three preprandial rapid-acting insulin is ideal and mimics the physiological insulin secretion. The initial total dosage of insulin/day is 0.6 units/kg body weight.
- *Blood glucose levels monitoring*: Self monitoring of blood glucose (SMBG) or monitoring blood glucose by caretaker of the patients is effective in improving the glycemic control in T2DM and to some extent in T1DM. SMBG can be considered in select older patients depending upon their cognitive abilities.

Comprehensive Geriatric Screening for Vascular Complications[17]

Microvascular

- *Diabetic retinopathy*: Screening for diabetic retinopathy and other ocular disease common in older people with diabetes such as cataract, glaucoma and macular degeneration should be done periodically by experienced ophthalmologist.

- *Diabetic nephropathy:* CKD is common in older people. ESRD is frequent among older diabetics with irregular glycemic control. Persistent micro-albuminuria in a diabetic is an important indication of ongoing diabetic nephropathy and ACEI/ARBs should be helpful medications in such patients.
- *Diabetic neuropathy and diabetic foot disease*: Various types of neuropathy including autonomic neuropathy do occur in long standing diabetic patients with poor glycemic control. Regular inspection of the feet, trophic ulcers and either painful or painless neuropathy may occur.

Macrovascular/Cardiovascular Complications

- CVD is the most common cause of mortality in patients with diabetes regardless of age. Lifestyle modification, weight reduction, regular exercise and smoking cessation are needed.
- Screening of CVD in diabetics with longer duration (more than 10 years of diabetes) is essential and includes ECG, stress testing, Doppler Echo at rest and at exercise (Dobutamine Echo) and if necessary coronary angiography (CAG) or CT coronary angiography to find out significant CAD.
- The treatment modalities such as coronary angioplasty or coronary artery bypass graft can be advised depending upon the angiographic findings. The echo-Doppler study shows in long standing diabetes the status of LV diastolic or systolic function or both. Diastolic dysfunction with preserved left ventricular ejection fraction (>50%) with or without HF which is fairly common in older patients. This might be a predictor of early mortality.
- The basic principle that we learnt from landmark trials like UK prospective diabetes study (UKPDS), Action to control cardiovascular risk in diabetes (ACCORD), A dose evaluation of a vasopressin antagonist in CHF patients undergoing exercise (ADVANCE) and Veterans affairs diabetes trial (VADT) is that heart disease prevention in the diabetic population is possible with improved glycemic control only when the glucose lowering measures (pharmacologic and nonpharmacologic) are started early in the course of diabetes and continued on long-term, may be 10 years or more.
- Aggressive and intensive glycemic control (HbA1C <6%) is harmful and may actually increase the mortality compared to people on standard glycemic control (HbA1C <7%).[18,19] Recently a Japanese trial reported results of multifactorial intervention versus standard care in about 1,000 patients aged more than or equal to 65 years (mean 72 years). After 6 years, no difference in mortality or CV events was found as in ADVANCE and VADT studies.[20] In a recent study of patients on intensive control from UK General Practice Research Database, there was a U-shaped association between HbA1C and mortality. Lowest hazard ratio for death was at an A1C of about 7.5%. Low as well as high mean values of A1C were associated with increased mortality and CV events.[21]

Final philosophy in managing elderly patients with diabetes of varying duration is "individualizing the treatment and holistic care plan".

This is especially important while treating the older diabetics in:

- Critical care unit admitted for sepsis, toxic shock, etc. on parenteral nutrition or in ICCU for MI, cardiogenic shock.

- Perioperative management for various surgical procedures. The basic aim should be "no hyperglycemia and no hypoglycemia". The blood glucose levels should be kept less than 180 mg/dL and should be monitored throughout day and night. Insulin infusion at appropriate dosage should be used along with other critical care measures. Use of glucose insulin potassium regime although commonly used in India has not been shown to be beneficial in a large study (CREATE).[22]

Lipid Lowering in Older Diabetics

There are no large trials of lipid-lowering interventions especially in older adults. ADA (2015) recommendations are:

- A screening lipid profile is reasonable at the time of first diagnosis of diabetes and at the initial medical evaluation.
- For the age group of 40–75 years which includes quite a number of older adults (≥65 years), a moderate to high intensity statin depending upon number of CVD risk factors.
- In the age group of more than or equal to 75 years, statin is advised depending upon the CVD risk factors which include LDL-C (≥100 mg/dL), high BP, smoking and overweight/obesity. Overt CVD includes those with previous CV events or ACS (Table 3).

Combination therapy (statin + fibrate and statin + niacin) has not been shown to provide additional CV benefit above statin therapy alone and hence is not generally recommended (ADA Standards of Medical Care 2015). A statin therapy should be backed up by lifestyle interventions, diet reduction of saturated fat intake, trans fat USF intake and cholesterol intake, and increasing the omega-3 fatty acids and viscous fiber intake (oats, legumes and citrus).

Table 3: Guidelines (ADA 2015)

Age group	*CVD risk factors*	*Recommended statin dose*
40–75 years	• None • CVD risk factors + • Overt CVD +	• Moderate • High • High
>75 years	• None • CVD risk factors + • Overt CVD +	• Moderate • Moderate–high • High

Blood Pressure Control in Elderly Diabetics

Benefits for older adults with diabetes have been inferred from the trials of older adults including but not limited to those with diabetes. Lowering the BP from very high levels (>170 mm Hg) to moderate targets (SBP <150 mm Hg and DBP <80 mm Hg) reduces CV risk in older diabetics. No benefits have been shown to systalic blood pressure (SBP) targets more aggressive than less than 140 mm Hg and that low diastolic blood pressure (DBP) less than 70 mm Hg may be a risk factor for mortality in this elderly diabetic population.

Aspirin use in Older Adults with Diabetes

In the absence of contraindications, aspirin therapy should be offered to virtually all older adults with diabetes and known CVD (secondary prevention); however the benefits of aspirin for primary prevention of CVD events have not been thoroughly elucidated in older adults with diabetes. The dosage of aspirin could be 75–162 mg/day orally. Dual anti-platelet therapy (aspirin 75 mg + clopidogrel 75 mg) is reasonable up to a year after an ACS event.

Recommendations

- Older adults with diabetes and with functional and cognitive intactness and with significant life expectancy should receive diabetes care and goals similar to those for younger adults.
- Glycemic goals in some older people may be relaxed and individualized but severe hypoglycemia should be avoided.
- CVD risk factors should be treated; HTN and hyperlipidemia should be treated. Aspirin use is beneficial in secondary prevention.
- Screening for diabetes complications should be individualized and treated. Depression screening in older diabetic patients should be done on priority. In the absence of contraindications, MF should be the first line. Alternatively short-acting SUs like glipizide or gliclazide or a meglitinide like repaglinide. DPP-4 inhibitors can also be considered.[2,17]

SUMMARY

The management of hyperglycemia in older adults with diabetes should be considered seriously by the clinician, the patient and the family. Progression from IGT to the present stage of T2DM and/or with its complications can be prevented effectively by life style interventions and appropriate pharmacologic interventions. The changing body physiology with aging, various geriatric syndromes in diabetes should be thoroughly understood. The various drugs including the OHAs and newer insulins, nutrition requirements of the older people and various comorbidities that can occur in the life of a diabetic particularly the elderly and with poor glycemic control have to be taken care of with periodic monitoring of blood glucose levels. Emergencies and critical care situations may land the older diabetics in ICUs and they have to be managed appropriately.

Hence diagnosis, treatment and overall management of elderly diabetic population call for an expertise apart from experience in the geriatric care, diabetic care and CV care.

REFERENCES

1. International Diabetes Federation. IDF Diabetes Atlas. 6th edition. Belgium: International Diabetes Federation; 2013. pp. 11-6.
2. ADA Standards of Medical Care in Diabetes-2015. Diabetes Care. 2015;38(Suppl 1):567-9.
3. Harris MI, Flegal KM, Cowie CC. Prevalence of diabetes, IFG and IGT in US adults. Third National Health And Nutritional Examination Survey (NHANES)1988-1994. Diabetes Care. 1998;21:518-24.
4. Radha Reddy, K M Prasanna Kumar. Diabetes in Elderly: In: Chandalia HB (Ed). RSSDI Text Book of Diabetes. 3rd edition. New Delhi: Jaypee Brothers Medical Publishers; 2014. pp 1186-96.
5. Ramchandran A, Shehalatha C, Dharmaraj D, et al. Prevalence of glucose intolerance in Asian Indians. Diabetes Care. 1992;15:348-55.
6. Baruah M, Kalra S, Mathew J, et al. Diabetes in the Elderly: Critical appraisal in management. Intern J Clin Cases Invest. 2010;1(4):7-14.
7. Ahmed H, Abdel Hafiz, Sinclair AJ. Management of type 2 diabetes in older people. Diabetes Ther. 2013;4:13-26.

8. Bawa SS, Sehagal V, Kalra S, et al. Management of type 2 diabetes in geriatric population: current perspectives. J Pharm Biochem Sci. 2014;6(3):151-7.
9. Kirkman MS, Venessa JB, Clark N, et al. Diabetes in older adults: a consensus report. J Amer Geriat Soc AGS JAGS. 2012;60:2342-56.
10. UK Prospective Diabetes Study (UKPDS) Group. Effect of intensive blood glucose control with Metformin on complications in overweight patients with type 2 diabetes (UKPDS-34). Lancet. 1998;352:854-65.
11. Nissen SE, Wolski K. Effect of rosiglitazone on the risk of myocardial infarction and death from cardiovascular causes. N Engl J Med. 2007;356:2457-71.
12. Dormandy JA, Charobonnel B, Eckland DJ, et al. Secondary prevention of macrovascular events in patients with type 2 diabetes in the prospective pioglitazone clinical trial in macrovascular events (PROACTIVE study): a randomized controlled trial. Lancet. 2005;366:1279-89.
13. Neumann A, Weill A, Ricordan P, et al. Pioglitazone and risk of bladder cancer among diabetic patients in France: A population-based Cohort study. Diabetologia. 2012;55:1953-62.
14. Saremi A, Schwenke D. Reduction in the carotid IMT progression in IGT and metabolic syndrome patients (ACTNOW study): Presented at ADA 71st scientific sessions.
15. Mazone I, Meyer PM, Fenistein SB, et al. Effect of Pioglitazone compared with glimepiride on carotid IMT in type 2 diabetes. JAMA. 2006;296:2572-81.
16. Scirica BM, Bhatt DL, Braunwald E, et al. Saxagliptin and cardiovascular outcome in patients with type 2 diabetes. NEJM. 2013;369:1317-26.
17. McCulloch D, Munsi M. Treatment of type 2 diabetes in the older patients. Official Reprint for UpToDate. Published by Wolters Kluwer; 2014, pp 6-16.
18. Gerstein HC, Miller M, Byrington RP, et al. Action to control cardiovascular risk in diabetes study group (ACCORD). Effects of intensive lowering of glucose in type 2 diabetic patients. NEJM. 2008;358:2545-59.
19. Skyler JS, Bergenstal R, Bonow RO, et al. Intensive glycemic control and the prevention of CV events. Implications of ACCORD, ADVANCE and VADT Trials: A position statement of ACC, AHA and ADA. Daibetes Care. 2009;32:187-92.
20. Araki A, Iimuro S, Sakurai T, et al. Japanese Elderly Diabetes Intervention Trial Study Group. Long term multiple risk factor intervention in Japanese Elderly Patients. Geriatric Gerontology Int. 2012;12(Suppl 1):7-17.
21. Curie CJ, Peters JR, Tynam A, et al. Survival a function of HbA1C in people with type 2 diabetes: A retrospective Cohort Study. Lancet. 2010;375:481-9.
22. Yusuf S, Mehta SR, Xie C, et al. Effects of reviparin, a low-molecular-weight heparin, on mortality, reinfarction, and strokes in patients with acute myocardial infarction presenting with ST-segment elevation. JAMA. 2005;293(4):427-35.

27

CHAPTER

Diabetes Education as a Pillar of Prevention and Care

Sarita Bajaj, Tanushree Chawla

PRESENT STATUS OF DIABETES IN INDIA

The global prevalence of diabetes mellitus is 366 million, which is expected to rise to 552 million (a 51% increase) by 2030. More than 60% of world's population with diabetes resides in Asia, of which two nations; India and China contribute the largest. The large scale DiabCare Asia study designed to describe and investigate diabetes control, management and complication status in patients with diabetes from Asian countries, reported that approximately half the patients living with diabetes in India at present have poor glycemic control and the age of onset of type 2 diabetes is earlier in Indians. The estimated number of people living with diabetes in India as of 2012 is 61.3 million which is expected to rise to 101.2 million (an alarming 65% increase) by 2030 implicating that every fifth person with diabetes in the world would be an Indian, which is quite a disturbing figure.

Till date, an estimated 77.2 million people in India and 280 million world-wide suffer from prediabetes contributing to the future burden of diabetes. The Asian Indian phenotype and lifestyle associated with urbanization essentially contributes to this distressing rise in prevalence of Diabetes Mellitus in India. It is not just a disease of the upper class; in fact recent surveys indicate diabetes at present affects staggering 10–16% of urban population and 5–8% of rural population in India.

The chronic nature of disease is not only physically and emotionally demanding for the patient but also a financial burden on the patient because of the cost of primary therapy as well as of associated complication treatment. The total cost of expenses on diabetes and its complications also puts enormous pressure on our economy.

ROLE OF DIABETES EDUCATION IN MANAGEMENT OF DIABETES

There has been a lot of contemplation on the positive role of health education, self-care, lifestyle modification and community participation in the management of diabetes and its complications thereby reducing disease burden on the society. Various trials have provided evidence for the same.[1]

It has been published in recent studies that a weight loss of 3–5% is likely to result in clinically meaningful reductions in triglycerides, blood glucose and A1C.[2] However, the 2013 Obesity Guidelines noted achieving more weight loss (10%) will also reduce blood pressure, improve low-density lipoprotein cholesterol and high-density lipoprotein cholesterol, and reduce the need for medications required to control cardiometabolic risk.[2]

Look AHEAD (Actions for Health in Diabetes) trial provides evidence, specific to diabetes, that an intensive lifestyle intervention can achieve a 5–10% weight loss and can improve sleep apnea quality-of-life indices, achieve cardiometabolic biomarker improvements and reduce need for medications.[3-6]

The Diabetes Prevention Program (DPP),[9] a landmark National Institutes of Health/National Institute of Diabetes and Digestive and Kidney Diseases, clinical multicentric trial, provided the best evidence that individuals at high risk for type 2 diabetes can prevent or delay the onset of the disease by modest weight loss and physical activity.[10] The study subjects were randomly assigned to either metformin group or to the lifestyle intervention group where they received intensive one-on-one training in behavior modification, including proper nutrition and increased physical activity.[8] The results were extremely positive for the lifestyle intervention group. With modest weight loss, i.e. at least 7% of body weight through a healthy, low-fat, low-calorie diet and increased physical activity, i.e. 150 minutes/week the risk of progression to type 2 diabetes was found to be significantly reduced by 58%. Which was true for all ethnic groups and it was also found that subjects above 60 years of age had an even greater. Reduction of 71%, a 10-year follow-up study found that the subjects in the lifestyle intervention arm maintained a decreased risk of diabetes by 34% even after a decade after trials conclusion and yet again, individuals above 60 years of age demonstrated a greater reduction in the risk of progression to diabetes by 49%.[7]

Groundbreaking results of this trial helped to recognize the importance of self-care in the management of diabetes but the cost of intensive individual counseling was quite high, but it was established that community-based approach can be very cost effective.

The American Association of Clinical Endocrinologists emphasizes the importance of patients becoming active and knowledgeable participants in their care. Likewise, WHO has also recognized the importance of patients learning to manage their diabetes. The American Diabetes Association had reviewed the standards of diabetes self-management education and found that there was a four-fold increase in diabetic complications for those individuals with diabetes who had not received formal education concerning self-care practices.

All the above evidence suggest that sustained health education plays a vital role in management of the disease and can help in reduction of the risk of complications, comorbidities and even delay progression of prediabetics to diabetics. This can effectively help in reducing the social and economic burden associated with the disease in a simple and safe method.

Barriers in Diabetes Management

The underestimation of diabetes education by the physicians as well as the dependence of the patient on the health professional is the major impediment in management. It has to be emphasized that diabetes is largely a preventable disease and more than the drugs, simple lifestyle modifications by the patient can help to decrease the disease burden.

Role of the patient has to be reversed from that of being a passive partner in management of the disease to an active one. Communication plays a crucial role. Developing an interpersonal relationship with the patient will help in understanding the patient's attitude toward his problem, impediments in adopting the recommended lifestyle modification advise and developing realistic targets on the individual basis.

Another fundamental problem is the difficulty in outreaching to the remote areas and maximum number of people. This can be overcome by telemedicine and education over telephonic conversation. Large number of people can be approached at the same time. It has been suggested by various studies, with the help of the local health practitioner and professionals, telemedicine can be an effective measure to reach out to people in the remotest area.

Ignorance is another major concern. Awareness about the disease and benefits of healthy lifestyle shall be extended to all by the means of posters, pamphlets, media, newspaper, messaging services and various health-related user friendly apps. Organizing diabetes awareness camps with providing incentives like free glucose monitoring, blood pressure recording, etc. may also prove beneficial.

Components of Diabetes Health Education

To encourage self-care behavior is an essential component of medical care provided to the diabetics. The patient should be given appropriate knowledge about his illness, and counseling directed toward lifestyle modification shall be started immediately with first contact. And to sustain this behavior reinforcement is essential that is with every clinical visit the importance of lifestyle changes shall be assertively communicated to the patient and the family members equally. Information regarding identification and management of certain preventable life-threatening complications, like hypoglycemia, shall be conveyed to the patient as well as the family members.

Health education for diabetes includes the following aspects—

Education about the Disease Process

Patients must be educated about progressive nature of the disease. Educating them about the severity of the disease, its association with various complications, which have a linear relationship with the degree of hyperglycemia. Thus emphasizing the importance of continuous vigilance and maintenance of normoglycemia at all times.

Lifestyle Modification[13]

- Dietary advice and physical exercise are two essential components of the education program.
- Dietary advice cannot be a blanket advice, i.e. one for all.
- Diet plan has to be individualized taking into account the food habits, quantity as well as quality of work, available resources.
- The associated comorbid conditions may restrict the exercise capacity of the person; therefore the exercise regimen has to be customized.

- Though in absence of any comorbidities every individual shall be advised for at least 30 minute of brisk walk every day.

Self-care Behavior

- Diabetes foot care and wound care are important aspects. Complications such as diabetic nephropathy and diabetic neuropathy put the foot at increased risk of complications.
- All diabetics shall take adequate foot care. They should avoid walking bare foot, use of proper foot wear and daily inspection of the foot for unnoticed wounds.

Self-monitoring of Blood Glucose

It has been shown that self-monitoring of blood glucose is associated with better glycemic control. The frequency of blood glucose measurement is determined by the type of regimen, the level of blood glucose before the initiation of treatment and the presence of complications. Maintenance of records of self-glucose measurement can help the physician better understand the adequacy of the treatment regimen and allows patient to assess the adequacy of the drugs, diet and physical activity and make appropriate changes on their own.[7]

Skill Development

To enhance the level of active participation of the patient in the self-management of the disease, appropriate skills have to be developed which will help them combat various situation like fasting states as observed by Muslims in Ramadan without developing any complications. Adequate training needs to be given to the patient and his family members for identification and management of hypoglycemia which is an easily preventable though fatal complication.

Compliance with Medications

Strong association of severity and duration of hyperglycemia with the development of the microvascular and macrovascular complications is well established. Patient shall be emphasized about the importance of adherence with the medications and maintaining near normal glucose range.

Major factors leading to nonadherence include cost of the treatment, regimen complexity, patient's emotional well-being, and patient's perceptions of medication side effects and medication-related intrusions on activities of daily living.

Elimination of the Misconceptions

Misconceptions related to disease process, use of insulin. For instance keeping insulin as a last resort for management of diabetes and using it as weapon to deal with nonadherence with medications has resulted in development of superfluous fear about insulin in the minds of people.

The major barriers in the path of sustaining this behavior are lack of time, lack of interest on the part of the physician as well as the patient, lack of motivation, and lack of adequate resources and funding.

Essential Aspects of Diabetes Prevention Program Development[7]

Only providing information is not sufficient, the patients have to be imparted adequate skills to cope with the day-to-day problems they face when living with diabetes.

This will require an integrated approach with trained staff, i.e. a health educator, nurse, dietician and pharmacist.

Diabetes prevention programs need to be developed which would have a patient centric approach and along with community participation. To device these programs patient attitude, illness-related behavior and patients disease perception have to be studied intensively so that they can be effectively delivered. It has been shown that programs developed based on this approach are very efficacious for the first 6 months.[12]

These programs shall be interactive sessions with workshops, group discussions and scenario-based learning. It is established that group sessions are more effective than one-on-one interaction. It provides an empathizing environment to the patient, an opportunity to share their experiences and innovative personal methods to combat with the disease. It helps them to understand the motives for their current behavior. The patients could relate to each other and makes it easier for them to acquire the knowledge and skills from their equals.[7,11]

The health professionals involved in imparting the health education through these programs should equally be motivated toward their goal and should have adequate expertise for the same. One important aspect is development of communication skills which plays a major role in developing a healthy and assertive patient and health professional relationship. Without which the imparted education may not be imbibed properly and all the efforts put in may become futile.

There should be continued medical education for the physicians to keep abreast with the latest guidelines pertaining to the management of the disease. The concept of negotiated curriculum is strongly recommended, i.e. subject matter shall be of personal interest which forms a strong motivation for patient participation.

Government needs to play an active role in health education by formulating programs for diabetes health education and training programs for development of skills in the health professionals. Adequate funding is also a concern.

Working Model for a Diabetes Education Program[8]

The programs should be based on the adult education theories. The various theories focus on five domains of learning in which change may take place: knowledge, skills, understanding, attitudes and application. This model should be used as a framework for directing patient education (process) and intervention goals (outcomes) within the trial.

First and foremost step in developing a program shall be laying down its organizational structure, defining its goals, the target population and enlisting the resources available. Formation of an advisory committee to ensure quality. It should include health professionals, individual with diabetes and community representatives.

A coordinator with academic or experiential preparation in chronic disease care and management shall be designated to oversee the planning, implementation and evaluation of diabetes self-management education. The instructors should be well versed with recent advancements in the diabetes education. Regular continuing education in the field of diabetes management and education shall be provided to the instructors. The content areas shall be determined by assessment of needs of the individuals with diabetes and prediabetes. The educational interventions and self-management strategies should be developed collaboratively by the patient and the educator.

Follow-up programs form the foundation. Defining outcomes and patient-defined goals and record keeping helps in an assessment of effectiveness of the program. Appropriate techniques shall be devised to measure these outcomes at regular intervals.

Continuous revision of the program shall be done to improve the quality of the program.

Sustaining the Advantage of the Diabetes Education

Reinforcement of the knowledge provided forms an essential component of diabetes education. Without continuous education, there is a gradual decline in the self-care behavior. Therefore, contact with the healthcare provider at regular interval is extremely important to help retain the self-care behavior in the patients.[14]

Patient's records, like body weight, body mass index, blood pressure, neuropathic screening records and electrocardiograms, shall be adequately maintained in the form of graphs to provide a visual analog to patient to self-assess their progress over the period of time. It helps patient to make appropriate changes to their management regimen.

DIABETES EDUCATION IN INDIA: ESSENTIAL COMPONENTS

India being a resource poor country and widespread demographic, cultural, educational and language differences pose a definite challenge in spreading awareness about diabetes.

A strategy utilizing both conventional (dramas, skits, newspaper, TV, etc.) and nonconventional (internet, short message service, mobile phone apps, etc.) modes of communication must be adopted to maximize the reach of diabetes education programs. Cost-effectiveness of telemedicine-based multidisciplinary care in achieving glycemic targets and providing continuous education may be considered. Titration of insulin and oral drugs in this program precludes the need for physical visits to the hospital and avoids hypoglycemia even in patients on insulin therapy. Popular figures and community leaders can prove to be an invaluable part of such awareness programs for popularizing insulin therapy. The inauguration of a program on "Changing Diabetes in Children" by former President APJ Abdul Kalam is an example of increasing awareness through public personalities. The program observed huge media coverage and increased awareness among public from all the states of India about the needs of children with type 1 diabetes. Similarly, Changing Diabetes Barometer, a public-private-partnership program launched in five states of India to improve lives of people with diabetes observed an increased awareness and glycemic control in patients from all these states after diabetes awareness programs. As media plays a pivotal role in the dissemination of information, sensitizing mass media personnel about the importance and the factual details of insulin will help in the dissemination of accurate information on insulin use.

CONCLUSION

Various diabetes trials have shown that diabetes education targeting a change in behavior of the patients may lead to a significant reduction in the progression of the disease and development of complications associated with it. Consequently leads to reduction in the hospitalization as well as morbidity and mortality related to the disease process, and thereby leading to a reduction in the economic and social burden.

An integrated multidisciplinary patient-centered approach is required for effective communication of the behavioral changes in the diabetics. In addition, the state should realize the financial benefits from the information provided to patients with type 2 diabetes and support such interventional programs.

Whilst education can empower patients to take on greater responsibility for the management of their disease, they cannot achieve long-term success without the cooperation of health professionals who can support and facilitate achievement of patients' goals. This role demands a greater understanding of the theories underlying patient education and the communication skills required to promote such autonomy. The responsibility for management of the disease resides with patients and the primary role of the health professional becomes one of supporter and educator.

REFERENCES

1. Srivastava SR, Srivastava PS, Ramasamy J, et al. Role of self-care in management of Diabetes Mellitus. J Diabetes Metabol Disord. 2013;12:4.
2. Toledo FGS, Ruppert K, Huber KA, et al. Efficacy of the telemedicine for reach, Education, Access, and Treatment (Treat) Model for Diabetes Care. Diabetes Care. 2014;37:E179-80.
3. Judith Wylie-Rosett. Weight-loss intervention by Telephone: Lessons Learned. Diabetes Care. 2014;37:2078-80.
4. Funnel MM, Brown TL, Childs BP, et al. National standards for diabetes self-management Education. Diabetes Care. 2011;34(1):S89-96.
5. Formosa C, G Alfred, Chokalingam N, et al. The importance of diabetes Foot Care Education in a Primary Care Setting. J Diabetes Nursing. 2012;16(10):410-4.
6. Cooper HC, Booth K, Gill G. Patients' perspectives on diabetes health care education. Health Edu Res. 2003;18(2):191-206.
7. Steinsbekk A, Rygg L, Lisulo M, et al. Group based diabetes self-management education compared to routine treatment for people with type 2 diabetes mellitus. A systematic review with meta-analysis. BMC Health Serv Res. 2012;12:213.
8. Green LW, Brancati Fl, Albright A, et al. Primary prevention of type 2 diabetes: integrative public health and primary care opportunities, challenges and strategies. Fam Pract. 2012;29:i13-23.
9. DPP Research Group. Reduction in the incidence of type 2 diabetes with lifestyle intervention or metformin. N Engl J Med. 2002;346:393-403.
10. Jensen MD, Ryan DH, Apovian CM, et al. AHA/ACC/TOS Guideline for the management of overweight and obesity in adults: A Report of the American College of Cardiology/American Heart Association Task Force on Practice Guidelines and the Obesity Society. Circulation. 2013.
11. Kuna ST, Reboussin DM, Borradaile KE, et al; Sleep AHEAD Research Group of the Look AHEAD Research Group. Long-term effect of weight loss on obstructive sleep apnea severity in obese patients with type 2 diabetes. Sleep. 2013;36:641-9A.
12. Wing RR, Bolin P, Brancati Fl, et al. Look ahead research group. Cardiovascular effects of intensive lifestyle intervention in type 2 diabetes. N Engl J Med. 2013;369:145-54.
13. Williamson DA, Rejeski J, Lang W, et al. Impact of a weight management program on health-related quality of life in overweight adults with type 2 diabetes. Arch Intern Med. 2009;169:163-71.
14. Annuzzi G, Rivellese AA, Bozzetto L, et al. The results of look ahead do not row against the implementation of lifestyle changes in patients with Type 2 Diabetes. Nutr Metab Cardiovasc Dis. 2014;24:429.

28
CHAPTER

Future Research and Newer Advancement in Diabetes

Samar Banerjee

INTRODUCTION

It is an acceptable fact that effective invention and researches in the subject of diabetes have led to many useful major advances, which has really added to the benefit of patient treatment. To mention some of them are faster-acting and longer-acting insulin analogs, oral antidiabetic agents with minimal or zero level hypoglycemia, smallest blood glucose meters even fitted with mobile phones and insulin pumps to help patients with their diabetes management.[1]

The important major developments of the last four decades are as follows:[2,3]

- In 1967, a laser treatment therapy focusing on affected arterioles for retinopathy was developed. This revolutionized the management of retinopathy, a deadly complication of diabetes that sometimes can lead to blindness. The laser accurately targets damaged parts of the retina, with minimal involvement of the surrounding tissues and helps to control the complication, thus improving a person's sight.
- Till 1969, there was no available method for a person with diabetes to test his or her own blood sugar level and to have an immediate report based on which he could adjust his antidiabetic drugs on spot. Then the Ames Company devised the Eyetone meter. The device was heavier one, weighed 3 pounds, cost $650 and initially was only available to physicians. A year later, patients could buy their own. Now the blood glucose meters are far less expensive, far lighter in weight and more readily available and usable at any time and any place.
- After a decade, in 1979, the hemoglobin A1C test was developed. This test allowed doctors and patients to track average blood sugar levels, giving a much clearer understanding of how well the treatment was working. Now small sized machines are available for testing A1C with very quick results.
- In the same year in 1979, the first insulin pump was invented, but it was very bigger in size and was inconvenient for most people, because it required to be carried around in a backpack. Today insulin pumps are about the size of a match box.
- In the 1980s and 1990s, genetic engineers created new types of insulin to replace the pig or cow insulin that had been standard treatment until then. These "monocomponent" insulins

were considered superior to earlier types, because they were more apt to mimic human insulin.

- Also in the 1980s and 1990s, the very-short-acting analog insulins were developed. These could be injected just 15 minutes before a meal and even after meals if required, giving patients more freedom in timing their meals.
- At the beginning of this century, new, long-acting insulin was introduced called glargine. This insulin has a 24-hour action period, but no peaks and valleys, making more stable blood sugar control possible for some. Subsequently long-acting insulins, like detemir, degludec glargine U300, are introduced with more longer duration of action and better bioavailability.

MORE HOPE FOR FUTURE ADVANCES

In 2006, the US government spent $1.1 billion on diabetes research and treatment. The Juvenile Diabetes Research Foundation (JDRF) and the American Diabetes Association also maintain funds and resources to improve in diabetes research. The work currently under way holds great promise for finding even more new and improved treatments for the disease.[4]

Specific targets of the researches are including the following:

- Prevention, early detection and early intervention
- Islet cell transplantation
- Immunology and immune-genetics to aid in risk identification and potential new treatments
- New treatments to prevent vascular, cardiac and neuronal damage
- Continuous glucose meters to minimize the need for so many finger pricks to test blood sugar levels
- Implantable glucose meters along with implantable pumps.

GENE RESEARCH TOOL IN TYPE 2 DIABETES

The spectrum of genetic research is expanding vastly, as more genes and gene variations are discovered and studied. Many genes have already been isolated with some important diseases and conditions, such as cancers, heart disease and diabetes. Gene variations that signal disease sequences are of special interest to scientists and they are called single nucleotide polymorphisms (SNPs). Of more than 20,000[6] genes in the human genome, it has been slow going for scientists as they are trying through them to find out which SNPs are responsible for chronic diseases that affect us.[5]

Until now, the process of finding the genes and gene clusters responsible for diabetes is very difficult and is like the trying to find needles in a haystack. A new software tool, developed at Michigan Technological University, may make finding genes and gene clusters that have a marked effect on complicated diseases easier. This tool has enabled scientists to pinpoint 11 gene variations,[7] or SNPs, that are associated with type 2 diabetes. The software is helping the scientists to investigate on a more specific array of genes. It is able to narrow the selection from the thousands of genes that make up the human genome down to a more manageable group of the genes and gene variations most likely to be linked to the specific disease. The test is further supported by using statistical methods to detect which variations act individually and which ones act in combination.

INNOVATIVE INSULIN PATCH-PEN

The patch-pen is a small plastic device that is designed to be worn on the skin like a bandage and dispenses rapid acting-insulin for up to 3 days and needs no batteries, electronics or infusion sets. It holds up to 200 units of insulin and is used as a bolus-only device.

ARTIFICIAL PANCREATIC TISSUE FOR ISLET CELL TRANSPLANTS

One of the problems associated with islet cell transplants is the length of time the cells survive in the body after transplant. Researchers have developed a cellular structure that resembles the environment of the pancreas that helps preserve islet cells, allowing them to survive significantly longer while also producing much more insulin.

IMPLANTABLE GLUCOSE SENSOR

Research workers have developed an implantable glucose sensor. This sensor is able to continuously monitor glucose for over a year without removal or maintenance. The encapsulated device showed no rejection by surrounding tissue for more than 500 days. Daily finger prick for multiple times may thus be avoided.

GLUCOSE SENSING TATTOO TO MONITOR GLUCOSE

Tattoos are no longer only body art. Scientists are developing a semipermanent medical tattoo that would give you reliable blood sugar readings and eliminate painful finger sticks.

CELL REPRODUCTION BY IMPLANTED CELL POUCH

Implanted cell pouch may eventually be an alternative to insulin injections. Researchers have developed a device that functions as an organ-like structure that is implanted under the skin. The pouch would contain insulin-producing islet cells that are protected from the body's natural immunity response while at the same time being able to deliver insulin to the body.

RESEARCH ON VACCINATIONS

The dream of diabetes vaccine is expected to be available within a few years. A vaccine that would arrest or slow the autoimmune response that destroys insulin-producing cells may soon be a reality. The Diamyd vaccine, now entering a Phase III clinical trial in both the US and Europe, has shown very promising results in both Phase I and II clinical trials.

ARTIFICIAL PANCREAS RESEARCH

The artificial pancreas research is effectively progressing. The JDRF is partnering with Animas Corporation to develop the first-generation artificial pancreas. This is exciting news because it could become the prototype of a fully automated diabetes management system that completely self-regulates the flow of insulin, much like a healthy pancreas.

NEWER ANTIDIABETIC DRUGS

There is a tremendous need for new antidiabetic treatments for the growing incidence of type 2 diabetes mellitus (T2DM) globally. A chronic disease, like diabetes, requires long-term medical attention and is also an expensive disease to treat. Obesity is closely related to type 2 diabetes, medications that target long-term weight reduction, also improve the diabetic state. Moreover drugs, which treat comorbid conditions, are in demand. Currently, many researchers are focused on developing diabetes therapies that can tackle multiple complications that follow the disease, particularly heart-related illnesses.

Global Diabetes Drug Market

The global increase in the incidence of diabetes numbers and increased medical innovation suggest that there is tremendous scope for drug developers and their investors. At least 235 different diabetes-related drugs were the subject of published clinical trials as of 2010. Analysts estimate the market for diabetes drugs that treat type 2, and potentially cure type 1, at about $25 billion worldwide, and that it will reach $45 billion by 2015. Several companies are investing in the diabetes-related drug development pipeline; primarily for type 2 since upward of 90% of diabetics have this type.[9]

In the Pipeline

Major pharmaceutical companies including Novo Nordisk, Abbott Laboratories, Merck, Sanofi-Aventis, Johnson & Johnson, Roche and Bayer lead the diabetes drug and device market. Additionally new innovative companies are involved in drug discovery and innovative delivery methods as well.

As of March 2012, Alkermes, a biotech company headquartered in Dublin, Ireland, with R&D facilities in Waltham, Massachusetts, had two diabetes drugs in Phase II trials. They are Medisorb and AIR insulin. Medisorb is a sustained-release injectable, and AIR is an inhalable insulin. Key areas for development include drugs that decrease insulin resistance, regenerate or prevent β-cell loss, target cardiovascular issues, have limited dosing requirements, and reduce neuropathies and associated pain. Sodium-glucose cotransporter-2 inhibitors, a promising new class of oral antidiabetic drug and the furthest along in development work on the kidney through insulin-independent mechanisms and theoretically reduce the risk for weight gain associated with current antidiabetes drugs.

Imeglimin [(6R)-(+)-4-dimethylamino-2-imino-6-methyl-1, 2, 5, 6-tetrahydro-1, 3, 5, triazine hydrochloride] is a new tetrahydrotriazine-containing class of oral antidiabetic agents, the glimins. In preclinical studies, imeglimin has been shown to reduce excessive hepatic glucose production, increase glucose uptake in skeletal muscle, and improve insulin secretion in response to glucose Imeglimin targets the mitochondria and is compatible with other drugs, which counter insulin resistance or enhance insulin secretion and β-cell protection. Imeglimin is effective as monotherapy in achieving glycemic control, and has shown a favorable tolerability profile in two Phase IIa studies compared with metformin, with no serious adverse events. The preclinical data shows that imeglimin acts on both insulin-resistant organs and βcells. The effects of imeglimin have been investigated as an add-on to therapies targeting the liver (with metformin) and β cell (with DPP-4 inhibitor). In a recently published add-on trial, imeglimin was shown to improve glycemic control in people with type 2 diabetes that was inadequately controlled by metformin monotherapy.[10]

Newer Drugs

The drug like 11β-hydroxysteroid dehydrogenase type 1 inhibitors inhibit an enzyme responsible for activating cortisone to cortisol, which minimizes the antiglycemic effects of cortisol.

Glycogen phosphorylase inhibitors inhibit the enzymes responsible for hepatic (liver) gluconeogenesis, the generation of glucose from noncarbohydrate enzymes, such as lactate, glycerol and glucogenic amino acids, and lower hepatic glucose output thus controlling the fasting blood glucose. The drugs like glucokinase activators activate a key enzyme to increase hepatic glucose metabolism. Though the mechanism of action is unknown, G-protein–coupled receptor 119 agonists induce insulin release and increase secretion of glucagon-like peptide-1 (GLP-1) and gastric inhibitory peptide (Box 1).

Box 1: Newer drugs

Glimins	Mechanism of action[8] reduce excessive hepatic glucose production, increase glucose uptake in skeletal muscle, and improve insulin secretion in response to glucose Imeglimin targets the mitochondria.
11β-hydroxysteroid dehydrogenase type 1 inhibitors	An enzyme responsible for activating cortisone to cortisol, which minimizes the antiglycemic effects of cortisol.
Glycogen phosphorylase inhibitors	Inhibit the enzymes responsible for hepatic (liver) gluconeogenesis.
G-protein–coupled receptor 119 agonists	Induce insulin release and increase secretion of glucagon-like peptide-1 and gastric inhibitory peptide.
Protein tyrosine phosphatase 1B inhibitors	Sustained insulin and leptin release.

Protein tyrosine phosphatase 1B inhibitors are being explored as a possible oral therapeutic target for glycemic control and weight management through sustained insulin and leptin release. Long-acting GLP-1 analogs and long-acting gliptins once a week are under trial.

Biopharmaceutical research companies are developing near 200 medicines to treat diabetes and related conditions stimulating the formation of insulin producing cells. Some of the ventures are discussed as follows. A potential class treatment for type 1 diabetes is planned to stimulate and enhance the regeneration of insulin-producing β cells in the islets. The treatment is a human peptide consisting of the bioactive part of a gene responsible for regenerating pancreatic islets. In diabetes, there are often too few insulin-producing islets to keep up with the demand for insulin, and regeneration of β cells are the true solution both for type 1 and type 2 diabetes.

Facilitating Glucose Regulation

A potential medicine in development for type 2 diabetes is a gut sensory modulator delivered directly to the stomach where it intensifies the body's natural food-driven signals that facilitate glucose regulation. The medicine, a delayed-release formulation of metformin (a medicine used to treat diabetes alone or in combination with other medicines), targets the lower gut to avoid systemic absorption in the blood stream, making it potentially useful to diabetes patients with renal impairment who are unable to use metformin due to the risk of building metformin up in the blood (lactic acidosis).

Controlling the Inflammation

Inflammation plays an important major role in all the stages of atherothrombosis. This effect starts from the initiation of endothelial injury to the formation of plaque/thrombus in the coronary arteries. This finally manifest into cardiovascular diseases such as acute myocardial infarction and stroke events. Inflammation is also known to be an important contributor to β-cell dysfunction and apoptosis in T2DM patients. Any action to delay the progression of inflammation will help in the prevention of long-term cardiovascular risks. Of the inflammatory molecules, interleukin-1 (IL-1) plays a major role in atherothrombosis. There are evidence to support the contribution of IL-1β isoform-mediated inflammation in atherogenesis and plaque progression, worsening of β-cell function in the islets, and disease progression.

One promising anti-inflammatory approach with potential relevance for cardiovascular disease is inhibition of the proinflammatory cytokine IL-1β. Canakinumab is a human monoclonal IL-1β antibody of the IgG1/k isotype. It blocks the interaction of this cytokine with its receptors and results in specific neutralization of the bioactivity of IL-1β, but does not prevent the binding of the natural inhibitor IL-1Ra to the IL-1 receptor, nor the binding to IL-1α. Canakinumab targets IL-1β-dependent inflammation and potentially preserve or improve the pancreatic β-cell function and inhibit the progression to atherothrombosis in the coronary arteries of T2DM patients who are at a high risk of developing cardiovascular disease.[11]

Early Diabetes Breakthroughs

Basic research is important to finding new treatments and possibly a cure for diabetes. Recent research discoveries offer hope that they can one day lead to new effective treatments. Some of the new discoveries include:

- Researchers at the Harvard Stem Cell Institute discovered a hormone that can stimulate production of insulin-secreting pancreatic β cells up to 30 times the normal rate in mice. These new cells only produce insulin when the body needs it, potentially leading to a natural regulation of insulin.

- Scientists at London's Imperial College have manipulated a patient's own stem cells into insulin-secreting cells.
- Further research aims to inject patients with 100% of insulin-producing cells that would release insulin for up to 1 year. Other scientists at the Walter and Eliza Hall Institute of Medical Research in Australia have isolated stem cells from the pancreas and turned them into insulin producing cells for the treatment of type 1 diabetes.
- A type 1 diabetes vaccine created by researchers at Stanford University shuts down certain segments of the human immune system. Most vaccines aim to boost the immune system to fight a virus, but the Stanford vaccine turns off portions of the immune system that are malfunctioning.
- Researchers at the University of Tokyo have identified a molecule that functions similarly to the hormone adiponectin, which is secreted by fat cells and helps to regulate glucose and insulin effectiveness. But the hormone was destroyed by the digestive system when taken orally. The new molecule can be taken orally and was found to be effective when studied in mice.
- Doctors at Boston Children's Hospital have isolated a pathway in animals that triggers T cells to attack the pancreas. With more research, the newly discovered pathway could lead to better treatments or even a cure for type 1 diabetes.

CONCLUSION

Though in the field of diabetes many new inventions have happened, it is far behind the real target. We are looking forward to the future for effective contribution of the researches, which will really improve the life of a diabetic. Drugs which can efficiently lower the blood glucose and insulin resistance with minimal side effects and regenerate β-cell function and prevent the complications are the final answer.

REFERENCES

1. "Diabetes Research" [2006]. [online] eMedTV.com website. Available from http://diabetes.emedtv.com/diabetes/diabetes-research.html. [Accessed August 2015].
2. Diabetes Stories: Personal Tales of Diabetes Through the Decades. Oxford Centre for Diabetes, Endocrinology & Metabolism, 2005 Oral History of Diabetes. 21 Sept. 2007.
3. Einhorn D. [2004]. "Advances in Diabetes for the Millennium: Insulin Treatment and Glucose Monitoring." [online] Medscape.com. website. 2004. Medscape. 21 Sept. 2007. (subscription) Available from http://www.medscape.org/viewarticle/488996>. Accessed August 2015
4. Irbina I. [2006]. "Rising Diabetes Threat Meets a Falling Budget". [online] NYtimes.com. website. Available from NYtimes.com. [Accessed September 2007].
5. Kalayoglu M. [2007]. "Laser Photocoagulation Systems for Diabetic Retinopathy and Other Retinal Disorders". [online] Medcompare.com. website. Available from Medcompare.com. [Accessed September 2007].
6. The Science Behind the Human Genome Project 2008. [online] Human Genome Project Information Archive website. Available form http://www.ornl.gov/sci/techresources/Human_Genome/project/info.shtml. [Accessed August 2015].

7. Satley M. [1996]. “History of Diabetes”. [online] DiabetesHealth.com. website. Available from http://www.diabeteshealth.com/read/1996/11/01/715.html. [Accessed September 2007].
8. “Joslin Research Sections”. Joslin Diabetes Center. 2007. Joslin.org. 22 Sept. 2007 <http://www.joslin.org/732_1206.asp>.
9. Goodrich M. [2008]. Researchers Link 11 Genetic Variations to Type 2 Diabetes. [online] MichiganTech News/Media website. Available from http://www.admin.mtu.edu/urel/news/media_relations/673. [Accessed August 2015].
10. Fouqueray P, Leverve X, Fontaine E, et al. Imeglimin—a new oral anti-diabetic that targets the three key defects of type 2 diabetes. J Diabetes Metab. 2011;2:126.
11. Howard C, Noe A, Skerjanec A, et al. Safety and tolerability of canakinumab, an IL-1β inhibitor, in type 2 diabetes mellitus patients: a pooled analysis of three randomised double-blind studies. Cardiovasc Diabetol. 2014;13:94.

INDEX

Page numbers followed by *f* refer to figure and *t* refer to table.

E